Management of Chronic Conditions in the Foot and Lower Leg

Content Strategist: Rita Demetriou-Swanwick
Content Development Specialists: Catherine Jackson/Nicola Lally
Project Manager: Umarani Natarajan
Designer/Design Direction: Christian Bilbow
Illustration Manager: Jennifer Rose
Illustrator: Antbits

Management of Chronic Conditions in the Foot and Lower Leg

Edited by

Keith Rome BSc(Hons), MSc, PhD, FCPodMed, SRCh

Professor in Podiatry and Co-Director, Health and Research Rehabilitation Institute, Department of Podiatry, School of Rehabilitation and Occupation Studies, Faculty of Health and Environmental Sciences, Auckland University of Technology, Auckland, New Zealand

Peter McNair DipPhysEd, DipPT, MPhEd(Distn), PhD

Professor of Physiotherapy and Director, Health and Rehabilitation Research Institute, Auckland University of Technology, Auckland, New Zealand

Foreword by

Christopher Nester BSc(Hons), PhD

Professor, Research Lead: Foot and Ankle Research Programme, School of Health Sciences, University of Salford, Salford, UK

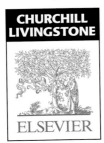

CHURCHILL LIVINGSTONE

ELSEVIER

Edinburgh   London   New York   Oxford   Philadelphia   St Louis   Sydney   Toronto   2015

CHURCHILL
LIVINGSTONE
ELSEVIER

ISBN 978 0 7020 4769 5

British Library Cataloguing in Publication Data
A catalogue record for this book is available from the British Library

Library of Congress Cataloging in Publication Data
A catalog record for this book is available from the Library of Congress

ELSEVIER your source for books, journals and multimedia in the health sciences
www.elsevierhealth.com

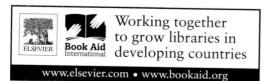

Working together to grow libraries in developing countries

www.elsevier.com • www.bookaid.org

The publisher's policy is to use **paper manufactured from sustainable forests**

Printed in China

Contents

Preface

The interpretation of the patient's history, the extraction of information from key laboratory and clinical tests, along with the decision-making process to find the best treatment solution for the patient's predicament, is a challenging but enjoyable endeavour for the clinician.

Nevertheless, in the past decade, there has been rapid growth in research activity focused upon risk factors, diagnosis, and treatment. In some instances, the growth has been bewildering and hence particularly difficult for clinicians to stay abreast of current thinking in each aspect of practice, and subsequently be confident in their decisions.

The book includes the following clinical conditions: osteoarthritis, rheumatoid arthritis, gout, stress fractures of the lower leg, Achilles tendinopathy, rearfoot entities, forefoot entities, and cerebral palsy. Thus not all conditions that might be encountered are covered. However, we believe that the book provides a sufficiently detailed account of a set of disorders that encompasses key changes to pathology in muscle, tendon, and joints that might be found across the majority of conditions affecting the lower leg, foot, and ankle. Our choice of material reflects discussions with clinicians, clinical researchers, and senior students concerning those conditions that would be most valuable to them. Furthermore, these enquiries extended to the level of complexity and comprehension that they wished to see in such a text. As a result, the book is not written as an early undergraduate text but rather for those close to being qualified or already in practice.

Each chapter is organized into sections that are consistent across the book, thus enhancing the ease that the book can be read. These sections include predisposing factors, diagnosis, impairments, function, quality of life, and management strategies. We have asked our authors to provide not only a discussion of the latest advances, but also to be thought provoking and to consider the less straight-forward features of each condition and provide suggestions for new paths of research. Each chapter is further supported by additional commentary from an internationally renowned researcher who highlights the key elements of the work and provides a supplementary perspective of the particular clinical condition.

Given the aforementioned growth in knowledge concerning these conditions, it seemed logical to find a group of authors who were highly regarded for their research and or clinical contributions to their respective professions. We are very thankful to our authors for sharing their expertise. They have devoted a large amount of their time, for which we are very appreciative and grateful. The authors represent a broad spectrum of professions, and all recognize that for the patient to receive the best possible care an interdisciplinary approach to their treatment is required, and this attitude is apparent throughout the book.

We wish to thank the people that we have worked with at Elsevier for their patience, support and kind attitude in all aspects of the publication process. Their advice and standards of excellence have been invaluable in bringing this book to completion. Finally, we thank those who read the book as it evolved for their critical comments and ideas for improving its content and presentation.

Keith Rome
Peter McNair

Foreword

Anyone working in or interested in healthcare provision, health policy, or health-related research will already understand the major factors that will shape the nature of health and wellbeing in the future. That you will have heard a great deal about 'the aging population', the increase in 'long-term conditions', and the 'obesity epidemic' and so on should not blunt the very real impact that these issues will have on the lives of everyone. Much of future healthcare need will be shaped by these issues, but also by some of the activities that healthy people choose to engage in: running and triathlons remain the fastest growing sports in the world, and so we look set to challenge our musculoskeletal systems to the maximum whether we are healthy or live with the daily challenges of a chronic condition. Understanding the underlying causative mechanisms, the identification of and management of chronic conditions is already an imperative in practice, but it is an area that, given the issues above, will only grow.

Thankfully, researchers and clinicians have been busy on these topics for a considerable time. More fortunately still for you, the need for research-led information and data to support management of chronic conditions has clearly energized the editors and authors of this book. This book is therefore timely but has also saved any reader a huge amount of time and resource that would otherwise be required to access such a diverse range of clinical conditions in such depth, and selecting so appropriately only the most pertinent and quality literature.

This book is also of the highest standard and makes a welcome addition to the current texts on chronic conditions of the lower limb and foot. It is research and scholarship led throughout but bridges undergraduate and postgraduate knowledge and experience in a very accessible way. Whilst it can be a practical tool that can inform daily decision making in practice, it will also support those building policy and management strategies more broadly in the clinical areas covered.

That the editors have drawn upon an international and multiprofessional authorship in each of the areas applauds the clear commitment to quality and trustworthy information. The inclusion of reviewer commentaries is a useful change in style and assists further in the reader contextualizing the information provided. It also builds trust in the information in each chapter.

That the editors used their relationships with clinical colleagues to shape the focus and style of the book reflects their commitment to meeting the real needs of people working in practice, and their commitment to research knowledge informing the care patients receive. A broad view of the needs of patients is offered throughout, a welcome departure from traditional texts that narrowly define objectives in too-clinical terms. Inclusion of specific sections on impairments, function, and quality of life reflect this ethos, since it seeks to connect clinical realities to real-world patient experiences. Furthermore, patient-reported outcome measures and health behaviour strategies are a consistent feature of this text.

Through this text, therefore, the authors are seeking to support clinicians and researchers in doing their current roles to the highest standards and shape knowledge in the musculoskeletal community that best prepares it for the future. Indeed, statements on 'future directions' are a key feature of this text and will help you seek further niche information from the related literature. As such, this book can strongly support your current professional development and underpin the quality and relevance of future service and policy developments too.

Professor Christopher Nester

List of Contributors

Kim Bennell BAppSc, PhD
Professor and Director, Centre for Health Exercise and Sports Medicine, Department of Physiotherapy, University of Melbourne, Melbourne, Australia

Peter Brukner MBBS, FACSP
Sports Physician, Olympic Park Sports Medicine Centre, Melbourne; Associate Professor in Sports Medicine, Department of Physiotherapy, University of Melbourne, Melbourne, Victoria, Australia

Vivienne Chuter BPod(Hons), PhD
Senior Lecturer, Podiatry, School of Health Sciences, Faculty of Health and Medicine, The University of Newcastle, Callaghan, NSW, Australia

Michael Corkill MBChB, FRACP
Rheumatologist, Clinical Director, Waitemata DHB Rheumatology Services, North Shore Hospital, Takapuna, North Shore City, Auckland, New Zealand

Mark W. Creaby BSc(Hons), PhD
School of Exercise Science, Australian Catholic University, Australia; and Centre for Health, Exercise & Sports Medicine, University of Melbourne, Australia

Mike Frecklington BHSc(Hons), MPhil
Lecturer, Department of Podiatry, School of Rehabilitation and Occupation Sciences, Faculty of Health and Occupation Sciences, Auckland University of Technology, Auckland, New Zealand

Fiona Hawke BAppSci(Hons), PhD
Lecturer in Podiatry, Faculty of Health and Medicine, University of Newcastle, Callaghan, NSW, Australia

Peter McNair DipPhysEd, DipPT, MPhEd(Distn), PhD
Director of the Health and Rehabilitation Research Institute, Professor in Physiotherapy, Auckland University of Technology, Auckland, New Zealand

Shannon E. Munteanu BPod(Hons), PhD
Senior Lecturer, Department of Podiatry, Faculty of Health Sciences, School of Allied Health, LaTrobe University, Bundoora, Victoria, Australia

David Rice BHSc, PhD
Lecturer and Senior Research Officer, Health and Rehabilitation Research Institute, Auckland University of Technology, Auckland; Audit, Quality and Research Officer, Waitemata Pain Services, Department of Anaesthesiology and Perioperative Medicine, North Shore Hospital, Auckland, New Zealand

Keith Rome BSc(Hons), MSc, PhD, FCPodMed, SRCh
Professor in Podiatry and Co-Director Health and Research Rehabilitation Institute, Department of Podiatry, School of Rehabilitation and Occupation Studies, Faculty of Health and Environmental Sciences, Auckland University of Technology, Auckland, New Zealand

N. Susan Stott MBChB, PhD, FRACS
Professor of Paediatric Orthopaedic Surgery, Department of Surgery, Faculty of Medical and Health Sciences, University of Auckland, Auckland, New Zealand

Bill Vicenzino BPhty, GradDipSportsphyty, MSc, PhD
Professor in Sports Physiotherapy, School of Health and Rehabilitation Sciences; Physiotherapy, University of Queensland, St Lucia Campus, Brisbane, Australia

Anita Williams BSc(Hons), PhD
Senior Lecturer and Post Graduate Research Student Co-ordinator, School of Health Science, Orthotics and Podiatry, University of Salford, Salford, UK

List of Commentary Writers

Robert L. Ashford DPodM, BA, BEd, MA, MMedSci, PhD, MChS, FCpodMed, FFPM, RCPS
Director of Postgraduate Research Degrees, Faculty of Health, Birmingham City University, City South Campus, Birmingham, UK

Mario Bizzini MSc, PhD, PT
Research Associate, FIFA – Medical Assessment & Research Centre Schulthess Clinic Lengghalde, Zürich, Switzerland

Roslyn N. Boyd BSc, BAppSc, MSc, PhD, PGRad
Professor of Cerebral Palsy and Rehabilitation Research; Scientific Director, Queensland Cerebral Palsy and Rehabilitation Research Centre, School of Medicine, University of Queensland, Brisbane, Australia

Nicola Dalbeth MBChB, MD, FRACP
Consultant Rheumatologist and Associate Professor, Department of Medicine, University of Auckland, Auckland, New Zealand

Phillip S. Helliwell MA, DM, PhD, FRCP
Senior Lecturer in Rheumatology, Leeds Institute of Molecular Medicine, Section of Musculoskeletal Disease, University of Leeds, UK

Tim Kilmartin PhD, FCPodS
Consultant Podiatric Surgeon, Hillsborough Private Clinic, Belfast and Ilkeston Hospital, Ilkeston, Derbyshire; Lecturer, School of Podiatry, Ulster University, Derry, UK

Karl B. Landorf DipAppSc, Grad Cert Clin Instr, GradDipEd, PhD, FFPM, RCPS
Senior Lecturer and Research Co-ordinator, Department of Podiatry, Faculty of Health Sciences, La Trobe University, Bundoora, Victoria, Australia

Nicola Maffulli MD, MS, PhD, FRCP, FRCS, FFSEM
Professor of Musculoskeletal Disorders, Consultant Orthopaedic Surgeon, University of Salerno, Salerno, Italy; Honorary Professor of Sport and Exercise Medicine, Queen Mary University of London, London, UK

Chapter 1

Osteoarthritis of the Ankle Joint

Peter McNair and David Rice

Chapter Outline

INTRODUCTION

Osteoarthritis (OA) is the most common form of arthritis. While the main characteristic of OA is a loss of articular cartilage, it is apparent that as the disease progresses a number of additional joint structures including the subchondral bone, capsule, ligaments, synovial membrane, and periarticular muscles are affected to varying degrees (Madry et al. 2012). With this progression, joint pain together with reduced physical, emotional, and social wellbeing commonly occurs (Busija et al. 2013). Furthermore, OA has a notable financial impact on the individual, and on direct and indirect costs associated with diagnosis and treatment (Bozic et al. 2012; Le et al. 2012). Due to improved health practices and medical advancements that can potentially increase our lifespans, OA is also forecast to increase in prevalence (Zhang and Jordan 2010).

Estimations of the prevalence of OA differ and the accuracy of the estimates is confounded by the lack of a standardized definition for OA, and the use of different clinical and radiological criteria to grade disease severity. In a review of epidemiological data based on radiological findings, Lawrence et al. (2008) reported the prevalence of OA at the hip or knees to be approximately 18–25% for men and 19–30% for women over 45 years old. In those over 60 years, the prevalence at the knee increased to 31% for men and 42% for women. These figures are likely to be conservative, as studies have tended to collect data up to the age of 75 years only. At the ankle joint, the prevalence of the OA has been reported to be between 1 and 13% (Cole and Kuettner 2002; Glazebrook et al. 2008).

OA can be divided into primary and secondary types. Primary OA is idiopathic and generally affects those from middle age onwards. In the lower limb, the hip and knee joints are most affected by primary OA;

however, a minority of patients present with primary OA at the ankle joint. Most patients with ankle OA have secondary osteoarthritis, which, as the name implies, occurs following an initial insult to the joint. Examples include infection, trauma, and dysplasia. At the ankle joint, OA is most associated with previous trauma (Valderrabano et al. 2009) and may present in up to 70% of cases attending a hospital orthopaedic department with chronic ankle pain (Saltzmann et al. 2005).

PREDISPOSING FACTORS

General Risk Factors

General risk factors for OA have been most extensively studied at the knee and hip joints. Of note, there is an increased risk of OA associated with increasing age (Felson et al. 1987). Furthermore, a gender effect is apparent, with an increased risk for women (Lawrence et al. 2008). Genetic polymorphisms associated with OA have also been identified (Dai and Ikegawa 2010; Lanyon et al. 2000). In addition, studies have highlighted increased mechanical loading on the joint as an important risk factor for OA. Increased loading is multifactorial and may reflect body mass increases (Felson et al. 1988; Hochberg et al. 1995), as well as the extent and intensity of participation in manual work (Jenson 2008a, 2008b; Kaila-Kangas et al. 2011), and some sporting activities (Kujala et al. 1995; Spector et al. 1996).

Anatomy and Biomechanical Loading at the Ankle Joint

Certain anatomical and biomechanical features of the ankle joint are thought to increase the risk of developing OA. For instance, the articular cartilage is thinner (1.0–1.5 mm) compared with the knee joint (1.7–2.6 mm) (Adam et al. 1998; Shepherd and Seedhom 1999). Furthermore, the area of the articular cartilage is considerably smaller (~350 mm^2) than in the hip or knee joints (~1100 mm^2) (Brown and Shaw 1983; Ihn et al. 1993; Kimizuka et al. 1980). In a study that utilized magnetic resonance and fluoroscopic imaging, Wan et al. (2006) showed that ankle joint contact was less than 50% of total possible cartilage area throughout the stance phase of gait (Figure 1-1). Contact areas during walking gait were lowest at footstrike and

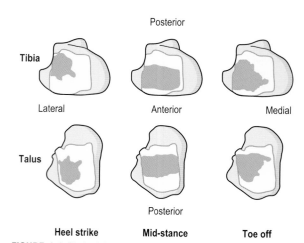

FIGURE 1-1 Typical in-vivo cartilage contact areas in the ankle during the stance phase of gait. (Reprinted from Wan L, de Asla RJ, Rubash HE, Li G, 2006. Determination of in-vivo articular cartilage contact areas of human talocrural joint under weightbearing conditions. Osteoarthritis Cartilage 14(12):1294–1301 with permission from Elsevier.)

greatest at mid-stance. In contrast, the landing forces are largest at footstrike. Vertical ground reaction forces of 1–2 BW during walking rise to 2–3 BW during jogging, and in activities such as landing from a jump can reach as high as 10 BW (McNair and Prapavessis 1999; Zadpoor and Nikooyan 2011). Furthermore, rates of loading are considerable during such tasks and have been associated with chronic lower limb disorders (Zadpoor and Nikooyan 2011). The combination of these forces with a limited joint contact area results in high levels of stress being placed on the articular cartilage, increasing the risk of damage.

During physical activity, the deformation in the articular cartilage can be considerable. Waterton et al. (2000) reported a 0.6 mm change in the thickness of knee articular cartilage over a day of normal loading. More acute changes were observed by Boocock et al. (2009), who noted 4–6% deformation in articular cartilage at the knee after 5000 steps of jogging, which took approximately 30 minutes to complete. Given the closer proximity of the ankle to initial ground reaction forces at footstrike, and the lesser motion available at the ankle joint to absorb energy, deformation of cartilage at the ankle joint is likely to be higher than that observed at the knee joint. Cartilage deformation occurs primarily through the movement of water and the extracellular matrix; depending upon the intensity and volume of the physical activity being performed, the shock absorption potential of the cartilage may be reduced. In turn, the likelihood of damage occurring to the more exposed chondrocytes and collagen fibres may be increased, ultimately affecting the integrity of the articular cartilage.

Although the features mentioned above may indicate a greater propensity for OA at the ankle joint, some authors (Cole and Kuettner 2002; Poole et al. 1994) have suggested that the architecture of the articular cartilage together with the processes of synthesis and repair influence whether a joint is more or less prone to the development of OA (Cole and Kuettner 2002). Undoubtedly, biomechanical properties of the tissue reflect biochemical content and processes operating within the articular cartilage (Treppo et al. 2000). Comparisons of knee and ankle cartilage show that cellular communication may be enhanced at the ankle joint, with the majority of chondrocytes being found in clusters (Schumacher et al. 2002). In contrast, knee chondrocytes were more likely to be isolated single cells, particularly in the superficial zone of the cartilage. Furthermore, Cole and Kuettner (2002) found that ankle joint chondrocytes have enhanced matrix synthesis rates and lesser responses to catabolic cytokines, thus making the ankle joint more resistant to cartilage degeneration. Such differences combined with differences in the content of glycosaminoglycans (GAGs), collagen, and water were indicative of the ankle joint cartilage being stronger, stiffer, and better suited to resisting the effects of loading (Figure 1-2).

Previous Trauma

A history of fracture in close proximity or directly affecting the ankle joint has been identified as an important risk factor for the development of OA (Figure 1-3). In a large retrospective cohort with ankle OA, Valderrabano et al. (2009) reported that the most commonly associated fracture was a malleolar fracture (39%). In a prospective cohort study, Lindsjo (1985) reported that, following such fractures, the level of joint laxity at the time of operation affected the subsequent likelihood of OA. At 2 to 6 years post fracture, OA was present in 4, 12, and 33% of Weber-classified A, B, and C fractures respectively. Also of note was that

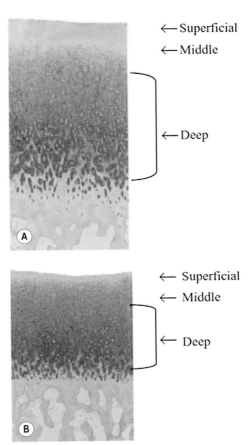

FIGURE 1-2 Example of articular cartilage at the knee compared with the ankle joint. Histological sections of full-thickness articular cartilage and subchondral bone from the femur (A) and talus (B) of a 52-year-old man that were stained with Safranin O and fast green. The relative positions of the superficial, middle and deep layers of the cartilage are shown (original magnification=4×). (Reprinted from Kuettner KE, Cole AA, 2005. Cartilage degeneration in different human joints. Osteoarthritis Cartilage 13(2):93–103 with permission from Elsevier.)

the degree of bone fragmentation at the time of injury was directly related to the presence of OA at follow-up. Other studies (Takakura et al. 1998) have highlighted the relationship between limb alignment following fracture and the subsequent development of OA.

Chondral (Figure 1-4) and osteochondral lesions are common following ankle trauma, often combined with ligamentous sprains (Hembree et al. 2012). Compared with the tibia, these lesions are most often observed in the talus (see Figure 2.3), and it is speculated (Elias et al. 2009) that the concave nature of the

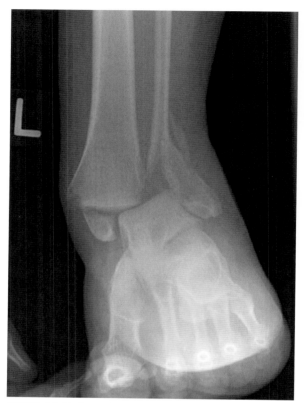

FIGURE 1-3 Radiograph of an ankle with a stage-3 pronation–abduction ankle fracture, showing lateral comminution with bending failure of the fibula after an abduction stress. (Reprinted with permission from Siegel J, Tornetta P. Extraperiosteal plating of pronation–abduction ankle fractures. J Bone Joint Surg Am 2007 Feb; 89-A(2):276–281. http://jbjs.org/.)

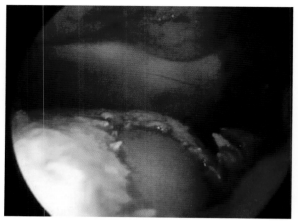

FIGURE 1-4 Chondral lesion of the talus after a stage-IV supination–external rotation fracture, as seen at arthroscopy prior to surgical reduction. The lesion exceeds 50% of the cartilage depth, and the subchondral bone is visible (a grade-IV lesion). (Reprinted with permission from Stufkens SA, Knupp M, Horisberger M, Lampert C, Hintermann B. Cartilage lesions and the development of osteoarthritis after internal fixation of ankle fractures: a prospective study. J Bone Joint Surg Am 2010 Feb; 92(2):279–286. http://jbjs.org/.)

talar dome promotes the likelihood of greater compressive shear forces occurring. During arthroscopy, Taga et al. (1993) noted that eight of nine patients who had sprained their ankle joint had also sustained chondral lesions. Interestingly, seven of these patients had isolated anterior talofibular ligament ruptures. Choi et al. (2013) examined the characteristics of chondral and osteochondral lesions at the ankle. These authors noted that chondral lesions were more frequently observed in teenagers and young adults, whereas osteochondral injuries were more evident in those over 40 years of age. The maturity of the interface between calcified and uncalcified regions of the cartilage was thought to be responsible for this observation.

When quantifying chondral and osteochondral lesions, it has been found that the majority of patients have lesions that are less than 150 mm² (Choi et al. 2013). In a large cohort, Elias et al. (2007) noted that 63% of lesions were in the medial talar dome whereas 33% affected the lateral aspect. In both instances, these lesions were observed in the central region of the dome, which is contrary to a traditional viewpoint (Barnes and Ferkel 2003) that they are most often observed anterolateral or posteromedial. Elias et al. (2007) speculated that the predominance of injuries on the medial aspect resulted from an impact of the medial tibial plafond and the medial talar dome during an inversion-type injury.

Ligament injury has also been associated with ankle OA. Up to 85% of ankle sprains that progress to OA damaged the lateral ligamentous complex and involved a hyperinversion injury at the joint (Valderrabano et al. 2006). Ankle sprains may lead to OA via multiple mechanisms. Firstly, as mentioned above, forces associated with ankle sprains may also induce chondral and/or osteochondral lesions. In addition, ligament damage itself may affect not just collagen fibrils, but also sensory receptors contributing to proprioception, and hence one's ability to control subsequent joint motion via reflex and feed-forward mechanisms (Armstrong et al. 2008). Additionally, poor healing of ligamentous and capsular structures may lead to joint laxity (Hubbard and Hicks-Little 2008). Increased laxity that cannot be adequately controlled by muscle activity leads to an abnormal pattern of motion within the joint. In turn, this may lead to altered joint loading, which places excessive stresses on the articular cartilage in a repetitive manner. A study by Tochigi et al. (2008) involving cadavers indicated that sequential cutting of ligamentous restraints at the ankle can lead to linear increases in articular cartilage contact stresses that could accelerate cartilage degeneration. More recently, in a small cohort, Bischof et al. (2010) utilized three-dimensional magnetic resonance imaging (3D MRI) modelling and fluoroscopy to show that, during walking, individuals with lateral ankle instability had increased contact strains (~30% greater), with peak strains located more anteriorly and medially than in ankles with intact ligaments. Though not at the ankle, more direct measurements have examined synovial fluid and articular cartilage shortly after injury (Pickvance et al. 1993), and observed increased levels of cytokines and catabolic enzymes that influence the integrity of the cartilage matrix. Some of these catabolic enzymes have been shown to remain at elevated levels within the joint for many years, ultimately influencing the onset and progression of OA (Lohmander et al. 1993).

The timeframe from a sprain injury to end-stage OA is different according to the nature of the injuries originally sustained. Valderrabano et al. (2006) noted a 35-year latency for those who had sustained lateral ligament injuries, versus 28 years for a medial ligament injury. Interestingly, these authors also reported that the latency for a single severe sprain was significantly less (26 years) compared with those who had sustained recurrent sprains of lesser severity (38 years). The most likely reason for this finding is the magnitude of loading at the time of the initial sprain.

Limb Alignment

Limb malalignment may also contribute to the development of ankle OA (Figure 1-5). Valderrabano et al. (2009) noted that the majority of subjects developing OA of the ankle joint were more likely to have a varus

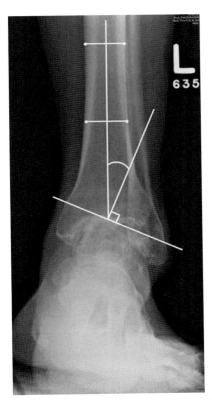

FIGURE 1-5 Example of a radiographic assessment to determine the coronal plane alignment of the ankle joint. (Reprinted from Queen RM, Carter JE, Adams SB, Easley ME, DeOrio JK, Nunley J, 2011. Coronal plane ankle alignment, gait, and end-stage ankle osteoarthritis. Osteoarthritis Cartilage 19(11):1338–1342 with permission from Elsevier.)

alignment. Other authors (Fortin et al. 2002) have highlighted cavovarus foot deformity and genu varum as contributing to degenerative changes. Recently, Knupp et al. (2009) utilized SPECT/CT to observe early degenerative changes in individuals with chronic varus- or valgus-aligned hindfeet that had not responded to conservative management. These authors found that radioisotope signals were greater in the medial regions of the talus and tibia in those with varus malalignment, whereas increased signals on the lateral regions were observed in those with valgus malalignment. In respect to valgus malalignment, Knupp et al. (2009) observed a trend toward greater signal levels in the talonavicular and subtalar joints. Potential contributors to such changes include genu valgum, severe pes planus, and acquired flatfoot deformity.

DIAGNOSIS

HISTORY

In addition to recording a standard clinical history, the clinician should pay particular interest to previous joint trauma and how it was treated, given the high prevalence of post-traumatic OA at the ankle. As indicated earlier, alignment problems are often associated with a history of lower leg fracture. Similarly, at end-stage OA, Valderrabano et al. (2009) noted that two-thirds of patients with a previous history of recurrent lateral ligament sprains had varus malalignment, and all patients with a history of medial or combined ligament damage had valgus malalignment.

PHYSICAL EXAMINATION

Pain

Pain is the primary symptom affecting those with OA at the ankle. Although pain can be assessed as a stand-alone question, for instance as a Visual Analogue Scale (VAS), it often forms a part of a multidomain questionnaire [e.g. American Orthopedic Foot and Ankle Society (AOFAS) scales or the Short Form-36 (SF-36)]. Using a VAS, Valderrabano et al. (2007a) and Pagenstert et al. (2011) reported individuals with end-stage OA ankle joints to have an average score of 7/10. In a similar group of patients, Glazebrook et al. (2008) reported a mean score of 33 for the bodily pain component of the SF-36 compared with US and Canadian populations' normative scores of 50–52. In a large epidemiological study, Valderrabano et al. (2009) observed that individuals with primary OA at the ankle joint experienced significantly less pain (6.1/10) than those with secondary and post-traumatic OA (6.9–7.0/10).

Apart from pain intensity, other characteristics of ankle OA pain have not been well defined. At the knee and hip joints, studies (Gooberman-Hill et al. 2007; Hawker et al. 2008) have examined sensory descriptors and how pain affects function, sleep, and mood. These have identified variations in pain sensations and intensity levels across joints at different stages of OA severity. They have also identified the priorities of

patients and the degree of concern that they have for different elements of pain and their subsequent effect on quality of life. Without doubt, studies focused upon OA at the ankle joint are required to provide a broader appreciation of the pain experience in this population.

Swelling

With OA, perennial inflammation is often apparent, and this is evident clinically by the observation of swelling at the joint. Pagenstert et al. (2011) measured swelling at the ankle joint using a categorical grading system and found patients with end-stage OA had a mean score of 2, which was indicative of 'ankle swelling with tightened skin without wrinkles'. Taga et al. (1993) noted that a chondral injury was nearly always associated with swelling at the joint irrespective of whether the patient's condition was acute or chronic.

IMAGING

The most popular form of imaging for OA is radiography, yet it is well known that OA can be present well before observations can be seen on radiographs (Wright et al. 2006) and the relationship between the damage evident on radiographs and the symptoms is often incongruous (Dieppe et al. 1997; Hannan et al. 2000). The most common scale for grading OA severity on radiographs is that of Kellgren and Lawrence (1957), which focuses upon joint space narrowing and the presence of osteophytes. Other scales such as those of Tanaka et al. (2006) and van Dijk et al. (1997) have also been used at the ankle joint. A recent study by Moon et al. (2010) that examined reliability across these scoring systems showed that they have fair to moderate reproducibility in patients with mid-stage OA. Recent work by Nosewicz et al. (2012) highlighted the complexity of radiographic assessments at the ankle joint, particularly where varus and valgus malalignment was present.

Both computerized tomography (CT) and magnetic resonance imaging (MRI) can provide evidence of small focal lesions in cartilage (Ragozzino et al. 1996). In MR images, the loss of smooth contours to articular cartilage, the presence of surface irregularities and synovitis, together with changes in cartilage thickness can provide evidence of OA (Recht et al. 2005). The appearance of articular cartilage can be further enhanced by MRI arthrography. This technique involves an injection of a contrast solution either directly into the joint or indirectly by intravenous administration of gadolinium prior to scanning (Cerezal et al. 2008).

Depending upon the sequence utilized, MRI scans can also provide evidence of subchondral bone lesions, bruising, oedema, and fractures, all of which can be present with OA. Conventional bone isotope scans can also provide information concerning metabolic processes in subchondral areas. More recently, combined single-photon emission CT and conventional CT has been shown to provide greater resolution and more sensitive measurement of subchondral bone metabolism (Knupp et al. 2009).

IMPAIRMENTS

Range of Motion (ROM)

Ankle OA is associated with reduced joint ROM. Compared with a mean of 56° in control limbs, Valderrabano et al. (2007a) and Pagenstert et al. (2011) noted total range of motion in plantar-dorsiflexion to be reduced to 16° and 21° respectively in patients with end-stage ankle OA. Valderrabano et al. noted that individuals with primary OA at the ankle joint had greater total range of plantar-dorsiflexion (28°) compared with those with secondary and post-traumatic OA (20–22°). In other planes of motion, Schenk et al. (2011) reported that total ROM for pronation/supination was a mean of 24° in patients with end-stage ankle OA.

In the accessory displacements that occur with joint rotations, losses are also evident. For instance, Hubbard et al. (2009) used instrumented testing procedures in which a load of 125 N was applied to the ankle joint, and they reported a 35% loss in anterior displacement, but no significant difference for posterior displacement. These observations were considered indicative of the increased stiffness that patients with OA often describe. In contrast, it has been observed that just over 50% of patients presenting with moderate ankle OA who have had a history of ankle sprains continue to display increased laxity when subject to anterior drawer and inversion/eversion stress tests (Valderrabano et al. 2006).

Strength

Strength deficits are notable in muscles acting in all planes of motion at the arthritic ankle joint. For instance, Valderrabano et al. (2007a) reported that those with end-stage ankle OA had 38% deficits in isometric dorsi- and plantarflexion, and a mean 2 cm difference in calf circumference across legs, the latter providing a crude indication of muscle atrophy. During maximal effort voluntary contraction, electromyographic analyses showed reduced muscle activation in medial gastrocnemius, tibialis anterior, and peroneus longus muscles. In a lesser-affected cohort with ankle OA (grade 1–2), Hubbard et al. (2009) noted 18–20% strength deficits in plantar- and dorsiflexion, and 28–35% deficits in eversion and inversion when compared with the unaffected side. Interestingly, when compared with matched controls, Hubbard observed much greater deficits in strength: 55–60% deficits in isometric plantar- and dorsiflexion, inversion, and eversion. Such findings provide indirect evidence for central nervous system pathways being affected, leading to the occurrence of cross-limb activation deficits (Rice and McNair 2010), and/or an overall increase in disuse in individuals with OA that leads to atrophy in the unaffected limb. Utilizing MRI, Wiewiorski et al. (2012) reported increased fatty infiltration in muscles acting in all planes of motion at the ankle joint. Interestingly, although there was a trend indicative of reduced cross-sectional area in all muscles too, individual analyses indicated that this was significant in the soleus only.

Gait

Gait analysis of individuals with end-stage ankle OA shows that spatiotemporal parameters such as velocity, cadence, and stride length are reduced. Shih et al. (1993) showed that the single-leg stance phase was reduced while the double-leg stance increased, and that these changes were more apparent as the severity of OA increased. Valderrabano et al. (2007b) and Brodsky et al. (2011) reported mean values for the above parameters of 0.80–1.1 m/s, 101–105 steps per minute, and 0.94–1.26 m respectively (Brodsky et al. 2011). The age of patients at the time of testing is likely to affect the absolute values presented. Generally though, spatiotemporal gait parameters are reduced by 10–20% compared with age- and gender-matched control subjects. Interestingly, Valderrano et al. (2007b) observed that by 12 months after joint replacement these parameters were not significantly different from those in control subjects.

Joint ROM during gait may also be affected. Early work by Stauffer et al. (1977) showed a 50% reduction in dorsiflexion during early stance phase, while Brodsky et al. (2011), reported reduced ankle plantarflexion at footstrike and in late stance with maximum motion reaching 3–4°. Valderrabano et al. (2007b) noted reduced total plantarflexion (38%) together with reductions of 28% and 20% in inversion and adduction respectively. At 12 months after joint replacement, these authors noted adduction and inversion motion was not significantly different from controls; however, plantarflexion continued to be less (23%). Recently, Kozanek et al. (2009) utilized a fluoroscopic technique to examine the interactions of the tibiotalar and subtalar joint during gait. At the tibiotalar joint, these authors noted that between footstrike and mid-stance OA ankles dorsiflexed ~2° whereas normal ankles plantarflexed ~9°. At the subtalar joint, there were no differences across the groups. From mid-stance to toe-off at the tibiotalar joint, a small but significant difference in the pattern of motion was observed with eversion of ~2° in OA ankles compared with inversion of ~2° in normal ankles. More notable differences were observed at the subtalar joint where there was minimal rotation in arthritic ankles and ~12° of internal rotation in normal ankles. Similarly, whereas normal ankles plantarflexed (~9°) and inverted ~11°, arthritic ankles dorsiflexed ~3° and everted ~3°. Such changes in those with OA most likely reflect the increased stiffness and loss of ROM at these joints, and are likely to have a notable effect not only upon the ability to absorb energy generated by ground reaction forces at footstrike, but also the ability to generate forces in the propulsive phase of gait.

Some authors (Brodsky et al. 2011; Valderrabano et al. 2007b) have examined kinetic parameters during gait such as ankle joint moments and power in patients with ankle OA. Valderrabano et al. (2007b) reported 14% and 44% reductions in plantarflexion and adduction moments respectively, while joint power was reduced by 58% compared with control subjects. Although Brodsky et al. (2011) and Valderrabano et al. (2007b) have noted similar improvements in these parameters following joint replacement, the latter compared improvements 12 months after joint replacement with controls, and observed that plantarflexion and adduction moments had increased to 89% and 55% of control values, while joint power remained at 63% of control values. The limited improvement in the adduction moment and joint power was thought to reflect ongoing muscle strength deficits. In respect to ground reaction forces, Shih et al. (1993) and Valderrabano et al. (2007b) noted no significant changes in the landing forces at footstrike, but significantly reduced vertical ground reaction forces (10–20%) in the latter part of stance, which is associated with push-off.

Balance

Given the combination of muscle atrophy and soft-tissue damage that occurs in capsular and ligamentous structures together with perennial inflammation in those with ankle OA, there are likely to be changes in the afferent signals providing information concerning joint position and motion. Hubbard et al. (2009) assessed balance while standing on a force plate, and noted that no subjects with grade 1–2 OA of the ankle could stand on one leg to undertake the test, and in bilateral stance increased deviations in sway magnitude and velocity were observed compared with matched controls. More recently, in a small cohort using a clinical test that categorized ability to stand for 10 seconds in different stances, McDaniel et al. (2011) observed that, irrespective of pain, age, gender, BMI, and co-morbidities, poorer balance was mildly associated with severity of joint space narrowing at the ankle joint.

FUNCTION

There are a number of scales that can be used to evaluate function in patients with ankle OA. The most popular are the AOFAS scales and they include a combination of signs, symptoms, and function, providing an overall assessment of the joint. However, their psychometric properties have been questioned (Button and Pinney 2004). The Foot Function Index (FFI) has a more specific focus that includes questions concerning pain, disability, and activity restriction (Budiman-Mak et al. 1991, 2006). Domsic and Saltzman (1998) modified the FFI to be more suited to individuals with

OA. Similarly, the Western Ontario and McMaster Universities Arthritis Index (WOMAC), which is a condition-specific questionnaire, is focused upon OA but has been most often used for the knee and hip joints. Scales that can be utilized across the lower limb but are not specific to OA include the Musculoskeletal Functional Assessment (Martin et al. 1996) and the Lower Limb Task Questionnaire (LLTQ) (McNair et al. 2007). A number of other scales focus more on activity, including the Foot and Ankle Ability Measure (FAAM) (Martin et al. 2005), University of California Los Angeles (UCLA) activity scale (Zahiri et al. 1998), Activities Rating Scale (Marx et al. 2001), and the International Physical Activity Questionnaire (Button and Pinney 2004). Research to support their psychometric properties is varied.

Table 1-1 shows typical scores from the above-mentioned questionnaires in individuals with ankle OA. Overall, they indicate that individuals with moderate to end-stage ankle OA have moderate difficulty during prolonged standing (i.e. over 1 hour), undertaking walking for even moderate distances (one block), or moving up and down stairs or across slopes. They are not commonly active in sports other than swimming and cycling and these are usually performed at a light recreational level or for the purposes of maintaining fitness (Naal et al. 2009; Valderrabano et al. 2006). Participation in high-impact sports such as jogging, tennis, and soccer is rare and may be associated with notable joint pain (Naal et al. 2009; Valderrabano et al. 2006).

QUALITY OF LIFE

Studies examining quality of life in individuals with ankle OA indicate substantial differences compared with the general population of a similar age. For instance, in end-stage ankle OA, Glazebrook et al. (2008) noted that in the physical component summary section of the SF-36 subjects were approximately 2 standard

TABLE 1-1 Typical Scores Observed for a Range of Common Scales in Individuals with Ankle Osteoarthritis

Scale	Sample Size	Disease Severity	Total Score Mean (SD)	Total Score Range	Pain Subscale Mean (SD)	Disability Subscale Mean (SD)	Reference
AOFAS AHFS	70 (post-traumatic OA)	End-stage (KL n/a)	26.7 (6.7)	12–42	—	—	Bonnin et al. (2009)
AOFAS AHFS	15 (primary OA)	End-stage (KL n/a)	31.8 (6.6)	17–39	—	—	Bonnin et al. (2009)
AOFAS AHFS	15 (post-instability OA)	End-stage (KL n/a)	24.6 (6.0)	17–35	—	—	Bonnin et al. (2009)
AOFAS AHFS	117	End-stage (KL n/a)	35.6 (14.0)	—	11.9 (11.4)	—	Madeley et al. (2012)
FFI	117	End-stage (KL n/a)	50.4 (18.1)	—	52.1 (20.5)	60.1 (22.4)	Madeley et al. (2012)
AOS	117	End-stage (KL n/a)	57.6 (17.2)	—	53.4 (18.3)	63.1 (20.8)	Madeley et al. (2012)
AOS	15 (group A) 13 (group B)	Moderate to end-stage (KL grade II–IV)	64.1 (12.8) 52.5 (18.7)	— —	58.8 (16.3) 51.9 (14.6)	69.4 (12.1) 52.9 (18.7)	Cohen et al. (2008)
WOMAC	15 (group A) 13 (group B)	Moderate to end-stage (KL grade II–IV)	55.9 (15.1) 45.9 (17.5)	— —	53.4 (16.6) 45.9 (17.3)	55.9 (15.6) 43.6 (19.3)	Cohen et al. (2008)

AOFAS AHFS=American Orthopedic Foot and Ankle Society ankle–hindfoot score, FFI=Foot Function Index, AOS=Ankle Osteoarthritis Scale, WOMAC=Western Ontario and McMaster Universities Arthritis Index, OA=osteoarthritis, KL=Kellgren Lawrence.

deviations below US and Canadian population-based norms, with a score of 29 compared with 50. They were also notably lower in subsection scores associated with social (score 37) and emotional wellbeing (score 39). However, in the general health and the mental health summary components, OA patients' scores were only slightly lower than population-based norms. Of note, Glazebrook et al. noted minimal differences in SF-36 scores across gender and those aged under and over 60 years. Such findings reflect those found at the hip and knee joint. In a review of SF-12 and SF-36 findings on non-traumatic disorders of the hip and knee, Van de Waal et al. (2005) reported on the extent to which patients with end-stage knee and hip OA were below reference populations: −3.1 standard deviations (SD) for physical function component, −1.9 SD for bodily pain, −1.2–1.5 for vitality and social functions, and −0.4–0.8 SD in general health, mental health, and emotion. Given that 0.5 SD is regarded as the threshold for important differences (Norman et al. 2003), it is apparent that OA has a substantial impact on health-related quality of life.

MANAGEMENT STRATEGIES

Where possible, this section refers to studies conducted in individuals with ankle OA. However, most studies examining the efficacy of treatment for OA have been performed at the knee, hip, and hand joints. Until such time as studies are specifically performed in individuals with ankle OA, one can only extrapolate possible effects from studies involving other joints.

PHARMACOLOGICAL STRATEGIES
Acetaminophen

Acetaminophen is widely recommended as a first-line drug of choice in the management of pain due to OA (AAOS 2008; Hochberg et al. 2012; Jordan et al. 2003; NICE 2008; Zhang et al. 2008). The precise mechanisms by which acetaminophen relieves pain are not well understood, but appear to involve descending serotonergic pathways that modulate nociceptive processing at a spinal cord level (Anderson 2008). A meta-analysis involving 5986 patients demonstrated that acetaminophen significantly reduces pain associated with OA of the hip and knee (Towheed et al.

2006). However, the effect was small when compared with placebo. Acetaminophen undergoes metabolism in the liver and may lead to the urinary excretion of a number of toxic metabolites. It should therefore be used with caution in patients with liver or kidney disease, and in patients who consume even moderate amounts of alcohol (Harvey and Hunter 2010).

Non-steroidal Anti-inflammatory Drugs

Oral non-steroidal anti-inflammatory drugs (NSAIDs) are commonly recommended in the management of OA (AAOS 2008; Hochberg et al. 2012; Jordan et al. 2003; NICE 2008; Zhang et al. 2008). NSAIDs inhibit the release of prostaglandins and have both analgesic and anti-inflammatory effects (Harvey and Hunter 2010). In a recent meta-analysis, NSAIDs were shown to be more effective (SMD 0.25) than acetaminophen in reducing pain associated with OA of the knee and hip (Towheed et al. 2006). There does not appear to be a difference in pain-relieving effect between different types of NSAIDs, all being equally effective (Bjordal et al. 2004; Watson et al. 2000). The use of NSAIDs is associated with an increased risk of adverse events in the gastrointestinal, renal, and cardiovascular systems (Harvey and Hunter 2010). Gastrointestinal events can be reduced with the concurrent use of a proton pump inhibitor (Lai et al. 2006; Scheiman et al. 2006). Compared with non-selective NSAIDs, NSAIDs that are cyclo-oxygenase-2 (COX-2) selective inhibitors have been shown to reduce adverse gastrointestinal events (Silverstein et al. 2000), but may increase the risk of cardiovascular events (Harvey and Hunter 2010). Due to the risks associated with their use, some OA guidelines have recommended that oral NSAIDs are administered at the lowest effective dose for the shortest time possible (Jordan et al. 2003; NICE 2008; Zhang et al. 2008).

Topical NSAIDs are recommended in both US (AAOS 2008; Hochberg et al. 2012) and international guidelines (Zhang et al. 2008) for the management of mild to moderate OA pain in superficial joints, and are recommended ahead of oral NSAIDs in recent European guidelines (Jordan et al. 2003; NICE 2008). The existing data support the short-term analgesic efficacy of topical diclofenac, ketoprofen, and ibuprofen formulations in patients with OA affecting one or more superficial joints (Altman and Barthel 2011). The effect size for pain relief is similar to that of oral NSAIDS (Zhang et al. 2010). Compared with oral NSAIDs, topical NSAIDs have a much lower systemic absorption and are thought to reduce the risk of adverse gastrointestinal, renal, and cardiovascular events. A number of trials (Sandelin et al. 1997; Simon et al. 2009; Tugwell et al. 2004) that have directly compared with topical and oral NSAIDs have shown superior tolerability for the topical agent, particularly with respect to gastrointestinal complaints. The most common adverse events with the use of topical NSAIDs are local skin reactions at the site of application. These include dry skin, dermatitis, pruritus, and rashes and are typically of a mild nature (Altman and Barthel 2011).

Opioids

For patients who have contraindications or a poor analgesic response to acetaminophen and NSAIDs, most OA guidelines support the use of opioids (Hochberg et al. 2012; Jordan et al. 2003; NICE 2008; Zhang et al. 2008), including tramadol (Hochberg et al. 2012). Tramadol is an analgesic that reduces pain by acting as a weak opioid agonist and inhibiting the reuptake of serotonin and norepinephrine (noradrenaline) (Cheng and Visco 2012). Due to its effects on the serotonergic system, acetaminophen consumption can have a synergistic pain-relieving effect with tramadol, allowing a lower dose of tramadol to be effective (Harvey and Hunter 2010). Despite this, the analgesic effect of tramadol in the treatment of OA appears to be relatively modest (Howes et al. 2011). A recent meta-analysis (Cepeda et al. 2006) of 11 randomized controlled trials involving patients with hip and knee OA demonstrated that, compared with placebo, patients receiving tramadol or tramadol and acetaminophen had an average absolute reduction in pain of 8.5 mm on a 0–100 mm VAS. Amongst patients taking tramadol, 21% reported an adverse event serious enough to stop treatment, compared with 8% in the placebo group – a number needed to harm of eight patients. Tramadol's most common side effects include nausea, vomiting, flushing, constipation, drowsiness, tiredness, and headache (Cheng and Visco 2012; Harvey and Hunter 2010; Howes et al. 2011). Tramadol has been associated with an increased risk of serotonin syndrome if used with selective serotonin reuptake inhibitors and is contraindicated in

patients with epilepsy as it lowers the threshold for seizures (Harvey and Hunter 2010).

The use of stronger opioids (e.g. codeine, oxycodone) may be appropriate in OA patients with severe intractable pain who have not responded to other analgesics including tramadol (Hochberg et al. 2012; Zhang et al. 2008). However, strong opioids are not recommended as a first-line treatment for OA-related pain due to their addiction potential, risk of adverse events, and lack of disease-modifying effects (Harvey and Hunter 2010). In addition, long-term use of opioids may be associated with a paradoxical increase in pain sensitivity due to drug-induced neuroplastic changes in the nervous system (Angst and Clark 2006; Mao 2002). With respect to analgesic efficacy, a recent systematic review (Nuesch et al. 2009) has been conducted on 10 studies examining the short-term use of oral and transdermal opioids in the treatment of knee and hip OA. The opioids used in these studies included oxycodone, codeine, oxymorphone, morphine, and transdermal fentanyl patches. Compared with placebo, an overall pooled effect size of −0.36 was found in favour of opioids. Subgroup analysis did not show any differences in effect size for the type of opioid tested or the method of delivery (oral versus transdermal). Across all studies, 35% of patients taking opioids were found to have a reduction in pain of 50% or more (treatment responders) compared with 31% of patients taking placebo medication. Those receiving opioid therapy were four times as likely to withdraw due to adverse events compared with those taking placebo.

Local Intra-articular Injections

Corticosteroids. Intra-articular corticosteroid injection is widely recommended in the treatment of OA-related pain (AAOS 2008; Hochberg et al. 2012; Jordan et al. 2003; NICE 2008; Zhang et al. 2008), particularly if oral analgesics fail to provide adequate pain relief (Hochberg et al. 2012; NICE 2008) or in the case of an acute flare-up in pain (Jordan et al. 2003). Corticosteroids have both anti-inflammatory and immunosuppressive effects (Pekarek et al. 2011), with imaging studies providing evidence of a reduction in synovitis and joint effusion (Ostergaard et al. 1996). Meta-analyses (Bellamy et al. 2005; Godwin and Dawes 2004) examining the efficacy of intra-articular corticosteroid injection in patients with

OA of the knee have demonstrated significant pain relief compared with placebo injection. However, the analgesic effects are typically short-lived, with benefits lasting an average 1–4 weeks after the initial injection (Bellamy et al. 2005: Godwin and Dawes 2004). At the foot and ankle, a single-arm prospective cohort study (Ward et al. 2008) followed 18 patients with OA ($n=12$) and RA ($n=6$) for 1 year after intra-articular corticosteroid injection (methylprednisone acetate; 90 ± 40 mg total dose) into one or more of the joints. An average of 2.0 ± 0.6 joints were injected with 90 ± 40 mg of methylprednisolone acetate. In agreement with studies in other joints, the maximum therapeutic benefit occurred at 4 weeks before slowly declining over time. However, statistically significant improvements in the foot and ankle outcome score were observed up to 6 months after the injection. Adverse events are rare following intra-articular corticosteroid injection, but include a temporary flare-up in pain (2–15%), subcutaneous atrophy (0.6%), and joint infection (0.001–0.03%) (Courtney and Doherty 2005; Schumacher and Chen 2005). Clinically, there is some concern that repeated corticosteroid injections may lead to a faster rate of OA progression. However, this conjecture is not supported by the existing evidence (Raynauld et al. 2003; Roberts et al. 1996).

Hyaluronic Acid. Intra-articular injection of hyaluronic acid (HA) is recommended as a second-line treatment in some OA guidelines (Hochberg et al. 2012; Jordan et al. 2003; Zhang et al. 2008) but not others (AAOS 2008; NICE 2008). Intra-articular HA injection increases the viscosity of synovial fluid in OA joints by replacing lost hyaluranon content (Sun et al. 2009). This increase in viscosity is thought to aid in shock absorption, thereby protecting the damaged joint from adverse mechanical loading (Sun et al. 2009). In addition, HA may have anti-inflammatory and anti-catabolic effects on articular cartilage (Sun et al. 2009). HA injection is one of the few pharmacological interventions that has been specifically examined in patients with ankle OA. A recent meta-analysis (Chang et al. 2013) of HA injections in patients with ankle OA included data from 354 subjects in four randomized controlled trials (three studies of HA injection versus saline injection, one study of HA injection versus exercise), one comparative study (HA injection plus arthroscopy versus arthroscopy alone) and four single-arm prospective cohort studies (HA injection only). The number of HA injections ranged from one to five, with molecular weights of 500 to 6000 kDa and 1 mL to 2.5 mL doses per injection. The length of follow-up ranged from 3 to 18 months. Across all studies, a large pooled effect size [2.01 (95% confidence interval (CI), 1.27–2.75)] was reported in the improvement of pain scores from baseline following HA injection. However, large improvements in pain were also observed following saline (placebo) injection, with subsequent analysis suggesting that as much as 87% of the positive treatment effects of HA may be attributed to the placebo effects of injection (Chang et al. 2013). A transient post-injection flare in pain is reported in ~10% of patients receiving HA injection for ankle OA and is more common when high-molecular-weight HA is used (Chang et al. 2013).

Glucosamine

Two international guidelines (Jordan et al. 2003; Zhang et al. 2008) recommend the use of glucosamine sulphate in the management of hip and knee OA. One of these (Zhang et al. 2008) stipulates that the use of glucosamine should be abandoned if no substantial benefit is seen after 6 months. In contrast, other guidelines (AAOS 2008; Hochberg et al. 2012; NICE 2008) do not recommend glucosamine in the management of OA. Glucosamine is an amino sugar that is present in high quantities in the extracellular matrix of articular cartilage. It has been suggested to have both analgesic and disease-modifying effects in OA, reducing pain and slowing the progression of joint space narrowing (Khosla and Baumhauer 2008). The ingestion of glucosamine is thought to have an anabolic effect, stimulating the production of HA and GAGs that are essential in the maintenance and repair of articular cartilage (Khosla and Baumhauer 2008). In addition, glucosamine may have anti-inflammatory and anti-catabolic effects, inhibiting the action of cytokines and enzymes involved in the breakdown of cartilage (Khosla and Baumhauer 2008; Sherman et al. 2012). Many of the physiological effects of glucosamine have been demonstrated in vitro using various culture systems and formulations of glucosamine (Henrotin et al. 2012). Importantly, the concentrations of glucosamine used in these studies were typically 'supra-physiological', in most cases 100–2000 times the maximum realistic plasma concentration (10 μm) that could be expected after a typical 1500 mg dose of glucosamine sulphate in humans (Henrotin et al. 2012). Vlad et al. (2007) performed a meta-analysis of 15 trials that have compared glucosamine with placebo in the treatment of OA-related pain. A pooled effect size of −0.35 was observed in favour of glucosamine. Smaller effect sizes were observed for trials that were industry independent and in those that adequately concealed the allocation of participants to treatment and placebo groups. There was no evidence supporting the clinical efficacy of glucosamine hydrochloride, only glucosamine sulphate. This is reflected in the OA management guidelines as none recommend the use of glucosamine hydrochloride. Interestingly, there is no chemical or structural reason for the apparent difference in clinical efficacy of these formulations, as both glucosamine hydrochloride and glucosamine sulphate are broken down in the acid environment of the stomach to produce the active ingredient glucosamine (Henrotin et al. 2012). A recent meta-analysis (Lee et al. 2010) concentrated on the disease-modifying effects of glucosamine in OA as measured by the rate of joint space narrowing observed on radiograph. These authors concluded that glucosamine sulphate was not effective at reducing joint space narrowing after 1 year of treatment, but produced a small to moderate protective effect on minimum joint space narrowing after 3 years. These findings were based on the results of two studies. Glucosamine is generally considered to be safe, with no major side effects reported. However, it should be used with caution in those with an allergy to shellfish and, as typical doses provide up to 30% of the recommended daily intake of salt, caution is warranted in individuals with hypertension and renal dysfunction (Henrotin et al. 2012).

Chondroitin Sulphate

Two international guidelines (Jordan et al. 2003; Zhang et al. 2008) recommend the use of chondroitin sulphate in the management of hip and knee OA. One of these (Zhang et al. 2008) stipulates that the use of chondroitin should be abandoned if no substantial benefit is seen after 6 months. In contrast, other guidelines (AAOS 2008; Hochberg et al. 2012; NICE 2008) do not recommend chondroitin in the management of

OA. Chondroitin sulphate is a constituent of articular cartilage, with its properties conveying much of the resistance to cartilage compression (Lee et al. 2010; Reichenbach et al. 2007). In addition, chondroitin is thought to suppress the expression of various pro-inflammatory cytokines, thus reducing cartilage catabolism (Sherman et al. 2012). As with glucosamine, chondroitin is claimed to provide both pain-relieving and disease-modifying effects. In respect to pain relief, Reichenbach et al. (2007) performed a meta-analysis on 20 trials examining the pain-relieving effects of chondroitin compared with placebo in individuals with hip and knee OA. They observed an overall pooled effect size of −0.75 in favour of chondroitin. However, large differences were observed between trials, which could be explained by small sample sizes, a lack of intention-to-treat analysis, and failure to adequately conceal the allocation of participants to treatment and placebo groups. When analysis was restricted to methodologically sound trials ($n = 3$) with adequate sample size, the effect size of chondroitin on joint pain diminished to zero. With respect to chondroitin's potential disease-modifying effects, recent meta-analyses (Lee et al. 2010; Reichenbach et al. 2007) have found significant small to moderate protective effects of chondroitin on the rate of joint space narrowing. There are no major side effects associated with the use of chondroitin (Reichenbach et al. 2007; Sherman et al. 2012).

Other Analgesic Agents

Topical application of capsaicin is recommended as a first-line treatment for OA-related pain in two guidelines (Jordan et al. 2003; Zhang et al. 2008) and as a second-line treatment in two others (Hochberg et al. 2012; NICE 2008). Capsaicin contains the active ingredient from chili peppers and is applied to the skin in a cream or patch where it produces a strong localized burning sensation. The analgesic effects of capsacian are thought to relate to a reversible degeneration of cutaneous nociceptive fibres (Anand and Bley 2011), effectively desensitizing the treated area (Altman and Barthel 2011; Anand and Bley 2011). A single application may lead to nerve degeneration that lasts for weeks or even months afterwards (Anand and Bley 2011). Topical capsaicin has been shown to reduce pain in knee and hand OA. To date, five RCTs

(Altman et al. 1994; Deal et al. 1991; Gemmel et al. 2003; McCarthy and McCarty 1992; McCleane 2000) have been conducted, with sample sizes ranging from 14 to 200. The duration of intervention ranged from 4 to 12 weeks and concentrations of 0.015% to 0.075% capsaicin were applied one to four times per day. In all trials, capsaicin led to a significant reduction in pain compared with a placebo cream. After 4 weeks, a 33% reduction in pain severity was reported, compared with a 20% reduction in the placebo group (Deal et al. 1991), and after 12 weeks the comparable reductions were 54% and 38% (Altman et al. 1994). Adverse events associated with capsaicin use are usually minor but may include localized burning pain and erythema that can be intolerable for some patients (Altman and Barthel 2011). Across 16 studies examining the efficacy of capsaicin in 1556 patients with a variety of chronic pain conditions, 13% of capsaicin-treated patients were reported to have withdrawn owing to adverse events, compared with 3% of patients who received a placebo intervention (Mason et al. 2004).

PHYSICAL STRATEGIES

The fundamental principles for conservative management of OA are similar across the joints of the lower limb. Given the impairments and loss of function presented above, it is essential that these are assessed and an individualized rehabilitation programme prescribed. In respect to exercise, there is very little research that has been centred on OA at the ankle joint. Most studies have focused upon OA affecting the knee joint.

The benefits of improving muscle performance in individuals with OA are thought to be multifaceted. Such improvements can lead to (1) enhanced shock absorption by muscles, (2) improved phasing and reflex activation of muscle activation, thus lessening stress on articular cartilage during gait activities, and (3) improved proprioception and balance. The overall aim of exercise is to improve function and reduce pain. In addition, there are indirect effects associated with continuing to exercise regularly that include reducing levels of depression and anxiety, which often present in patients with chronic pain conditions, and lessening the likelihood of cardiovascular co-morbidities, which are often apparent in those with OA of the lower limb.

A Physical Activity Guidelines Advisory Committee report to the US Department of Health and Human Services (2008) has provided guidelines concerning physical activity for those individuals with disabilities. This report made specific mention of exercise for those with OA with the guidelines recommending that adults should get at least 150 minutes of moderate-intensity or 75 minutes of vigorous-intensity aerobic activity per week. Vigorous activity is defined as that in which heart and breathing rate are elevated to the point where conversation is hard. Furthermore, it was recommended that individuals also undertake strength training of moderate or high intensity on 2 or more days per week. These recommendations are very similar to those of the American College of Sports Medicine that individuals aged 50–64 with chronic conditions such as arthritis need to undertake moderately intense cardiovascular exercise for 30 minutes a day, 5 days a week *or* undertake vigorously intense cardio exercise for 20 minutes a day, 3 days a week, *and* undertake 8–10 strength-training exercises (8–12 repetitions of each exercise) twice a week. This amount of exercise is considerable. Ham et al. (2009) reported that, on any given day in the USA, only 29% of men and 22% of women aged 40–75 years participate in physical activity for longer than 30 minutes, and this activity included a combination of sports, exercise, and recreational activities. Notably, activity levels were decreased when individuals were overweight or obese, which is not uncommon in those with OA. Furthermore, as indicated in previous sections, individuals with OA can have notable pain, disability, poor self-efficacy, and depression. Hence the likelihood of these individuals meeting the guidelines seems unrealistic. It is therefore important that exercise programmes for individuals with OA are progressive and modified to suit the sensitivity of the patient's symptoms, hence minimizing flare-ups at the damaged joint and ultimately leading to increased compliance. Additionally, it is advantageous to limit the presence of inflammatory exudate as it can adversely affect articular cartilage (Roemer et al. 2011) and, at least at the knee, as little as 10 mL of intra-articular swelling can lead to muscle activation deficits (Wood et al. 1988). Muscle activation deficits are clinically important as they reduce the effectiveness of strengthening exercises and can lead to long-lasting muscle weakness.

Our experience is that formal programmes in which older individuals (65+ years) go to a gym-like environment for their exercise are not always successful, with compliance being the main issue. Recent work by Grant (2008) noted that many older people have in their youth never exercised in a regular manner for the improvement of health. In those times, the physicality of their daily lives was sufficiently habitual. Grant et al. commented that some older adults thought exercising deliberately was 'an unusual way to spend my time' and 'boring' compared with undertaking hobbies. Thus it seems likely that elderly individuals are more likely to incorporate exercise/increased physical activity into their lives when it is purposeful (e.g. gardening, or walking greater distances or faster when going shopping or visiting people). Where formal exercise sessions are undertaken, these are likely to have improved attendance when they are run as a group session with participants being of a similar age, often incorporating opportunities for social engagement within/after the sessions thus allowing camaraderie to develop within the group.

Prescriptions recommended for increasing strength (Rhea 2004) suggest that loading levels of >60% 1 RM (repetition maximum) can be effective in individuals who have been relatively sedentary. A typical regimen that we employ when individuals start a strengthening programme is 3 sets at 15–20 RM with 2 minutes rest between each set. We find that higher loading levels introduced too early in sedentary individuals with OA can induce delayed-onset muscle soreness and flare-ups of pain and swelling in the joint. This regimen stays in place for 2–3 weeks and then the load is increased such that the person is performing three sets at 12 RM, ultimately aiming to attain loads of 8–10 RM for each set. Such a programme would be expected to lead to 20–25% improvements in strength. In patients with notable pain and joint swelling, it may be necessary to target muscle activation deficits using interventions such as cryotherapy (Rice et al. 2009) and transcutaneous electrical stimulation (Pietrosimone et al. 2011) in conjunction with resistance training.

For muscle endurance, which is focused on improving the aerobic metabolism of the muscle, the prescription involves 20–30 RM for three sets with rest breaks of 1 minute between sets. This prescription has been shown to increase repetitions to failure by 50–100% over 8 weeks (Campos et al. 2002). For stretching, the ideal prescription for gaining range of motion is unknown. In individuals with minimal losses in ROM, a single sustained stretch of 30 seconds per day, 5 days per week for 6 weeks has been shown to induce gains of 20–25% in ROM (Bandy et al. 1997). In elderly patients with limited dorsiflexion, Gajdosik et al. (2005) reported improvements in dorsiflexion ROM from 11° to 16° following an 8-week training programme of 10 15-second stretches of the plantarflexors performed three times per week. These authors also noted significant improvements in agility and speed of walking. Some research (Gajdosik 2006) has shown that dorsiflexion ROM is positively correlated with balance. There is also evidence (McNair et al. 2001) to suggest that dynamic stretching can be more beneficial than sustained holds at the end of range in reducing stiffness at a joint, stiffness in this context being resistance through the range of motion.

At the knee and hip joint, cardiovascular fitness in those with moderate to severe OA has been shown to be 55–70% that of matched subjects without osteoarthritis (Ries et al. 1995). Decreased cardiovascular fitness is associated with co-morbidities such as coronary heart disease (Sandvik et al. 1993), therefore it would be beneficial to target this element of fitness. Furthermore, as findings (Older et al. 1999) suggest that poor cardiovascular fitness in those individuals who are having surgery increases the risk of having complications and mortality, there is much to be gained from an exercise programme inclusive of aerobic fitness, particularly in older patients undergoing surgery for their OA. Despite concerns related to additional loading causing damage to articular cartilage, there is good evidence to support the use of aerobic exercise programmes involving gait activities to improve pain and cardiovascular fitness levels (Loew et al. 2012). Of note, Minor et al. (1989) reported ~20% improvements in peak VO_2 in poorly conditioned subjects with OA of the knee after walking and aquatic programmes of 12 weeks, where subjects exercised at 60–80% of their maximum heart rate.

Given that limb alignment issues can influence the pattern of loading on articular cartilage during gait activities, ankle foot orthoses (AFO) may be beneficial in providing improvements in alignment and limiting range of motion particularly in the sagittal plane, ultimately redistributing stress more evenly across the joint surface. Ideally, while restricting motion at the ankle joint, orthoses should allow motion at other joints, particularly in the mid- and forefoot. Using three-dimensional motion analysis, Huang et al. (2006) tested three different types of braces that varied in their size and the amount of movement restriction. In subjects with OA at the ankle joint, they found that a rigid brace was effective in reducing both sagittal and frontal plane motion compared with wearing standard shoes. They also reported that the HFO-R brace was most effective in allowing forefoot motion while reducing hindfoot motion, and hence recommended it for patients with OA of the ankle joint. Of note, John and Bongiovanni (2009) comment that compliance can be an issue particularly when braces are bulky and unattractive from a cosmetic perspective.

It is also apparent that shoes that have good shock absorption (Lafortune and Hennig 1992) will be beneficial in reducing the magnitude of the shock waves associated with the ground reaction force at footstrike. There are no studies that have explored the effects of shoe inserts upon biomechanical variables during gait or symptoms in individuals with ankle OA. However, there is evidence that these can reduce ground reaction forces and tibial accelerations during gait activities (Zhang et al. 2005), with research utilizing finite element modelling indicating that conformity of the insole is more important than the material utilized within the insert (Goske et al. 2006). Additionally, patients should be encouraged to exercise as much as possible on surfaces other than concrete pathways (Mohamed et al. 2005).

Patients who have post-traumatic OA as compared with primary OA are likely to be younger and hence more active, thereby placing greater loads upon the joint (Schenk et al. 2011). Thus education should also include discussion of the volume and type of exercise that they should perform. The presence of flare-ups in pain and swelling following exercise provides a guide as to the appropriate amount of exercise to be performed in a single session.

SURGICAL STRATEGIES

For focal lesions, surgery is focused upon the repair of the articular surface. Microfracture, which involves the perforation of the subchondral bone with drill holes, stimulates a bone marrow reaction that leads to fibrocartilaginous repair (Figure 1-6). It is generally the first choice for lesions that are less than 1.5 cm^2 (Choi et al. 2009). A recent review by Zengerink et al. (2010) indicated such procedures had an 85% success rate. However, although clinical outcomes are positive, the study of Lee et al. (2009) in arthroscoped patients 1 year after microfracture treatment found 40% to have abnormal tissue repair and a further 35% to have unhealed tissue, indicative of the need for a cautious return to work and sporting activities. An alternative surgical technique that can be utilized for larger lesions is autologous osteochondral transplantation (Figure 1-7). This involves harvesting plugs of cartilage and bone (often from the knee joint) that are inserted side by side within the damaged area. A biomechanical analysis using cadavers showed that force and pressure levels can be restored to near-normal levels following this procedure (Fansa et al. 2011). Of crucial importance is the congruence of the graft with the talar articular surface (Murawski and Kennedy 2013). Case series studies (Hangody et al. 2008; Paul et al. 2012) indicate good to excellent clinical results in the short and medium term, with between 5 and 15% of patients continuing to experience symptoms.

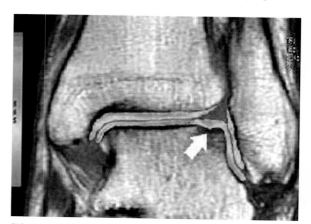

FIGURE 1-6 Microfracture at the ankle joint. Thirteen months following microfracture to the lateral margin of the talar dome, a coronal quantitative T2 map demonstrates diffuse short T2 values without colour stratification at the site of cartilage repair indicative of less normal/mature tissue. (Reprinted with permission of Sage Publications, from Murawski CD, Foo LF, Kennedy JG. A review of arthroscopic bone marrow stimulation techniques of the talus: the good, the bad, and the causes for concern. Cartilage 2010;1(2):137–144. All rights reserved. Copyright (2010). http://online.sagepub.com.)

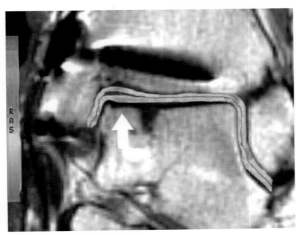

FIGURE 1-7 Autologous osteochondral transplantation at the ankle joint. Coronal quantitative T2 map of an autologous osteochondral plug transplanted into the medial margin of the talar dome showing normal colour stratification of T2 values, at the site of cartilage repair, indicative of relative normal cartilage. (Reprinted with permission of Sage Publications, from Murawski CD, Foo LF, Kennedy JG. A review of arthroscopic bone marrow stimulation techniques of the talus: the good, the bad, and the causes for concern. Cartilage 2010;1(2):137–144. All rights reserved. Copyright (2010). http://online.sagepub.com.)

Although realignment surgery is utilized for OA of the knee and hip joints, it is less often considered as a strategy to slow progression of cartilage damage at the ankle joint. However, it is a logical option for younger patients who have articular cartilage damage but wish to continue participating in vigorous athletic activity. The primary aim is to unload the damaged area and hence reduce pressure/stress (Friedman et al. 2001). Research has primarily focused upon osteotomy at the distal tibia, though it is apparent that additional surgery within the hindfoot is needed, particularly where fixed deformities or osteoarthritis are apparent in the subtalar joints (Pagenstert et al. 2007). Of key importance is whether hindfoot malalignment is fixed or mobile, the latter responding well to soft-tissue surgical techniques such as lengthening of tendons, tendon transfers, and ligament repair (Di-Domenico and Gatalyak 2012; Gibson and Prieskorn 2007). Good outcomes from realignment surgery have been observed in case series assessing reductions in pain and improvements in function in the short term (3–5 years) (Pagenstert et al. 2007; Takakura et al. 1998).

Traditionally, arthrodesis was the primary technique for surgical intervention in end-stage ankle OA. Arthrodesis involves fusion of the ankle joint using internal and external fixation. Numerous procedures have been described (Abidi et al. 2000), and generally the results suggest that pain is decreased and stability increased (Coester et al. 2001). At a 4-year follow-up (Thomas et al. 2006), gait analysis following arthrodesis showed that cadence and step length were reduced significantly, leading to ~25% decrease in gait velocity. Thomas et al. (2006) also reported considerable ROM reductions (20–70%) in the sagittal and frontal plane in the hindfoot and forefoot. In contrast, researchers (Wu et al. 2000) have observed increased ROM in hindfoot and the forefoot joints during gait, which have been thought to be compensating for loss of motion at the ankle joint per se. In some instances, arthritic changes in these articulations have subsequently been reported (Fuchs et al. 2003). Certainly the position and motion of joints that attach to the calcaneum must be considered if the optimal results for ankle joint procedures are to be attained (Gibson and Prieskorn 2007).

In recent years, there has been increased interest in joint replacement as an alternative to arthrodesis, particularly in light of improvements in function observed in the third-generation implants (Figure 1-8). These joints are categorized as being mobile bearing devices and have three components: a metal tibial and talar component, together with a polyethylene meniscus, which is not attached. For a review of the evolution of ankle joint replacements see Gougoulias et al. (2009). Notable improvements in gait parameters have been observed following joint replacement at the ankle. For instance, a recent study by Brodsky et al. (2011) showed walking velocity, cadence, and stride length to be increased by 20, 13, and 17% respectively. These changes reflected plantarflexion increases of 4–6°, improving motion at toe-off considerably with accompanying improvements in the plantarflexor moments and ankle joint power of 24–45%. Interestingly, ROM at the knee and hip during the gait cycle was also increased by 5–7°. The duration over which ankle joint replacements can be expected to remain functional varies between 70% and 98% over 3–6 years and from 80% to 95% at 8–12 years (Easley et al. 2011). A recent meta-analysis by Haddad et al. (2007) that compared arthrodesis with second-generation

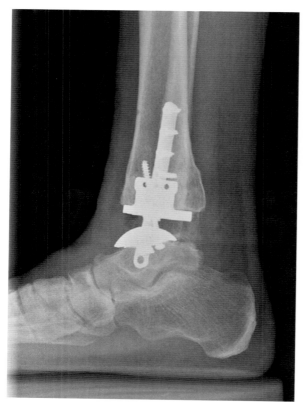

FIGURE 1-8 Total ankle joint replacement as seen on a radio-graph. (Reprinted with permission from Schweitzer KM, Adams SB, Viens NA, Queen RM, Easley ME, Deorio JK, Nunley JA. Early prospective clinical results of a modern fixed-bearing total ankle arthroplasty. J Bone Joint Surg Am 2013 95(11):1002–1011. http://jbjs.org/.)

joint replacements showed that AOFAS scores were similar: 75 versus 78 respectively. In a systematic review that focused upon currently used implants, Gougoulias et al. (2010) concluded that residual pain was commonly observed (23–60%), ROM improvement was small (0–14°), and satisfaction was rated at 8/10 by patients.

LIFESTYLE AND EDUCATION STRATEGIES

Education programmes are aimed at increasing the ability of patients to understand their condition, and manage it more effectively in various situations (social, physical, emotional) that commonly occur in their normal daily life. The key topics addressed in such programmes include the effects of OA on the body, treatments available, how to protect the joint and

maintain function, and instituting coping strategies. The findings of research in this area are mixed. Based on a meta-analysis of the literature, Devos-Comby et al. (2006) reported a minimal effect for self-management programmes upon physical outcomes and a small significant effect for improvement in psychological outcomes. The reported cost effectiveness of such programmes is also small (Lord et al. 1999; Lorig et al. 1993; Mazzuca et al. 1999). Consequently, Devos-Comby et al. (2006) called for more innovative and novel lifestyle and education strategies. In this respect, education based on pain neuroscience has been shown to be effective in individuals with other types of chronic musculoskeletal pain (Louw et al. 2011). This approach deliberately de-emphasizes tissue mechanics and pathology, instead focusing on increased nerve sensitivity as an explanation for the patient's pain. There is evidence that such a strategy can lead to immediate reductions in pain, catastrophizing, fear of movement/re-injury, and self-reported disability (Louw et al. 2011). These findings provide support for longer-term evaluations being undertaken, including in an OA population.

Recently there has been increasing interest in the effect of socioeconomic determinants on OA outcomes. These determinants include educational level, occupation, and wealth (individual and neighbourhood). It is apparent that individuals with OA who have lower socioeconomic status are likely to score worse on outcome questionnaires related to severity of OA pain and function (Juhakoski et al. 2008). Furthermore they are less likely to receive specialist consultation and joint replacement (Brennan et al. 2012; Ellis and Bucholz 2007). Numerous factors with varying levels of modification available might be responsible. These include the type of work in which these patients are employed and their ability to access health services easily. Furthermore, health literacy is important (Gordon et al. 2002) as it affects the ability of patients to understand their diagnosis and prognosis, as well as their perception of the risk associated with treatments and the effectiveness of various treatments (Hawker et al. 2004), particularly those involving the use of anti-inflammatory and other pain medications and what to expect from surgery. Further work is needed in this area. A recent review by Lowe et al. (2013) highlighted the dearth of research examining the effectiveness of education programmes for those with low literacy levels. The findings also indicated that only small effects in improving knowledge, self-efficacy, and wellbeing were apparent. Consideration should also be given to the possibility of general practitioners not being confident that patients with lower socioeconomic status can appreciate and adhere to the commitment associated with surgical and rehabilitation procedures, and thus being more restrictive in their treatment recommendations (van Ryn and Burke 2000).

The influence of neighbourhood factors is also apparent. Living in lower socioeconomic areas is associated with increased prevalence of self-reported and radiologically confirmed OA as well as increased symptoms (Callahan et al. 2011). Such findings highlight the importance of access to resources in the community, such as level walkways with good lighting, cycle paths, swimming pools, exercise equipment, community halls, and disabled parking. Such resources can affect rehabilitation potential and one's ability to commit to and maintain ongoing lifestyle changes associated with physical activity (Martin et al. 2012). Additionally, social support services are important, and their presence has been positively correlated with levels of function in those with OA (Ethgen et al. 2004). Such services include help with the performance of daily living activities, sharing of concerns and burden, and improvement in interactions with family and friends.

FUTURE DIRECTIONS

Irrespective of the lower limb joint affected, there are a number of paths that are being followed to improve the quality of life of individuals with OA. A number of risk factors such as body mass and physical activity levels are readily modifiable. However, in respect to the former, the ideal strategy to combat this global epidemic remains elusive, and requires a multifaceted approach involving not only targeting the individual's lifestyle and coping strategies but also bringing into effect government policies that ensure food-based corporations act responsibly in the content and marketing of their products. There are also notable links between obesity, metabolic syndrome, and inflammation. These conditions provide a systemic source for increased inflammation in addition to that emanating from the damaged joint, and subsequently there is a need to consider OA as a multisystem disease rather than an isolated joint problem.

In regard to physical activity, the current guidelines for physical activity in individuals with chronic conditions such as OA are demanding, and with the additional burden of pain as well as common issues of increased body weight, low self-efficacy, and depressed mood, it seems unlikely that these guidelines could be met without new innovative strategies for motivating people to start exercise as well as maintaining their compliance. This is particularly so for the older patient. Linked to this concern is the need to establish the most efficient exercise regimen to prescribe for the individual. At present, the right blend between local muscle endurance and strengthening exercises, together with more global exercise to aid balance and improve cardiovascular fitness, is not known. Yet to combine all in the same programme is likely to dilute their effect and render an overall programme less effective.

Advances in genetics may produce reliable markers that can identify patients at risk of osteoarthritis. These people can then be targeted with physical activity and education programmes as well as medications that optimize their time without symptoms and disability. Genetic markers might also identify those individuals who respond to a particular treatment but not others. In this respect, medical treatment will become much more customized to the individual.

Regarding medications, recent research focused on the chondrocyte's action in osteoarthritic joints suggests that drugs targeting the signalling pathways that sustain the inflammatory process have potential for arresting the loss of articular cartilage. As mentioned above, there is a need for medications that also target the systemic lower-grade inflammation associated with metabolic syndrome and obesity. More recent advances in our understanding of the mechanisms of chronic pain, including OA, suggest that drugs that act on the central nervous system by increasing the effectiveness of endogenous pain-inhibitory pathways or dampening the excitability of nociceptive pathways may have a role to play in the future management of OA-related pain.

There are many important decisions to be made by patients concerning treatment options and the inherent risks and benefits associated with their choice. Given the small improvements in understanding associated with current education and lifestyle programmes, there is a need to consider better-designed and more innovative approaches, particularly for those individuals with limited formal education. Combined with such programmes, additional community-based initiatives are needed to increase the number of quality of resources (physical and social) available to those with OA. This is particularly important for the very old and frail who will otherwise not fare well in remaining independent in their own homes.

At the ankle, because OA is often the result of trauma, usually sustained in young adults, the onset of OA is much earlier. Yet the treatment options, particularly those involving joint replacement, are limited by the lifespan of the current prostheses and the increased likelihood of a poor result when surgical revision is attempted. Thus technical advancements in materials to improve wear resistance and the ability of such devices to emulate more closely the motion of the ankle joint in vivo are needed.

Finally, there is a need for more research focused upon the nature and pattern of pain and how it changes as OA of the ankle progresses. In doing so, an appreciation of the burden of the disease can be better appreciated and rehabilitation can be honed to those problems of most concern to the patient.

INVITED COMMENTARY

This chapter presents an excellent overview of the relevant knowledge on ankle osteoarthritis (OA), ranging from predisposing factors, to diagnosis, and then to management strategies. The detection of primary OA, especially in its early stages, is often difficult because of the absence of signs and symptoms in the affected individuals. This represents a major challenge in research. Among the different predisposing factors, the increased joint loading (also related to high body weight/mass, and continuous participation in work and sports) may be the crucial factor. This 'loading factor' (added to anatomical or lower limb alignment issues) is also discussed to be one of the causes for development of stress fractures. Long-distance runners and soldiers (but not only) are some examples of individuals sustaining this type of overuse injuries. Can prevention play a role in this context? The answer is likely to be 'yes', despite the lack of scientific studies in the area. A healthy lifestyle, an individual-adapted regular fitness and/or sports participation, and compliance with exercise-based injury prevention programmes may contribute to 'better' joint function ('joint homeostasis' or 'envelope of function', as formulated by Dr Scott Dye). Stabilization and strengthening training for the core and lower extremity (including gluteal musculature), neuromuscular control and balance training – such interventions were recently found to have a protective reduction in knee joint loading in individuals with early knee OA.

After a detailed description of the most common diagnostic options, the authors discuss the various conservative (pharmacological and physical) and surgical treatment strategies in OA patients. Despite the advances in the pharmacological agents, the importance of physical activity (supported by strong scientific evidence) should be continuously promoted. It is also best for prevention of other co-morbidities (such as cardiovascular which is typically observed in OA patients). The documentation of pain, function, and quality of life with scientifically valid/reliable/responsive scales or questionnaires (as summarized in Table 1-1) represents an important aspect at all stages of rehabilitation (before/during and after).

The fact that a previous injury is an important predisposing factor for secondary OA indirectly highlights the role of optimal rehabilitation after the injury or surgery. In all situations, one of the goals should be to address the underlying causative factors. As an example, muscle strength deficits (often at the core, trunk, and pelvis level) or imbalances (quadriceps versus hamstring) need to be specifically addressed in the rehabilitation process. The treatment protocols should be individually targeted, and not only follow strictly schematic recommendations. If available, the use of 'progressive-loading treadmills' (Anti-Gravity Treadmill®; AlterG) allows for an individual dosage of joint loading, thus possibly helping the normalization of the homeostasis in the OA-affected joint(s).

When dealing with active exercising, one should not forget the possibility of water-based training. The properties of water offer an optimal exercising environment to unload the OA-affected lower limb joint(s). Clinical and empirical experiences often show that group activities (land- or pool-based) are stimulating and motivating situations for OA patients, because they are linked with a socializing component.

As pointed out in the 'Future directions' paragraph, and discussed here, the early detection of OA would represent a major step torward an optimal management of OA, while preventive measures (as an example through exercise-based programmes) may or should be the way to go, even in the absence of hard scientific evidence.

Mario Bizzini MSc, PhD, PT
Research Associate, Orthopaedics Lower Extremity,
FIFA – Medical Assessment and
Research Centre, Zurich, Switzerland

REFERENCES

AAOS, 2008. American Academy of Orthopaedic Surgeons clinical practice guideline on the treatment of osteoarthritis of the knee (non-arthroplasty), American Academy of Orthopaedic Surgeons, Rosemont, IL.

Abidi, N.A., Gruen, G.S., Conti, S.F., 2000. Ankle arthrodesis: indications and techniques. Journal of the American Academy of Orthopaedic Surgeons 8, 200–209.

Adam, C., Eckstein, F., Milz, S., et al., 1998. The distribution of cartilage thickness within the joints of the lower limb of elderly individuals. Journal of Anatomy 193 (2), 203–214.

Altman, R.D., Aven, A., Holmburg, C.E., et al., 1994. Capsaicin cream 0.025% as monotherapy for osteoarthritis: a double-blind study. Seminars in Arthritis and Rheumatism 23, 25–33.

Altman, R.D., Barthel, H.R., 2011. Topical therapies for osteoarthritis. Drugs 71, 1259–1279.

Anand, P., Bley, K., 2011. Topical capsaicin for pain management: therapeutic potential and mechanisms of action of the new high-concentration capsaicin 8% patch. British Journal of Anaesthesia 107, 490–502.

Anderson, B.J., 2008. Paracetamol (acetaminophen): mechanisms of action. Paediatric Anaesthesia 18, 915–921.

Angst, M.S., Clark, J.D., 2006. Opioid-induced hyperalgesia: a qualitative systematic review. Anesthesiology 104, 570–587.

Armstrong, B., Mcnair, P., Taylor, D., 2008. Head and neck position sense. Sports Medicine 38, 101–117.

Bandy, W.D., Irion, J.M., Briggler, M., 1997. The effect of time and frequency of static stretching on flexibility of the hamstring muscles. Physical Therapy 77, 1090–1096.

Barnes, C.J., Ferkel, R.D., 2003. Arthroscopic debridement and drilling of osteochondral lesions of the talus. Foot and Ankle Clinics 8, 243–257.

Bellamy, N., Campbell, J., Robinson, V., et al., 2005. Intraarticular corticosteroid for treatment of osteoarthritis of the knee. Cochrane Database of Systematic Reviews (2), CD005328.

Bischof, J.E., Spritzer, C.E., Caputo, A.M., et al., 2010. In vivo cartilage contact strains in patients with lateral ankle instability. Journal of Biomechanics 43, 2561–2566.

Bjordal, J.M., Ljunggren, A.E., Klovning, A., et al., 2004. Non-steroidal anti-inflammatory drugs, including cyclo-oxygenase-2 inhibitors, in osteoarthritic knee pain: meta-analysis of randomized placebo controlled trials. British Medical Journal 329, 1317.

Bonnin, M.P., Laurent, J.R., Casillas, M., 2009. Ankle function and sports activity after total ankle arthroplasty. Foot and Ankle International 30, 933–944.

Boocock, M., Mcnair, P., Cicuttini, F., et al., 2009. The short-term effects of running on the deformation of knee articular cartilage and its relationship to biomechanical loads at the knee. Osteoarthritis and Cartilage 17, 883–890.

Bozic, K.J., Stacey, B., Berger, A., et al., 2012. Resource utilization and costs before and after total joint arthroplasty. BMC Health Services Research 12, 73.

Brennan, S.L., Stanford, T., Wluka, A.E., et al., 2012. Utilisation of primary total knee joint replacements across socioeconomic status in the Barwon Statistical Division, Australia, 2006–2007: a cross-sectional study. British Medical Journal Open 2 (5), pii:e001310.

Brodsky, J.W., Polo, F.E., Coleman, S.C., et al., 2011. Changes in gait following the Scandinavian total ankle replacement. Journal of Bone and Joint Surgery, American Volume 93, 1890–1896.

Brown, T.D., Shaw, D.T., 1983. In vitro contact stress distributions in the natural human hip. Journal of Biomechanics 16, 373–384.

Budiman-Mak, E., Conrad, K., Stuck, R., et al., 2006. Theoretical model and Rasch analysis to develop a revised Foot Function Index. Foot and Ankle International 27, 519–527.

Budiman-Mak, E., Conrad, K.J., Roach, K.E., 1991. The Foot Function Index: a measure of foot pain and disability. Journal of Clinical Epidemiology 44, 561–570.

Busija, L., Buchbinder, R., Osborne, R.H., 2013. A grounded patient-centered approach generated the Personal and Societal Burden of Osteoarthritis model. Journal of Clinical Epidemiology 66, 994–1005.

Button, G., Pinney, S., 2004. A meta-analysis of outcome rating scales in foot and ankle surgery: is there a valid, reliable, and responsive system? Foot and Ankle International 25, 521–525.

Callahan, L.F., Cleveland, R.J., Shreffler, J., et al., 2011. Associations of educational attainment, occupation and community poverty with knee osteoarthritis in the Johnston County (North Carolina) osteoarthritis project. Arthritis Research and Therapy 13, R169.

Campos, G.E., Luecke, T.J., Wendeln, H.K., et al., 2002. Muscular adaptations in response to three different resistance-training regimens: specificity of repetition maximum training zones. European Journal of Applied Physiology 88, 50–60.

Cepeda, M.S., Camargo, F., Zea, C., et al., 2006. Tramadol for osteoarthritis. Cochrane Database Systemic Reviews (3), CD005522.

Cerezal, L., Llopis, E., Canga, A., et al., 2008. MR arthrography of the ankle: indications and technique. Radiologic Clinics of North America 46, 973–994, v.

Chang, K.V., Hsiao, M.Y., Chen, W.S., et al., 2013. Effectiveness of intra-articular hyaluronic acid for ankle osteoarthritis treatment: a systematic review and meta-analysis. Archives of Physical Medicine and Rehabilitation 94, 951–960.

Cheng, D.S., Visco, C.J., 2012. Pharmaceutical therapy for osteoarthritis. Physical Medicine and Rehabilitation 4, S82–S88.

Choi, G.W., Choi, W.J., Youn, H.K., et al., 2013. Osteochondral lesions of the talus: are there any differences between osteochondral and chondral types? American Journal of Sports Medicine 41, 504–510.

Choi, W.J., Park, K.K., Kim, B.S., et al., 2009. Osteochondral lesion of the talus: is there a critical defect size for poor outcome? American Journal of Sports Medicine 37, 1974–1980.

Coester, L.M., Saltzman, C.L., Leupold, J., et al., 2001. Long-term results following ankle arthrodesis for post-traumatic arthritis. Journal of Bone and Joint Surgery, American Volume 83-A, 219–228.

Cohen, M.M., Altman, R.D., Hollstrom, R., et al., 2008. Safety and efficacy of intra-articular sodium hyaluronate (Hyalgan) in a randomized, double-blind study for osteoarthritis of the ankle. Foot and Ankle International 29, 657–663.

Cole, A.A., Kuettner, K.E., 2002. Molecular basis for differences between human joints. Cellular and Molecular Life Sciences 59, 19–26.

Committee PAGA, 2008. Physical Activity Guidelines Advisory Committee report, US Department of Health and Human Services, Washington DC.

Courtney, P., Doherty, M., 2005. Joint aspiration and injection. Best Practice and Research in Clinical Rheumatology 19, 345–369.

Dai, J., Ikegawa, S., 2010. Recent advances in association studies of osteoarthritis susceptibility genes. Journal of Human Genetics 55, 77–80.

Deal, C.L., Schnitzer, T.J., Lipstein, E., et al., 1991. Treatment of arthritis with topical capsaicin: a double-blind trial. Clinical Therapeutics 13, 383–395.

Devos-Comby, L., Cronan, T., Roesch, S.C., 2006. Do exercise and self-management interventions benefit patients with osteoarthritis of the knee? A metaanalytic review. Journal of Rheumatology 33, 744–756.

Didomenico, L.A., Gatalyak, N., 2012. End-stage ankle arthritis: arthrodiastasis, supramalleolar osteotomy, or arthrodesis? Clinics in Podiatric Medicine and Surgery 29, 391–412.

Dieppe, P.A., Cushnaghan, J., Shepstone, L., 1997. The Bristol 'OA500' study: progression of osteoarthritis (OA) over 3 years and the relationship between clinical and radiographic changes at the knee joint. Osteoarthritis and Cartilage 5, 87–97.

Domsic, R.T., Saltzman, C.L., 1998. Ankle osteoarthritis scale. Foot and Ankle International 19, 466–471.

Easley, M.E., Adams, S.B., Jr., Hembree, W.C., et al., 2011. Results of total ankle arthroplasty. Journal of Bone and Joint Surgery, American Volume 93, 1455–1468.

Elias, I., Raikin, S.M., Schweitzer, M.E., et al., 2009. Osteochondral lesions of the distal tibial plafond: localization and morphologic characteristics with an anatomical grid. Foot and Ankle International 30, 524–529.

Elias, I., Zoga, A.C., Morrison, W.B., et al., 2007. Osteochondral lesions of the talus: localization and morphologic data from 424 patients using a novel anatomical grid scheme. Foot and Ankle International 28, 154–161.

Ellis, H., Bucholz, R., 2007. Disparity of care in total hip arthroplasty. Current Opinion in Orthopaedics 18, 2–7.

Ethgen, O., Vanparijs, P., Delhalle, S., et al., 2004. Social support and health-related quality of life in hip and knee osteoarthritis. Quality of Life Research 13, 321–330.

Fansa, A.M., Murawski, C.D., Imhauser, C.W., et al., 2011. Autologous osteochondral transplantation of the talus partially restores contact mechanics of the ankle joint. American Journal of Sports Medicine 39, 2457–2465.

Felson, D.T., Anderson, J.J., Naimark, A., et al., 1988. Obesity and knee osteoarthritis. The Framingham Study. Annals of Internal Medicine 109, 18–24.

Felson, D.T., Naimark, A., Anderson, J., et al., 1987. The prevalence of knee osteoarthritis in the elderly. The Framingham Osteoarthritis Study. Arthritis and Rheumatism 30, 914–918.

Fortin, P.T., Guettler, J., Manoli, A.I.I., 2002. Idiopathic cavovarus and lateral ankle instability: recognition and treatment implications relating to ankle arthritis. Foot and Ankle International 23, 1031–1037.

Friedman, M.A., Draganich, L.F., Toolan, B., et al., 2001. The effects of adult acquired flatfoot deformity on tibiotalar joint contact characteristics. Foot and Ankle International 22, 241–246.

Fuchs, S., Sandmann, C., Skwara, A., et al., 2003. Quality of life 20 years after arthrodesis of the ankle. A study of adjacent joints. Journal of Bone and Joint Surgery, British Volume 85, 994–998.

Gajdosik, R.L., 2006. Relation of age and passive properties of an ankle dorsiflexion stretch to the timed one-leg stance test in older women. Perceptual and Motor Skills 103, 177–182.

Gajdosik, R.L., Vander Linden, D.W., McNair, P.J., et al., 2005. Effects of an eight-week stretching program on the passive-elastic properties and function of the calf muscles of older women. Clinical Biomechanics 20, 973–983.

Gemmell, H.A., Jacobson, B.H., Hayes, B.M., 2003. Effect of a topical herbal cream on osteoarthritis of the hand and knee: a pilot study. Journal of Manipulative and Physiological Therapeutics 26 (5), e15.

Gibson, V., Prieskorn, D., 2007. The valgus ankle. Foot and Ankle Clinics 12, 15–27.

Glazebrook, M., Daniels, T., Younger, A., et al., 2008. Comparison of health-related quality of life between patients with end-stage ankle and hip arthrosis. Journal of Bone and Joint Surgery, American Volume 90, 499–505.

Godwin, M., Dawes, M., 2004. Intra-articular steroid injections for painful knees. Systematic review with meta-analysis. Canadian Family Physician 50, 241–248.

Gooberman-Hill, R., Woolhead, G., Mackichan, F., et al., 2007. Assessing chronic joint pain: lessons from a focus group study. Arthritis and Rheumatism 57, 666–671.

Gordon, M.M., Hampson, R., Capell, H.A., et al., 2002. Illiteracy in rheumatoid arthritis patients as determined by the Rapid Estimate of Adult Literacy in Medicine (REALM) score. Rheumatology 41, 750–754.

Goske, S., Erdemir, A., Petre, M., et al., 2006. Reduction of plantar heel pressures: insole design using finite element analysis. Journal of Biomechanics 39, 2363–2370.

Gougoulias, N., Khanna, A., Maffulli, N., 2010. How successful are current ankle replacements?: a systematic review of the literature. Clinical Orthopaedics and Related Research 468, 199–208.

Gougoulias, N.E., Khanna, A., Maffulli, N., 2009. History and evolution in total ankle arthroplasty. British Medical Bulletin 89, 111–151.

Grant, B., 2008. An insider's view on physical activity in later life. Psychology of Sport and Exercise 9, 817–829.

Haddad, S.L., Coetzee, J.C., Estok, R., et al., 2007. Intermediate and long-term outcomes of total ankle arthroplasty and ankle arthrodesis. A systematic review of the literature. Journal of Bone and Joint Surgery, American Volume 89, 1899–1905.

Ham, S.A., Kruger, J., Tudor-Locke, C., 2009. Participation by US adults in sports, exercise, and recreational physical activities. Journal of Physical Activity and Health 6, 6–14.

Hangody, L., Vasarhelyi, G., Hangody, L.R., et al., 2008. Autologous osteochondral grafting – technique and long-term results. Injury 39 (Suppl. 1), S32–S39.

Hannan, M.T., Felson, D.T., Pincus, T., 2000. Analysis of the discordance between radiographic changes and knee pain in osteoarthritis of the knee. Journal of Rheumatology 27, 1513–1517.

Harvey, W.F., Hunter, D.J., 2010. Pharmacologic intervention for osteoarthritis in older adults. Clinics in Geriatric Medicine 26, 503–515.

Hawker, G.A., Stewart, L., French, M.R., et al., 2008. Understanding the pain experience in hip and knee osteoarthritis – an OARSI/OMERACT initiative. Osteoarthritis and Cartilage 16, 415–422.

Hawker, G.A., Wright, J.G., Badley, E.M., et al., 2004. Perceptions of, and willingness to consider, total joint arthroplasty in a population-based cohort of individuals with disabling hip and knee arthritis. Arthritis and Rheumatism 51, 635–641.

Hembree, W.C., Wittstein, J.R., Vinson, E.N., et al., 2012. Magnetic resonance imaging features of osteochondral lesions of the talus. Foot and Ankle International 33, 591–597.

Henrotin, Y., Mobasheri, A., Marty, M., 2012. Is there any scientific evidence for the use of glucosamine in the management of human osteoarthritis? Arthritis Research and Therapy 14, 201.

Hochberg, M.C., Altman, R.D., April, K.T., et al., 2012. American College of Rheumatology 2012 recommendations for the use of nonpharmacologic and pharmacologic therapies in osteoarthritis of the hand, hip, and knee. Arthritis Care and Research (Hoboken) 64, 465–474.

Hochberg, M.C., Lethbridge-Cejku, M., Scott, W.W., Jr., et al., 1995. The association of body weight, body fatness and body fat distribution with osteoarthritis of the knee: data from the Baltimore Longitudinal Study of Aging. Journal of Rheumatology 22, 488–493.

Howes, F., Buchbinder, R., Winzenberg, T.B., 2011. Opioids for osteoarthritis? Weighing benefits and risks: a Cochrane Musculoskeletal Group review. Journal of Family Practice 60, 206–212.

Huang, Y.C., Harbst, K., Kotajarvi, B., et al., 2006. Effects of ankle–foot orthoses on ankle and foot kinematics in patient with ankle osteoarthritis. Archives of Physical Medicine and Rehabilitation 87, 710–716.

Hubbard, T.J., Hicks-Little, C., Cordova, M., 2009. Mechanical and sensorimotor implications with ankle osteoarthritis. Archives of Physical Medicine and Rehabilitation 90, 1136–1141.

Hubbard, T.J., Hicks-Little, C.A., 2008. Ankle ligament healing after an acute ankle sprain: an evidence-based approach. Journal of Athletic Training 43, 523–529.

Ihn, J.C., Kim, S.J., Park, I.H., 1993. In vitro study of contact area and pressure distribution in the human knee after partial and total meniscectomy. International Orthopaedics 17, 214–218.

Jensen, L.K., 2008a. Hip osteoarthritis: influence of work with heavy lifting, climbing stairs or ladders, or combining kneeling/squatting with heavy lifting. Occupational and Environmental Medicine 65, 6–19.

Jensen, L.K., 2008b. Knee osteoarthritis: influence of work involving heavy lifting, kneeling, climbing stairs or ladders, or kneeling/squatting combined with heavy lifting. Occupational and Environmental Medicine 65, 72–89.

John, S., Bongiovanni, F., 2009. Brace management for ankle arthritis. Clinics in Podiatric Medicine and Surgery 26, 193–197.

Jordan, K.M., Arden, N.K., Doherty, M., et al., 2003. EULAR Recommendations 2003: an evidence based approach to the management of knee osteoarthritis: report of a task force of the Standing Committee for International Clinical Studies Including Therapeutic Trials (ESCISIT). Annals of the Rheumatic Diseases 62, 1145–1155.

Juhakoski, R., Tenhonen, S., Anttonen, T., et al., 2008. Factors affecting self-reported pain and physical function in patients with hip osteoarthritis. Archives of Physical Medicine and Rehabilitation 89, 1066–1073.

Kaila-Kangas, L., Arokoski, J., Impivaara, O., et al., 2011. Associations of hip osteoarthritis with history of recurrent exposure to manual handling of loads over 20 kg and work participation: a population-based study of men and women. Occupational and Environmental Medicine 68, 734–738.

Kellgren, J.H., Lawrence, J.S., 1957. Radiological assessment of osteo-arthrosis. Annals of the Rheumatic Diseases 16, 494–502.

Khosla, S.K., Baumhauer, J.F., 2008. Dietary and viscosupplementation in ankle arthritis. Foot and Ankle Clinics 13, 353–361, vii.

Kimizuka, M., Kurosawa, H., Fukubayashi, T., 1980. Load-bearing pattern of the ankle joint. Contact area and pressure distribution. Archives of Orthopaedic and Traumatic Surgery 96, 45–49.

Knupp, M., Pagenstert, G.I., Barg, A., et al., 2009. SPECT-CT compared with conventional imaging modalities for the assessment of the varus and valgus malaligned hindfoot. Journal of Orthopaedic Research 27, 1461–1466.

Kozanek, M., Rubash, H.E., Li, G., et al., 2009. Effect of post-traumatic tibiotalar osteoarthritis on kinematics of the ankle joint complex. Foot and Ankle International 30 (8), 734–740.

Kuettner, K.E., Cole, A.A., 2005. Cartilage degeneration in different human joints. Osteoarthritis and Cartilage 13 (2), 93–103.

Kujala, U.M., Kettunen, J., Paananen, H., et al., 1995. Knee osteoarthritis in former runners, soccer players, weight lifters, and shooters. Arthritis and Rheumatism 38, 539–546.

Lafortune, M.A., Hennig, E.M., 1992. Cushioning properties of footwear during walking: accelerometer and force platform measurements. Clinical Biomechanics 7, 181–184.

Lai, K.C., Chu, K.M., Hui, W.M., et al., 2006. Esomeprazole with aspirin versus clopidogrel for prevention of recurrent gastrointestinal ulcer complications. Clinics in Gastroenterology and Hepatology 4, 860–865.

Lanyon, P., Muir, K., Doherty, S., et al., 2000. Assessment of a genetic contribution to osteoarthritis of the hip: sibling study. British Medical Journal 321, 1179–1183.

Lawrence, R.C., Felson, D.T., Helmick, C.G., et al., 2008. Estimates of the prevalence of arthritis and other rheumatic conditions in the United States. Part II. Arthritis and Rheumatism 58, 26–35.

Le, T.K., Montejano, L.B., Cao, Z., et al., 2012. Healthcare costs associated with osteoarthritis in US patients. Pain Practice 12, 633–640.

Lee, K.B., Bai, L.B., Yoon, T.R., et al., 2009. Second-look arthroscopic findings and clinical outcomes after microfracture for osteochondral lesions of the talus. American Journal of Sports Medicine 37 (Suppl. 1), 63S–70S.

Lee, Y.H., Woo, J.H., Choi, S.J., et al., 2010. Effect of glucosamine or chondroitin sulfate on the osteoarthritis progression: a meta-analysis. Rheumatology International 30, 357–363.

Lindsjo, U., 1985. Operative treatment of ankle fracture-dislocations. A follow-up study of 306/321 consecutive cases. Clinical Orthopaedics and Related Research 28–38.

Loew, L., Brosseau, L., Wells, G.A., et al., 2012. Ottawa panel evidence-based clinical practice guidelines for aerobic walking programs in the management of osteoarthritis. Archives of Physical Medicine and Rehabilitation 93, 1269–1285.

Lohmander, L.S., Hoerrner, L.A., Dahlberg, L., et al., 1993. Stromelysin, tissue inhibitor of metalloproteinases and proteoglycan fragments in human knee joint fluid after injury. Journal of Rheumatology 20, 1362–1368.

Lord, J., Victor, C., Littlejohns, P., et al., 1999. Economic evaluation of a primary care-based education programme for patients with osteoarthritis of the knee. Health Technology Assessment 3, 1–55.

Lorig, K.R., Mazonson, P.D., Holman, H.R., 1993. Evidence suggesting that health education for self-management in patients with chronic arthritis has sustained health benefits while reducing health care costs. Arthritis and Rheumatism 36, 439–446.

Lowe, W., Ballinger, C., Protheroe, J., et al., 2013. The effectiveness of musculoskeletal education interventions in people with lower literacy – a systematic review. Arthritis Care and Research (Hoboken) 65 (12), 1976–1985.

Louw, A., Diener, I., Butler, D.S., et al., 2011. The effect of neuroscience education on pain, disability, anxiety, and stress in chronic musculoskeletal pain. Archives of Physical Medicine and Rehabilitation 92 (12), 2041–2056.

McCarthy, G.M., McCarty, D.J., 1992. Effect of topical capsaicin in the therapy of painful osteoarthritis of the hands. Journal of Rheumatology 19, 604–607.

McCleane, G., 2000. The analgesic efficacy of topical capsaicin is enhanced by glyceryl trinitrate in painful osteoarthritis: a randomized, double blind, placebo controlled study. European Journal of Pain 4, 355–360.

McDaniel, G., Renner, J.B., Sloane, R., et al., 2011. Association of knee and ankle osteoarthritis with physical performance. Osteoarthritis and Cartilage 19, 634–638.

McNair, P.J., Dombroski, E.W., Hewson, D.J., et al., 2001. Stretching at the ankle joint: viscoelastic responses to holds and continuous passive motion. Medicine and Science in Sports and Exercise 33, 354–358.

McNair, P.J., Prapavessis, H., 1999. Normative data of vertical ground reaction forces during landing from a jump. Journal of Science and Medicine in Sport 2, 86–88.

McNair, P.J., Prapavessis, H., Collier, J., et al., 2007. The lower-limb tasks questionnaire: an assessment of validity, reliability, responsiveness, and minimal important differences. Archives of Physical Medicine and Rehabilitation 88, 993–1001.

Madeley, N.J., Wing, K.J., Topliss, C., et al., 2012. Responsiveness and validity of the SF-36, Ankle Osteoarthritis Scale, AOFAS Ankle Hindfoot Score, and Foot Function Index in ankle arthritis. Foot and Ankle International 33, 57–63.

Madry, H., Luyten, F.P., Facchini, A., 2012. Biological aspects of early osteoarthritis. Knee Surgery, Sports Traumatology, Arthroscopy 20, 407–422.

Mao, J., 2002. Opioid-induced abnormal pain sensitivity: implications in clinical opioid therapy. Pain 100, 213–217.

Martin, D.P., Engelberg, R., Agel, J., et al., 1996. Development of a musculoskeletal extremity health status instrument: the Musculoskeletal Function Assessment instrument. Journal of Orthopaedic Research 14, 173–181.

Martin, K.R., Schoster, B., Woodard, J., et al., 2012. What community resources do older community-dwelling adults use to manage their osteoarthritis? A formative examination. Journal of Applied Gerontology 31, 661–684.

Martin, R.L., Irrgang, J.J., Burdett, R.G., et al., 2005. Evidence of validity for the Foot and Ankle Ability Measure (FAAM). Foot and Ankle International 26, 968–983.

Marx, R.G., Stump, T.J., Jones, E.C., et al., 2001. Development and evaluation of an activity rating scale for disorders of the knee. American Journal of Sports Medicine 29, 213–218.

Mason, L., Moore, R.A., Derry, S., et al., 2004. Systematic review of topical capsaicin for the treatment of chronic pain. British Medical Journal 328, 991.

Mazzuca, S.A., Brandt, K.D., Katz, B.P., et al., 1999. Reduced utilization and cost of primary care clinic visits resulting from self-care education for patients with osteoarthritis of the knee. Arthritis and Rheumatism 42, 1267–1273.

Minor, M.A., Hewett, J.E., Webel, R.R., et al., 1989. Efficacy of physical conditioning exercise in patients with rheumatoid arthritis and osteoarthritis. Arthritis and Rheumatism 32, 1396–1405.

Mohamed, O., Cerny, K., Jones, W., et al., 2005. The effect of terrain on foot pressures during walking. Foot and Ankle International 26, 859–869.

Moon, J.S., Shim, J.C., Suh, J.S., et al., 2010. Radiographic predictability of cartilage damage in medial ankle osteoarthritis. Clinical Orthopaedics and Related Research 468, 2188–2197.

Murawski, C.D., Kennedy, J.G., 2013. Operative treatment of osteochondral lesions of the talus. Journal of Bone and Joint Surgery, American Volume 95, 1045–1054.

Naal, F.D., Impellizzeri, F.M., Loibi, M., et al., 2009. Habitual physical activity and sports participation after total ankle arthroplasty. American Journal of Sports Medicine 37, 95–102.

NICE. 2008. National Institute for Health and Care Excellence (NICE) Guideline: The care and management of osteoarthritis in adults. Online. Available: http://www.nice.org.uk/nicemedia/pdf/CG59NICEguideline.pdf.

Norman, G.R., Sloan, J.A., Wyrwich, K.W., 2003. Interpretation of changes in health-related quality of life: the remarkable universality of half a standard deviation. Medical Care 41, 582–592.

Nosewicz, T.L., Knupp, M., Bolliger, L., et al., 2012. The reliability and validity of radiographic measurements for determining the three-dimensional position of the talus in varus and valgus osteoarthritic ankles. Skeletal Radiology 41, 1567–1573.

Nuesch, E., Rutjes, A.W., Husni, E., et al., 2009. Oral or transdermal opioids for osteoarthritis of the knee or hip. Cochrane Database Systemic Reviews (4), CD003115.

Older, P., Hall, A., Hader, R., 1999. Cardiopulmonary exercise testing as a screening test for perioperative management of major surgery in the elderly. Chest 116, 355–362.

Ostergaard, M., Stoltenberg, M., Gideon, P., et al., 1996. Changes in synovial membrane and joint effusion volumes after intraarticular methylprednisolone. Quantitative assessment of inflammatory and destructive changes in arthritis by MRI. Journal of Rheumatology 23, 1151–1161.

Pagenstert, G., Horisberger, M., Leumann, A.G., et al., 2011. Distinctive pain course during first year after total ankle arthroplasty: a prospective, observational study. Foot and Ankle International 32, 113–119.

Pagenstert, G.I., Hintermann, B., Barg, A., et al., 2007. Realignment surgery as alternative treatment of varus and valgus ankle osteoarthritis. Clinical Orthopaedics and Related Research 462, 156–168.

Paul, J., Sagstetter, M., Lammle, L., et al., 2012. Sports activity after osteochondral transplantation of the talus. American Journal of Sports Medicine 40, 870–874.

Pekarek, B., Osher, L., Buck, S., et al., 2011. Intra-articular corticosteroid injections: a critical literature review with up-to-date findings. Foot (Edinb) 21, 66–70.

Pickvance, E.A., Oegema, T.R. Jr., Thompson, R.C. Jr., 1993. Immunolocalization of selected cytokines and proteases in canine articular cartilage after transarticular loading. Journal of Orthopaedic Research 11 (3), 313–323.

Pietrosimone, B.G., Saliba, S.A., Hart, J.M., et al., 2011. Effects of transcutaneous electrical nerve stimulation and therapeutic exercise on quadriceps activation in people with tibiofemoral osteoarthritis. Journal of Orthopaedic and Sports Physical Therapy 41, 4–12.

Poole, A.R., Ionescu, M., Swan, A., et al., 1994. Changes in cartilage metabolism in arthritis are reflected by altered serum and synovial fluid levels of the cartilage proteoglycan aggrecan. Implications for pathogenesis. Journal of Clinical Investigation 94, 25–33.

Queen, R.M., Carter, J.E., Adams, S.B., et al., 2011. Coronal plane ankle alignment, gait, and end-stage ankle osteoarthritis. Osteoarthritis and Cartilage 19 (11), 1338–1342.

Ragozzino, A., Rossi, G., Esposito, S., et al., 1996. [Computerized tomography of osteochondral diseases of the talus dome]. La Radiologia Medica 92, 682–686.

Raynauld, J.P., Buckland-Wright, C., Ward, R., et al., 2003. Safety and efficacy of long-term intraarticular steroid injections in osteoarthritis of the knee: a randomized, double-blind, placebo-controlled trial. Arthritis and Rheumatism 48, 370–377.

Recht, M.P., Goodwin, D.W., Winalski, C.S., et al., 2005. MRI of articular cartilage: revisiting current status and future directions. American Journal of Roentgenology 185, 899–914.

Reichenbach, S., Sterchi, R., Scherer, M., et al., 2007. Meta-analysis: chondroitin for osteoarthritis of the knee or hip. Annals of Internal Medicine 146, 580–590.

Rhea, M.R., 2004. Synthesizing strength and conditioning research: the meta-analysis. Journal of Strength and Conditioning Research 18, 921–923.

Rice, D., McNair, P.J., Dalbeth, N., 2009. Effects of cryotherapy on arthrogenic muscle inhibition using an experimental model of knee swelling. Arthritis and Rheumatism 61, 78–83.

Rice, D.A., McNair, P.J., 2010. Quadriceps arthrogenic muscle inhibition: neural mechanisms and treatment perspectives. Seminars in Arthritis and Rheumatism 40, 250–266.

Ries, M.D., Philbin, E.F., Groff, G.D., 1995. Relationship between severity of gonarthrosis and cardiovascular fitness. Clinical Orthopaedics and Related Research 313, 169–176.

Roberts, W.N., Babcock, E.A., Breitbach, S.A., et al., 1996. Corticosteroid injection in rheumatoid arthritis does not increase rate of total joint arthroplasty. Journal of Rheumatology 23, 1001–1004.

Roemer, F.W., Guermazi, A., Felson, D.T., et al., 2011. Presence of MRI-detected joint effusion and synovitis increases the risk of cartilage loss in knees without osteoarthritis at 30-month follow-up: the MOST study. Annals of the Rheumatic Diseases 70, 1804–1809.

Saltzman, C.L., Salamon, M.L., Blanchard, G.M., et al., 2005. Epidemiology of ankle arthritis: report of a consecutive series of 639 patients from a tertiary orthopaedic center. Iowa Orthopedic Journal 25, 44–46.

Sandelin, J., Harilainen, A., Crone, H., et al., 1997. Local NSAID gel (eltenac) in the treatment of osteoarthritis of the knee. A double blind study comparing eltenac with oral diclofenac and placebo gel. Scandinavian Journal of Rheumatology 26, 287–292.

Sandvik, L., Erikssen, J., Thaulow, E., et al., 1993. Physical fitness as a predictor of mortality among healthy, middle-aged Norwegian men. New England Journal of Medicine 328, 533–537.

Scheiman, J.M., Yeomans, N.D., Talley, N.J., et al., 2006. Prevention of ulcers by esomeprazole in at-risk patients using non-selective NSAIDs and COX-2 inhibitors. American Journal of Gastroenterology 101, 701–710.

Schenk, K., Lieske, S., John, M., et al., 2011. Prospective study of a cementless, mobile-bearing, third generation total ankle prosthesis. Foot and Ankle International 32, 755–763.

Schumacher, B.L., Su, J.L., Lindley, K.M., et al., 2002. Horizontally oriented clusters of multiple chondrons in the superficial zone of ankle, but not knee articular cartilage. Anatomical Record 266, 241–248.

Schumacher, H.R., Chen, L.X., 2005. Injectable corticosteroids in treatment of arthritis of the knee. American Journal of Medicine 118, 1208–1214.

Schweitzer, K.M., Adams, S.B., Viens, N.A., et al., 2013. Early prospective clinical results of a modern fixed-bearing total ankle arthroplasty. Journal of Bone and Joint Surgery, American Volume 95 (11), 1002–1011.

Shepherd, D.E., Seedhom, B.B., 1999. Thickness of human articular cartilage in joints of the lower limb. Annals of the Rheumatic Diseases 58, 27–34.

Sherman, A.L., Ojeda-Correal, G., Mena, J., 2012. Use of glucosamine and chondroitin in persons with osteoarthritis. Physical Medicine and Rehabilitation 4, S110–S116.

Shih, L.Y., Wu, J.J., Lo, W.H., 1993. Changes in gait and maximum ankle torque in patients with ankle arthritis. Foot and Ankle 14, 97–103.

Siegel, J., Tornetta, P., 2007. Extraperiosteal plating of pronation-abduction ankle fractures. Journal of Bone and Joint Surgery, American Volume 89-A (2), 276–281.

Silverstein, F.E., Faich, G., Goldstein, J.L., et al., 2000. Gastrointestinal toxicity with celecoxib vs nonsteroidal anti-inflammatory drugs for osteoarthritis and rheumatoid arthritis: the CLASS study: a randomized controlled trial. Celecoxib Long-term Arthritis Safety Study. Journal of the American Medical Association 284, 1247–1255.

Simon, L.S., Grierson, L.M., Naseer, Z., et al., 2009. Efficacy and safety of topical diclofenac containing dimethyl sulfoxide (DMSO) compared with those of topical placebo, DMSO vehicle and oral diclofenac for knee osteoarthritis. Pain 143, 238–245.

Spector, T.D., Harris, P.A., Hart, D.J., et al., 1996. Risk of osteoarthritis associated with long-term weight-bearing sports: a radiologic survey of the hips and knees in female ex-athletes and population controls. Arthritis and Rheumatism 39, 988–995.

Stauffer, R.N., Chao, E.Y., Brewster, R.C., 1977. Force and motion analysis of the normal, diseased, and prosthetic ankle joint. Clinical Orthopaedics and Related Research 127, 189–196.

Stufkens, S.A., Knupp, M., Horisberger, M., et al., 2010. Cartilage lesions and the development of osteoarthritis after internal fixation of ankle fractures: a prospective study. Journal of Bone and Joint Surgery, American Volume 92 (2), 279–286.

Sun, S.F., Chou, Y.J., Hsu, C.W., et al., 2009. Hyaluronic acid as a treatment for ankle osteoarthritis. Current Reviews in Musculoskeletal Medicine 2, 78–82.

Taga, I., Shino, K., Inoue, M., et al., 1993. Articular cartilage lesions in ankles with lateral ligament injury. An arthroscopic study. American Journal of Sports Medicine 21, 120–126, discussion 126–127.

Takakura, Y., Takaoka, T., Tanaka, Y., et al., 1998. Results of opening-wedge osteotomy for the treatment of a post-traumatic varus deformity of the ankle. Journal of Bone and Joint Surgery, American Volume 80, 213–218.

Tanaka, Y., Takakura, Y., Hayashi, K., et al., 2006. Low tibial osteotomy for varus-type osteoarthritis of the ankle. Journal of Bone and Joint Surgery, British Volume 88, 909–913.

Thomas, R., Daniels, T.R., Parker, K., 2006. Gait analysis and functional outcomes following ankle arthrodesis for isolated ankle arthritis. Journal of Bone and Joint Surgery, American Volume 88, 526–535.

Tochigi, Y., Rudert, M.J., Mckinley, T.O., et al., 2008. Correlation of dynamic cartilage contact stress aberrations with severity of instability in ankle incongruity. Journal of Orthopaedic Research 26, 1186–1193.

Towheed, T.E., Maxwell, L., Judd, M.G., et al., 2006. Acetaminophen for osteoarthritis. Cochrane Database Systemic Reviews (1), CD004257.

Treppo, S., Koepp, H., Quan, E.C., et al., 2000. Comparison of biomechanical and biochemical properties of cartilage from human knee and ankle pairs. Journal of Orthopaedic Surgery 18, 739–748.

Tugwell, P.S., Wells, G.A., Shainhouse, J.Z., 2004. Equivalence study of a topical diclofenac solution (pennsaid) compared with oral diclofenac in symptomatic treatment of osteoarthritis of the knee: a randomized controlled trial. Journal of Rheumatology 31, 2002–2012.

Valderrabano, V., Hintermann, B., Horisberger, M., et al., 2006. Ligamentous posttraumatic ankle osteoarthritis. American Journal of Sports Medicine 34, 612–620.

Valderrabano, V., Horisberger, M., Russell, I., et al., 2009. Etiology of ankle osteoarthritis. Clinical Orthopaedics and Related Research 467, 1800–1806.

Valderrabano, V., Nigg, B.M., Von Tscharner, V., et al., 2007a. J. Leonard Goldner Award. 2006. Total ankle replacement in ankle osteoarthritis: an analysis of muscle rehabilitation. Foot and Ankle International 28, 281–291.

Valderrabano, V., Nigg, B.M., Von Tscharner, V., et al., 2007b. Gait analysis in ankle osteoarthritis and total ankle replacement. Clinical Biomechanics 22, 894–904.

Van Der Waal, J.M., Terwee, C.B., Van Der Windt, D.A., et al., 2005. The impact of non-traumatic hip and knee disorders on health-related quality of life as measured with the SF-36 or SF-12. A systematic review. Quality of Life 14, 1141–1155.

Van Dijk, C.N., Verhagen, R.A., Tol, J.L., 1997. Arthroscopy for problems after ankle fracture. Journal of Bone and Joint Surgery, British Volume 79, 280–284.

Van Ryn, M., Burke, J., 2000. The effect of patient race and socio-economic status on physicians' perceptions of patients. Social Science and Medicine 50, 813–828.

Vlad, S.C., Lavalley, M.P., McAlindon, T.E., et al., 2007. Glucosamine for pain in osteoarthritis: why do trial results differ? Arthritis and Rheumatism 56, 2267–2277.

Wan, L., De Asla, R.J., Rubash, H.E., et al., 2006. Determination of in-vivo articular cartilage contact areas of human talocrural joint under weightbearing conditions. Osteoarthritis and Cartilage 14, 1294–1301.

Ward, S.T., Williams, P.L., Purkayastha, S., 2008. Intra-articular corticosteroid injections in the foot and ankle: a prospective 1-year follow-up investigation. Journal of Foot and Ankle Surgery 47, 138–144.

Waterton, J.C., Solloway, S., Foster, J.E., et al., 2000. Diurnal variation in the femoral articular cartilage of the knee in young adult humans. Magnetic Resonance in Medicine 43, 126–132.

Watson, M.C., Brookes, S.T., Kirwan, J.R., et al., 2000. Non-aspirin, non-steroidal anti-inflammatory drugs for osteoarthritis of the knee. Cochrane Database Systemic Reviews (2), CD000142.

Wiewiorski, M., Dopke, K., Steiger, C., et al., 2012. Muscular atrophy of the lower leg in unilateral post traumatic osteoarthritis of the ankle joint. International Orthopaedics 36, 2079–2085.

Wood, L., Ferrell, W.R., Baxendale, R.H., 1988. Pressures in normal and acutely distended human knee joints and effects on quadriceps maximal voluntary contractions. Quarterly Journal of Experimental Physiology 73, 305–314.

Wright, R.W., Boyce, R.H., Michener, T., et al., 2006. Radiographs are not useful in detecting arthroscopically confirmed mild chondral damage. Clinical Orthopaedics and Related Research 442, 245–251.

Wu, W.L., Su, F.C., Cheng, Y.M., et al., 2000. Gait analysis after ankle arthrodesis. Gait and Posture 11, 54–61.

Zadpoor, A.A., Nikooyan, A.A., 2011. The relationship between lower-extremity stress fractures and the ground reaction force: a systematic review. Clinical Biomechanics 26, 23–28.

Zahiri, C.A., Schmalzried, T.P., Szuszczewicz, E.S., et al., 1998. Assessing activity in joint replacement patients. Journal of Arthroplasty 13, 890–895.

Zengerink, M., Struijs, P.A., Tol, J.L., et al., 2010. Treatment of osteochondral lesions of the talus: a systematic review. Knee Surgery, Sports Traumatology, Arthroscopy 18, 238–246.

Zhang, S., Clowers, K., Kohstall, C., et al., 2005. Effects of various midsole densities of basketball shoes on impact attenuation during landing activities. Journal of Applied Biomechanics 21, 3–17.

Zhang, W., Moskowitz, R.W., Nuki, G., et al., 2008. OARSI recommendations for the management of hip and knee osteoarthritis, part II: OARSI evidence-based, expert consensus guidelines. Osteoarthritis and Cartilage 16, 137–162.

Zhang, W., Nuki, G., Moskowitz, R.W., et al., 2010. OARSI recommendations for the management of hip and knee osteoarthritis: part III: changes in evidence following systematic cumulative update of research published through January. 2009. Osteoarthritis and Cartilage 18, 476–499.

Zhang, Y., Jordan, J.M., 2010. Epidemiology of osteoarthritis. Clinics in Geriatric Medicine 26, 355–369.

Chapter 2

Rheumatic Diseases

Anita Williams and Michael Corkill

INTRODUCTION

'Rheumatic disease' is a term that encompasses the plethora of disorders that can affect any or many of the body's systems but predominantly affect the joints and connective tissues. Many of these disorders tend to be chronic and often people have variable symptoms, experiencing periods of both exacerbation and remission in relation to both the type and severity of these symptoms.

People with rheumatic diseases are generally managed within the specialty of rheumatology. Because the pathogenesis and the characteristics of some of these disorders are explained in terms of autoimmunity, they are also referred to as *autoimmune disorders*. Further, as inflammation is one of the results of this autoimmune response against specific structures of the musculoskeletal system, the term *inflammatory arthritis* is also used to describe them.

This chapter will concentrate on rheumatoid arthritis (RA). RA commonly affects the lower limb in relation to pain, activity limitation and disability, thereby impacting on people's quality of life. However, less common rheumatic diseases, for example, systemic lupus erythematosus (SLE), systemic sclerosis (scleroderma) and psoriatic arthritis also have various consequences for the lower limb, such as changes in foot structure and extra-articular complications involving the skin and vascular integrity. Hence, the management of foot problems is based on the same principles and with the same considerations as with RA.

RA is a chronic, systemic, inflammatory joint disease characterized by synovial inflammation and progressive articular destruction (Scott and Wolfe 2010). RA is the commonest inflammatory arthritis, with around 400 000 adults in the UK with RA and approximately 20 000 new cases every year (Symmons

2002). The prevalence of RA is approximately 0.8%, a risk that is doubled for relatives of confirmed cases (Hawker 1997), with the overall prevalence being higher for women (1.2%) than men (0.4%) – approximately two-thirds of new cases being women (Young et al. 2002). The average age of onset is 55 years and it has been observed that this is increasing for both men and women (Symmons 2005).

The systemic effects of RA are associated with increased morbidity and mortality. The median age of death in males and females is respectively 4 and 10 years earlier than the general population (Mitchell et al. 1986). Those most at risk are those with more severe disease and with the extra-articular complications of the disease such as infections and organ involvement (Faguer et al. 2013). Coronary heart disease is linked to inflammation of the blood vessels (Ahmad et al. 2012). Therefore, in addition to the usual risk factors of obesity, hyperlipidaemia and hypertension, RA is considered to be an independent risk factor for coronary heart disease (Kitas and Erb 2003). Further systemic features include interstitial lung disease, eye manifestations, rheumatoid nodules and distal polyneuropathy (Alam et al. 2011). The incidence of RA and the severity of complications are falling owing to earlier detection, earlier targeted therapy (Emery et al. 2002), earlier use of biologic therapies when traditional first-line management fails and changes in the classification criteria (Aletaha et al. 2010).

In addition to the effects that RA has on the individual, it has been identified that the annual direct and indirect costs of RA are estimated to be between £0.8 and £1.3 billion in the UK (Barrett et al. 2000). RA has been described by March and Lapsley (2001) as a 'time consuming disease' as everyday activities take much longer and certain activities have to be discontinued. Up to 4 out of every 10 working people suffering from RA find that within 5 years they can no longer work, with three-quarters being for reasons directly related to their condition (Young et al. 2002). Barrett et al. (2000) suggest that 1 in 7 people give up work within 1 year of diagnosis, one-third within 2 years and up to 60% within 10 years. However, Rat and Boissier (2004) highlight that more recent developments with early effective treatment may not only postpone and slow disease progression but also preserve an individual's ability to participate in work and recreational activities.

Foot Involvement In Rheumatoid Arthritis

The foot is the most common site of pathology in the early stages of RA (Shi et al. 2000) with many patients reporting foot symptoms at initial diagnosis and up to 100% of patients reporting foot problems within 10 years of disease onset (Grondal et al. 2008). An early study by Michelson et al. (1994) found that the frequency of foot symptoms was more common in the ankle than the forefoot, supporting the work by Spiegel and Spiegel (1982). In a Swedish study by Grondal et al. (2008) investigating 1000 patients with RA, 45% reported forefoot involvement, 17% reported hindfoot/ankle involvement and 9% reported both forefoot and hindfoot involvement at the start of the disease. Foot involvement becomes greater with disease progression (Michelson et al. 1994). In a study of 40 patients with RA and 40 controls, Göksel-Karatepe et al. (2010) reported the frequency of foot deformity, as evidenced by radiographs, was 79% in established disease (mean disease duration 15 years). Similarly, Grondal et al. (2008) found that 80% of patients, with established disease (median disease duration 10 years), reported current foot problems.

Even when the disease is in remission, patients with RA still report foot problems (Grondal et al. 2008). The suggested reason is that, in addition to the destructive nature of inflammation on the structures of the foot, stresses caused by abnormal mechanics have a large role to play (Michelson et al. 1994). For example, forefoot synovitis of the metatarsophalangeal (MTP) joints is a significant feature of both early and active disease, leading to deformities such as hallux valgus, forefoot widening, hammer and claw toes, and subluxation and dislocation of the joints (Spiegel and Spiegel, 1982). Soft-tissue structures are also affected, such as dysfunction of the posterior tibial tendon, which is associated with pes planus deformity (Barn et al. 2013).

The prevalence rates for pain and swelling of the MTP joints and walking disability are initially high and then often stabilize, but the prevalence and severity of forefoot joint damage increases over an 8-year course of RA (Spiegel and Spiegel 1982), highlighting a changing pattern in the aetiology of symptoms.

During the course of the disease, the number of involved forefoot joints increases and the severity of the lesions become more pronounced. The structural and functional changes associated with joint involvement directly affect gait and mobility (Hulsmans et al. 2000; Priolo et al. 1997; van der Leeden et al. 2008; Woodburn et al. 2002a), with an increase in forefoot pressures resulting in delayed heel lift, reduced 'toe contact' and an increased double-limb support time, together with a slower walking pace (Turner et al. 2006; Turner and Woodburn 2008; Woodburn et al. 2002a).

Structural changes to the joints increase pressure on specific areas of the foot such as the plantar MTP joint area, predisposing to callus formation. In a number of patients, foot ulceration can occur as a result of these pressures, particularly in cases with poor tissue viability (Firth et al. 2008). Furthermore, bacterial and fungal skin infections and nail pathologies are more prevalent in this patient group, adding to the serious risk of ulceration (Figure 2-1), infection spreading to the soft tissues and systemic infection. Additionally, the risk of infection is also increased if the patient's medical management includes immunosuppressive drugs (Otter et al. 2004; Wilske 1993).

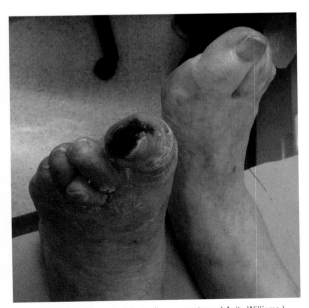

FIGURE 2-1 Ulcerated feet. (Image courtesy of Anita Williams.)

PREDISPOSING FACTORS

RA has been reported to be associated with different environmental risk factors, such as smoking, hormonal factors, diet, caffeine and infection (Oliver and Silman 2006). Studies indicate RA is perceived to be a multifactorial disease, generated by interactions between different genetic backgrounds and environmental factors (Söderlin et al. 2011). Besides atherosclerosis and lung cancer, smoking is considered to play a major role in the pathogenesis of autoimmune diseases. It has long been known that there is a connection between rheumatoid factor-positive rheumatoid arthritis and cigarette smoking. Recently, an important gene–environment interaction has been revealed; that is, carrying specific HLA-DRB1 alleles encoding the shared epitope and smoking establish a significant risk for anti-citrullinated protein antibody-positive rheumatoid arthritis (Baka et al. 2009).

Multiple studies demonstrate an increased cardiovascular risk associated with RA compared with the general population. Although part of this risk appears to be mediated by RA-specific factors, such as long-term inflammation, traditional cardiovascular risk co-morbidities also play an important role. Liao and Solomon (2013) reviewed the evidence from previous studies of the relationship between RA and traditional cardiovascular risk co-morbidities such as dyslipidaemia, obesity, insulin resistance and diabetes, hypertension, cigarette smoking and physical inactivity.

A recent study described patients' conceptions of the cause of their RA (Bergsten et al. 2011). Two major categories were identified. First were the consequences beyond personal control, such as being exposed to climatic changes or being considered to be genetically susceptible. Secondly were the consequences of strain, which were either work- or family-related. However, Sugiyama et al. (2010) in their meta-analysis of studies exploring the association between smoking and disease onset, concluded that smoking is a major risk factor for RA. A more recent study by Lahiri et al. (2012) added to this evidence by concluding that the risk is dose-related, stronger in males and especially strong for those who are anti-citrullinated peptide antibody positive. They also identified that after smoking cessation there is a latency of up to 20 years before returning to baseline risk.

DIAGNOSIS

CLASSIFICATION

The definition of RA is sometimes imprecise, but the term is normally used to describe a symmetrical, persistent, and destructive polyarthritis often associated with rheumatoid factor or with positive results in tests for anti-cyclic citrullinated peptide (anti-CCP) antibodies (Combe et al. 2007).

The 1987 classification criteria for RA were designed to improve the differential diagnosis of RA from other inflammatory joint diseases. They were adopted by the American College of Rheumatology (ACR) and have been widely used in RA studies (Arnett et al. 1988). However, the 1987 classification has not been helpful in achieving the goal of identifying patients who would benefit from early effective intervention. A systematic review of publications evaluating the performance of the ACR's 1987 clinical criteria found the sensitivity to early RA to be between 77% and 80%, with specificities between 33% and 77% based on pooled data (Banal et al. 2009).

In the new classification criteria by Aletaha et al. (2010), 'definite RA' is based on the confirmed presence of synovitis in at least one joint, absence of an alternative diagnosis that better explains the synovitis, and achievement of a total score of 6 or greater (of a possible 10) from individual scores in four domains: number and site of involved joints (score range 0–5), serological abnormality (score range 0–3), elevated acute-phase response (score range 0–1), and symptom duration (2 levels; range 0–1). This new classification system redefines the traditional paradigm of RA by focusing on features at earlier stages of disease, rather than defining the disease by its late-stage features.

This is important in achieving earlier diagnosis and institution of effective disease-suppressing therapy in order to prevent or minimize the occurrence of the undesirable sequel in relation to joint damage and the development of complications (Emery et al. 2002).

DIAGNOSTIC MARKERS

Rheumatoid factor (RF), an antibody recognizing the Fc or conserved portion of human antibodies, is present in 60–90% of RA patients with established RA, but in less than 50% of patients with early RA (Taylor et al. 2011). However, 3–5% of healthy adults also have serum RF and this figure increases to 10–30% in the elderly (Raptopoulou et al. 2007).

An alternative diagnostic test involves antibodies to keratin such as anti-cyclic citrullinated peptide antibodies. Anti-CCP is present in the serum of a portion of RA patients and has been identified in the serum of patients at all stages of RA: preclinical, early, and established (Taylor et al. 2011). In clinical research studies, anti-CCP antibodies were found in 55–69% of patients with RA (Kwok et al. 2005) and 65% of RA patients with late-onset RA (Lopez-Hoyos et al. 2004). Recent clinical trials suggest that anti-CCP is highly accurate in selectively identifying RA patients (Nikolaisen et al. 2007; Quinn et al. 2006) and is of particular diagnostic use in patients who are negative for RF (Quinn et al. 2006) and an indicator of prognosis (Bas 2005).

DISEASE ACTIVITY

Numerous RA disease activity measurement tools are currently available for use and include measures of RA disease activity, for example, the Patient (PtGA) and Provider (PrGA) Global Assessment of Disease Activity; the Disease Activity Score (DAS) and Disease Activity Score With 28-Joint Counts (DAS28); Simplified Disease Activity Index (SDAI); Clinical Disease Activity Index (CDAI); Patient Activity Score (PAS) and Patient Activity Score-II (PASII); Routine Assessment of Patient Index Data (RAPID); Rheumatoid Arthritis Disease Activity Index (RADAI) and Rheumatoid Arthritis Disease Activity Index-5 (RADAI-5); Chronic Arthritis Systemic Index (CASI); Patient-Based Disease Activity Score With ESR (PDAS1) and Patient-Based Disease Activity Score Without ESR (PDAS2); and Mean Overall Index for Rheumatoid Arthritis (MOI-RA). In this chapter, the Disease Activity Score (DAS) and Disease Activity Score with 28-Joint Counts (DAS28) will be reviewed. The other measures can be read about in a full review by Anderson et al. (2012).

The DAS and DAS28 combine single measures into an overall continuous measure of RA disease activity. Both the DAS and DAS28 have been extensively validated and are endorsed by the ACR and the European League Against Rheumatism (EULAR) RA as disease activity measurement in clinical trials (Aletaha et al. 2008). They are often considered the 'gold standard' by which to measure RA disease activity, with the majority of newer disease-activity-monitoring tools either based on or compared with the DAS28 (Anderson et al. 2012).

Although both the DAS and DAS28 are feasible to use in RA disease activity monitoring, the shorter DAS28 is more practical for regular clinical use (Anderson et al. 2012). The original DAS includes the number of painful joints calculated by the Ritchie Articular Index (RAI), a 44 swollen joint count (44 SJC), erythrocyte sedimentation rate (ESR), and a PtGA of disease activity or general health (GH) on a visual analogue scale (VAS). The DAS28 includes a 28-swollen joint count (28SJC), 28 tender joint count (28TJC), ESR, and a PtGA or GH assessment on a VAS (van Gestel et al. 1996).

For all DAS versions, the level of disease activity can be interpreted as remission (DAS < 1.6), low (1.6 ≤ DAS < 2.4), moderate (2.4 ≤ DAS ≤ 3.7), or high (DAS > 3.7); the level of disease activity can be interpreted as remission (DAS28 < 2.6), low (2.6 ≤ DAS28 < 3.2), moderate (3.2 ≤ DAS28 ≤ 5.1), or high (DAS28 > 5.1). However, alternative cut-off values for the DAS28 have been proposed that include a more stringent remission of ≤ 2.4 with a change of 1.2 (twice the measurement error) in either the DAS or DAS28 that is considered a significant change (Aletaha and Smolen, 2005). The EULAR response criteria classify patients as good, moderate, or non-responders, using both the change in DAS and level of DAS reached. Good response is defined as improvement in DAS > 1.2 and follow-up DAS ≤ 2.4; non-responders have improvement in DAS ≤ 0.6 or improvement > 0.6, but ≤ 1.2 and follow-up DAS > 3.7; all others are classified as moderate responders (Anderson et al. 2012).

BLOOD INVESTIGATIONS

Markers for inflammation, also known as acute phase markers of disease activity include erythrocyte sedimentation rate (ESR) and C-reactive protein (CRP). CRP is more sensitive than ESR to changes in inflammatory levels. Both are considered complementary to other test results such as clinical signs and factors identified in history taking.

Miller et al. (1983) suggested the rule for calculating normal maximum ESR values in adults (98% confidence limit) is given by a formula with men under 50 years old less than 15 mm/h; men over 50 years old less than 20 mm/h; women under 50 years old less than 20 mm/h, and women over 50 years old less than 30 mm/h (Wetteland et al. 1996). Values in excess of these provide one of the diagnostic criteria for RA (Aletaha et al. 2010) and, once diagnosed and treatment instigated, may indicate subsequent response to medical management. However, false positives may be present in those patients with RA who also have infections such as influenza. C-reactive protein (CRP) levels of 10 mg/L or lower are considered 'normal' with 100 mg/L and above indicating inflammation associated with inflammatory arthritis.

IMAGING

Imaging is considered to be the most objective measure of joint and soft-tissue damage associated with RA. Plain-film radiography has been the traditional imaging technique, but magnetic resonance imaging (MRI) and power Doppler musculoskeletal ultrasonography (MSUS) are increasingly being used.

Radiographs are often the first imaging used. However, their use is very limited in the very early stages of the disease because the focal point of the inflammatory process is the soft tissues rather than the bony structures (Turner et al. 2006). Erosions of the bone often do not appear until 1–2 years of disease duration, with the feet preceding the hands (Priolo et al. 1997). Hence, plain-film radiographs are more valuable when there is a need for quantifying the degree of joint damage. Radiographic characteristics in RA include soft-tissue swelling, juxta-articular osteopenia, bone erosions, joint space narrowing, cysts, joint subluxation, malalignment and ankylosis (Ravindran and Rachapalli 2011).

Erosions and joint space narrowing can be quantified using either the Larsen Index (Larsen et al. 1977) or the Sharp van der Hejde Score (van der Heijde 1999). The Sharp/van der Heijde indices involve each side of the MTP joints or interphalangeal (IP) joints being scored for erosions from 0 to 5 with a maximum of 10 for both sides of the joint, and for joint space narrowing from 0 to 4 with a maximum of four per joint. For the total Sharp/van der Heijde score, the erosions and joint-space-narrowing scores are added. The maximum total score for both feet adds up to 168. The Larsen method involves erosions and joint space narrowing as well as other signs of inflammation expressed in one score with a range from 0 (normal) to 5 (total mutilation of the joint). The scoring is based on the comparison with the standard film series (van der Heijde 1999). Typical median scores reported in the literature relating to the foot are Larsen and Sharp/van der Heijde scores of 1.0 and 4.0 respectively (Baan et al. 2011). The smallest detectable difference (SDD) is 5.0 for the Sharp/van der Heijde method and 5.8 for the Larsen/Scott method (Bruynesteyn et al. 2002). With the Sharp/van der Heijde method, the SDD of 5.0 corresponds closely with the minimal clinically important difference (MCID) of 4.6 (Bruynesteyn et al. 2002).

There is increasing use of MRI in both the diagnosis and monitoring of RA. The advantage of MRI over radiography, apart from the absence of ionizing radiation, is the superior imaging of the structures in RA, such as synovial tissue, tendons, sheaths, ligaments, bone, and cartilage (Baan et al. 2011). A recent MRI study has demonstrated that focal deficiencies attributed to plantar plate pathology of the lesser (second to fifth) MTP joints are common in the forefoot of patients with RA and associated with synovitis, bone oedema, and bone erosion (Siddle et al. 2012a). In a more recent study, MRI arthrography demonstrated pathology at 18 of 28 lesser MTP joints (64%) examined in 15 patients with RA (Siddle et al. 2012b). The authors reported that MRI arthrography abnormalities were associated with RA disease duration, forefoot deformity, Larsen score, subluxation, and peak plantar pressure. Unenhanced MRI had a sensitivity of 78% and specificity of 90% for detecting pathology compared with MRI arthrography.

An alternative to MRI is musculoskeletal ultrasound (MSUS) (Wakefield et al. 1999). Within the last decade, technological improvements in the diagnostic capacity of MSUS have led to an increasingly important role of this imaging modality in the evaluation and monitoring of patients with chronic inflammatory arthritis. MSUS is much more sensitive than clinical examination for detecting synovitis (Kane et al. 2003). Grey-scale MSUS with Doppler technique allows direct assessment of joint effusion and synovial hypertrophy, tenosynovitis, synovial and tenosynovial vascularity, tendon and ligament lesions, bone erosions and articular cartilage damage. MSUS is a routinely available, multiplanar, dynamic and non-invasive

imaging modality. It is portable, is relatively inexpensive and has high patient acceptability (Alcade et al. 2012). Colour Doppler (CD) and power Doppler (PD) techniques are also able to detect increased synovial vascularization (Alcalde et al. 2012).

HISTORY

Because of the genetic link for RA, Kallberg et al. (2007) suggested that it is useful to ascertain whether there is a family history of the condition. Age, gender and social habits such as smoking, general symptoms such as malaise, weight loss, mild fevers and night sweats should be considered (Oliver and Silman 2006), In addition, patients may commonly report fatigue (Hewlett et al. 2012) and depression (Palkonyai et al. 2007) early on in the disease (Lempp et al. 2011).

The characteristics of musculoskeletal pain can be particularly variable between individuals (Studenic et al. 2012). The duration of stiffness, particularly morning stiffness, is a marker of active disease and useful to monitor disease progression and the impact of interventions (Sierakowski and Cutolo 2011). The degree of morning stiffness appears to reflect functional disability and pain more than the traditional markers of inflammation such as joint counts and ESR in patients with early RA (Yazici et al. 2004). However, although established diagnostic criteria for RA include morning stiffness, it is not part of the more recent classification criteria developed to guide early treatment decisions (Aletaha et al. 2010).

CLINICAL EXAMINATION

The clinical signs of joint involvement in the foot may sometimes be subtle, with synovitis often being difficult to detect clinically in the MTP joints (Maillefert et al. 2003).

Inflammation of the synovium may produce separation of the toes known as the daylight sign (Figure 2-2). This results from the stretching and weakening of the joint capsule and loss of integrity of the collateral ligaments and plantar plate (Jaakkola and Mann 2004; Keenan et al. 1991).

The metatarsal squeeze test of the forefoot is considered to be a useful indicator of inflammation, but the sensitivity and specificity are not considered to be exceptional (67% and 89%). However, it is one of the components of the so-called 'trinity of signs' (Emery

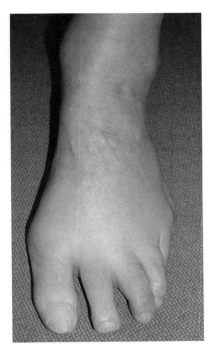

FIGURE 2-2 Early RA with daylight sign. (Image courtesy of Anita Williams.)

et al. 2002), which are considered to be vital as a first-line indicator of inflammatory joint disease. This set of signs is aimed to help non-specialist practitioners to make the clinical decision to refer for expert opinion should there be a suspicion of RA. They include patients presenting with metatarsalgia, a positive squeeze test, plus early morning stiffness of greater than 30 minutes in three or more swollen joints. A recent study evaluated the use of the metatarsal squeeze test with the DAS28 (de Jong et al. 2012). The DAS28 comprises a 28-joint count but excludes the joints of the feet. Agreement between the DAS and the DAS28-squeeze (82%) was significantly higher than agreement between the DAS and the DAS28 (76%). When assessing the group of patients who had arthritis of the forefeet only (22 patients and 46 assessments), the overall agreement between the DAS and the DAS28 was 40%, whereas agreement between the DAS and the DAS28-squeeze was 59% and that between the DAS and the DAS28-BCP disease state was 65%. Furthermore, the specificities of the DAS28-squeeze and the DAS28-BCP (80% and 81%, respectively) were higher

than that of the DAS28 (76%), while the sensitivities of the DAS28, DAS28-squeeze, and DAS28-BCP to identify true remission according to the Boolean criteria were 88%, 87%, and 81%, respectively. Adding the squeeze test of the forefeet to the DAS28 has value for a more-dependable classification of the disease state in patients with early RA.

IMPAIRMENTS AND FUNCTION

The typical impairments associated with RA are pain, limited range of motion in the joints of the feet and lower limb, and muscle weakness. These all contribute to a reduced capacity to walk effectively and efficiently, difficulty in climbing and descending stairs, and an inability to stand for periods of time. When these problems affect the person's ability to carry out the tasks related to work and recreation (Backman et al. 2004) then this has consequences for their quality of life (Whalley et al. 1997). Impairments are typically not evaluated individually, but are usually incorporated within questionnaires that contain sections on pain along with aspects of disability and function.

In respect of general disease status, there are composite tools that combine both objective and subjective measures to produce a single score. For example, the DAS (van der Heijde et al. 1990) incorporates the ESR, 44 swollen joint count and the RAI (Ritchie et al. 1968) with a subjective questionnaire, the Health Assessment Questionnaire (HAQ), which evaluates functional ability (Felson et al. 1993). However, the DAS does not provide a measure of foot involvement; thus patients may be at risk of ongoing joint damage if treatment decisions are made solely on the basis of the DAS (Bakker et al. 2012). Given that patients can report severe symptoms in their feet, and these general health tools omit the feet, it is vital that foot health assessment tools are used in combination with the general disease assessment tools.

Patient-reported Foot Pain, Function and Disability

Forefoot joint damage in the rheumatoid foot is related to increased pressure under the forefoot, especially pressure under the first and fourth MTP joints. High forefoot pressure is associated with pain during barefoot walking. A prolonged stance phase and delayed heel lift are related to disability in daily activities (van der Leeden et al. 2006). Specific tools for measuring the impact of foot pathology on foot pain, function and disability have been validated. However, only three are specific to people with RA-related foot problems (Foot Function Index – Budiman-Mak et al. 1991; Foot Impact Scale – Helliwell et al. 2005; Salford Arthritis Foot Evaluation Tool – Walmsley et al. 2012) and a further one still requires further validation for part B of the Salford Arthritis Foot Evaluation Tool (Walmsley et al. 2012).

Pain is the commonest problem facing patients with RA both generally and specifically related to their feet (Otter et al. 2010). Pain is most often measured using the VAS and rated on a scale of 0–10. It is a well-established measure of pain with good reliability and responsiveness and it correlates with many clinical variables (Wolfe and Michaud 2007). Inflammatory pain is reported early in the disease and hence pain scores can be high (for example, levels of 8–10 on a VAS), whereas later on in the disease reported pain may be associated with altered structure and increased pressures on the feet.

The Foot Function Index

The Foot Function Index (FFI) measures the impact of foot pathology on function with sections on pain, disability and activity restriction (Budiman-Mak et al. 1991). The index was developed as a means to establish the benefits of orthotic intervention in patients with established RA and has been widely used (Bal et al. 2006; de P Magalhães et al. 2006; Hodge et al. 1999; Woodburn et al. 2002a). The FFI has also been found to be effective where there is marked disability and activity limitation (Landorf and Keenan, 2002).

The index is composed of 23 items in total with each item rated using a 10 cm VAS. The FFI consists of three subscales, which are pain, disability, and activity limitation. The VAS scale of each item is anchored at each end with a verbal descriptor and is scored between 1 and 9. Test–retest agreement is reported to be high for the FFI total scores although it does vary for the subscale scores. It has been criticized for difficulty in completion and hence has been revised to a simpler version using a five-point scoring (Budiman-Mak et al. 2006). A recent notable change was the addition of a psychosocial subscale. Minimum detectable difference and minimum clinically important difference have not

been reported for the FFI-R, which limits its clinical usability (Riskowski et al. 2011).

However, The FFI has been used in research. Williams et al. (2007b) reported on a 12-week study to evaluate the value of a new footwear design based on 80 RA patients' opinions compared with a traditional footwear design. Mean pain scores significantly reduced from 63.0 at baseline to 36.2 after 12 weeks. The disability domain demonstrated a score of 45 at baseline and a significant reduction after 12 weeks to 25. The activity limitation domain demonstrated a significant reduction from 8 to 3.

The Manchester Foot Pain and Disability Questionnaire

The Manchester Foot Pain and Disability Questionnaire (MFPDQ) is both an evaluative and a discriminative questionnaire for use in population surveys for identifying and assessing levels of foot pain and disability (Garrow et al. 2000). The MFPDQ is composed of 19 items in total, distributed among three constructs represented as subscales, which are: functional limitation (6 items), pain intensity (11 items), and personal appearance (2 items). Each item pertains to the previous month and is scored using a three-point Likert-type rating scale with the response options: 'none of the time', 'on some days' and 'on most/every day(s)'. Although patients with RA were involved in the process of developing the MFPDQ, a ceiling effect was observed by Helliwell (2003). Evidence for the responsiveness of the MFPDQ has yet to be clearly demonstrated and provision for clinical interpretability is similarly lacking. Walmsley et al. (2010) suggested that this tool might be more useful in non-RA populations.

The Foot Health Status Questionnaire

The Foot Health Status Questionnaire (FHSQ) is both an evaluative and discriminative instrument developed for the assessment of foot health pre- and post-surgery, for the assessment of general foot health status and the efficacy of more conventional podiatric interventions (Bennett et al. 1998). It is composed of 13 items in total, each item with a five-point Likert response scale, divided into four domains: foot pain, foot function, footwear and general foot health. The subscales yield scores individually, ranging from 0 (best possible outcome) to 100 (worst possible outcome), which are summed together to produce an overall score. In order to calculate scores using the instrument, the purchase of proprietary software is necessary. Reliability for the FHSQ has been demonstrated in terms of both internal consistency and temporal stability for each of the subscales (Bennett et al. 1998). The pragmatic properties of the FHSQ are considered to be generally good and patient burden is low as the instrument provides clear completion instructions and requires only 3–5 minutes for completion. Typical mean scores for patients with RA in the following domains are foot pain (39); foot function (38); foot health (16) and general health (39).

The Foot Impact Scale

The Foot Impact Scale (FIS) was the first RA foot-specific measure (Helliwell et al. 2005). It was developed specifically to assess the rheumatoid foot, and has demonstrable measurement properties, such as reliability, construct validity, responsiveness, and wide applicability for the evaluation of the impact of RA on the feet (Bowen et al. 2010) and specific podiatric care package interventions (Siddle et al. 2012b). Constructs assessed by the FIS are closely allied with the domains of the World Health Organization (2013) International Classification for Disability, thereby creating a strong conceptual basis. The FIS is composed of 51 items in total, divided into two subscales: impairments/shoes (FISIF) (21 items) and activities/participation (FISAP) (30 items). Each item pertains to the present time and consists of a single brief statement anchored with a dichotomous response option, labelled 'true/false'. The test–retest reliability of the FIS is high [intraclass correlation coefficient (ICC) of 0.84] and it also demonstrates good concurrent validity relative to the Manchester Foot Pain and Disability Questionnaire (Garrow et al. 2000).

An elevated FISIF or FISAP score indicates greater foot impairment or activity limitation, respectively. Scores of ≤6 are considered mild, from 7–13 are considered moderate, and ≥14 are considered severe for the FISIF. For the FISAP, scores of ≤9 are considered mild, from 10–19 are considered moderate, and ≥20 are considered severe (Hooper et al. 2012). Score ranges were pragmatically derived by the division of the total score into approximate thirds. A previous study suggested a longitudinal change in either the

FISIF or FISAP total of 3 points in either direction to be clinically relevant (Turner et al. 2007). The FIS questionnaire with its foot-related disability subscales that differentiates disability from pain has been validated in patients with RA (Hooper et al. 2012).

The Salford Arthritis Foot Evaluation Tool

In their review of patient-reported measures, Walmsley et al. (2010) identified a need to develop an RA-disease and foot-specific tool with a greater emphasis on a bio-psychosocial conceptual basis. The Salford Arthritis Foot Evaluation (SAFE) (Walmsley et al. 2012) tool incorporates the development of items that have meaning to both the patient and clinician. It has a nomothetic scale (SAFE-Part A-19 items) that focuses on impairment, disability and footwear, and an idiographic scale (SAFE-Part B-42 items) that focuses on the impact, feelings and experiences of living with feet affected with RA. The SAFE-Part B allows patients to communicate clearly to clinicians how their lives are affected by RA involvement in their feet. The SAFE-Part A has strong evidence for convergent validity and test–retest reliability. However, Walmsley et al. (2010) acknowledge that the SAFE-Part B currently has no quantitative measurement properties, such as construct validity and test–retest reliability. There are no typical scores for patients with RA using this scale, as it is a new tool.

Gait

Even the most basic of activities such as walking become progressively more difficult with the progression of RA. The walking patterns of people with RA change in relation to the degree of joint involvement, joint motion, stiffness, altered muscle activity and stresses on the foot. The subtlety of some of these changes may not be evident when carrying out a clinical assessment in the early stages of the disease (Turner et al. 2006). Assessment of function in people with RA can, therefore, be supplemented using technology such as three-dimensional (3D) gait analysis (Woodburn et al. 2002a), measurement of temporal and spatial parameters (McDonough et al. 2001) and electromyography (Barn et al. 2012).

Gait Analysis. A systematic review of studies investigating walking abnormalities associated with RA

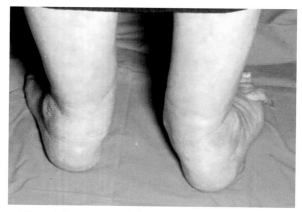

FIGURE 2-3 Severe valgus deformity of the rearfoot. (Image courtesy of Anita Williams.)

(Baan et al. 2012) demonstrated changes in gait such as a slower walk, longer double-support time, and avoidance of extreme positions. These changes were in relation to the frequently found static features in RA, for instance hallux valgus, pes planovalgus and hindfoot abnormalities (Figure 2-3). However, in a review, Barn et al. (2012) concluded that gait research should focus on more uniformity in methodology in order to produce more clinical applicable conclusions.

Traditionally, the basic gait parameters such as walking speed cadence and stride length have been measured with tape measures and stopwatches (Fransen and Edmonds 1999). Although such measures were considered to be reliable and responsive, newer technology has improved accuracy. Instrumented walkways embedded with pressure sensors record the spatial and temporal parameters and, through computer software algorithms provide walking speed, cadence, stride length, gait cycle time, double-limb support, angle and base and the timing of stance and swing phases of the gait cycle.

In respect of RA, the disease duration alone is not strongly predictive of changes in gait, with trends showing towards associations between decreased walking speed and stride length with increased disease duration (Turner and Woodburn 2008). However, we need to acknowledge other factors that affect this relationship, such as age and cardiovascular disease.

Previous studies (Isacson and Broström 1988; Jaakkola and Mann 2004; Locke et al. 1984; Platto et al. 1991) have explored abnormalities in gait parameters with their findings showing 50 and 90% changes compared with cohorts without pathology, even when adjusted for age and gender. In relation to specific foot impairments, Platto et al. (1991) concluded that rearfoot pain and deformity impeded walking more than those in the forefoot and showed stronger correlations with gait parameters. Keenan et al. (1991) found decreased velocity, shortened stride length, and reduced single-limb support time in those with disease duration averaging 25 years and pes planovalgus deformity. Similar results were found by Turner et al. (2003) in those with average disease duration of 7 years and pes planovalgus. These gait parameters are useful for understanding the impact of RA foot disease on gait and also for evaluating the success or otherwise of specific foot interventions such as orthoses and specialist footwear (Fransen and Edmonds 1997; Mac-Sween and Brydson, 1999; Mejjad et al. 2004).

The temporal and spatial gait parameters that represent the overall gait strategy of people with RA are that walking speed is slower and stride length, and step length and single limb support are reduced (Turner et al. 2003). These changes are notable compared with similar walking speed in healthy subjects (Turner et al. 2006; Turner and Woodburn 2008).

Kinematics

The effects of RA disease on the joints and surrounding structures are known to cause laxity in early disease and stiffness later in the course of the disease. These pathological changes affect joint kinematics, as do the compensatory mechanisms adopted to lessen symptoms. It has been demonstrated that pes planovalgus, excessive and prolonged eversion, coupled with internal leg rotation and dorsiflexion are the most common effects of the disease on the joints and related structures (Woodburn et al. 1999). Collapse of the medial arch with forefoot inversion, dorsiflexion and abduction are features of abnormal motion patterns that can be controlled with foot orthoses with a reduction in symptoms and a sustained improvement in foot kinematics (Woodburn et al. 1999). Excellent within-day reliability has been found for the inter-segment kinematics. Between-day reliability ranged from fair to good to excellent for kinematic variables and all ICCs were excellent; the standard error of the mean (SEM) ranged from 0.60° to 1.99°. The authors concluded that multisegmented foot kinematics could be reliably measured in RA patients with pes planovalgus (Baan et al. 2012).

Plantar Pressure

Plantar pressure distribution is a frequently used technique used to examine activities such as walking and stair climbing. Peak pressure and the pressure time integral are often higher in those with RA and are associated with impairments of pain, stiffness and deformity (van der Leeden et al. 2006). In those with decreased sensation of the feet, it is a useful tool in the detection of excessive forefoot loading before complications such as mechanical damage to the articular structures and extra-articular structures are manifested (Rosenbaum et al. 2006). In relation to the evaluation of foot interventions such as foot orthoses, plantar pressure assessment can provide information as to their effectiveness in the redistribution of pressure. In their study of RA and non-RA control participants, Li et al. (2000) observed that foot orthoses produced greater pressure redistributions and loading force relief in the RA patients than in control subjects.

Electromyography

It is suggested that loss of muscle function, as assessed with electromyography (EMG), contributes to the development of foot deformity (Barn et al. 2013). However, in RA patients, Barn et al. (2012) found that, although foot kinematics can be reliably measured, leg muscle EMG activity was less so. They found that the discrete temporal and amplitude EMG parameters were highly variable across all muscle groups but particularly poor for tibialis posterior and peroneus longus. The SEM ranged from 1% to 9% of stance and 4% to 27% of maximum voluntary contraction. In most cases, the 95% confidence interval crossed zero. Furthermore, the authors recommend that caution should be exercised when EMG measurements are considered to study disease progression or intervention effects.

QUALITY OF LIFE

Though objective measures such as joint ranges of motion and tender and swollen joint counts may be reliable, valid and integral to measuring outcomes in RA, they are limited in that they are based upon the biomedical model of disease, where outcomes are considered primarily in relation to the pathological processes of disease (Bowling 2001). In addition, such measures often do not permit patients to provide their own perspective of their health status, and this often differs to the perspective of the clinician (Hewlett 2003). It is therefore imperative that clinicians gain insight into patients' individual experience of these impairments in order to monitor the impact of the disease on their life and their perceptions of the success or otherwise of treatments.

In relation to the impact of feet problems on the patient's quality of life, it is known that they impact negatively (Otter et al. 2012). Living with feet affected by RA often results in diverse and multidimensional implications for the patient. These are in relation to physical capacity, mental resilience and general well-being (Walmsley et al. 2012) and in respect of how the physical changes in the feet affect overall body image (Williams and Graham 2012) creating restrictions for social activities through not being able to wear footwear of choice and style suitable to the occasion. The authors of two qualitative studies (Otter et al. 2012; Wickman et al. 2004) investigating women's experience of wearing specialist therapeutic footwear concluded that, unlike any other intervention, specialist therapeutic footwear replaces something that is normally worn and is part of an individual's body image. It has a negative impact on female patients' emotions and activities. Further, the participants of these two studies (Otter et al. 2012; Wickman et al. 2004) and a later study (Williams and Graham 2012) revealed how living with feet affected with RA had a huge impact on how they think that others see them in relation to personal and social roles. This often resulted in their declining invitations to social events and resulted in social isolation.

MANAGEMENT STRATEGIES

In working towards an overall goal of reducing symptoms, preventing structural damage and assisting a person with RA to live a full and fulfilling life, there is an increasing evidence base of a range of effective strategies. Many of these strategies overlap and can be implemented in parallel. These include medical strategies concerning diagnosis, prognosis and thera-peutics, psychosocial strategies of chronic disease management and self-help along with more specific strategies to deal with symptomatic body structures (such as the foot) or co-morbid risk factors (such as cardiovascular disease).

EARLY TREATMENT STRATEGIES IN RA

A series of differing studies of either placebo-controlled studies of disease-modifying anti-rheumatic drugs (DMARDs) or of delayed treatment with DMARDs has demonstrated the benefit of earlier treatment (Quinn et al. 2001). A small but important subset of previous studies has shown that the benefit of earlier treatment may last well beyond any delay in starting therapy (Lard et al. 2001; Nell et al. 2004; van Aken et al. 2004).

GOAL-DIRECTED TREATMENT STRATEGIES

Four seminal studies have been performed comparing differing treatment strategies. Each had a different design and their findings have not been replicated; nor can the results be pooled in a statistical sense. However, these studies have led to a much greater understanding and confidence in the approach to managing RA. Two trials (TICORA and FIN-RACo) used both differing treatments and differing protocols for intensification or change of therapy if an adequate response to treatment had not occurred. The CAMERA trial used the same medication, but with differing assessment and intensification protocols. The fourth trial (BESt) used similar assessments and cut-off points for intensification of therapy for each of the four differing treatment groups.

The TICORA study compared 'usual care' with a strategy aimed at achieving a prescribed level of disease control using a predetermined treatment pathway at monthly assessments (Grigor et al. 2004). The FIN-RACo study compared combination DMARD therapy with intensification of treatment at 3 months if less than a 50% improvement in two of three clinical variables (swollen join score, tender joint score, ESR) had occurred with monotherapy and intensification at a longer interval (6 months) at a lower level of response (25%) of the two/three variables (Mottonen et al. 1999). The CAMERA trial involved frequent (monthly) assessments with intensification of

therapy if remission was not achieved or less than 20% improvement had occurred between visits. These were compared with 3-monthly standard (for the time) clinical assessments (Verstappen et al. 2007). The fourth trial, the BESt trial, compared four treatment pathways [sequential monotherapy, step-up combination, step-down combination with high-dose glucocorticoid or step-down combination with a tumour necrosis factor (TNF) inhibitor)]. Assessments were undertaken and therapy was either intensified or reduced if the DAS44 changed by >2.4 or ≤2.4 respectively (Allaart et al. 2006).

PHARMACOLOGICAL STRATEGIES

The specific drugs used to treat RA fall into two broad categories: those that relieve symptoms and those that may slow or arrest the underlying disease process. Glucocorticoids are often considered separately, in part because of debate about their degree of disease-modifying effect and in part because of their very broad range of effects and side effects (Kirwan 1995). In addition, many patients with RA are treated with additional agents aimed at treating co-morbid conditions (such as osteoporosis, vascular disease, or sleep and mood disturbance) or to manage side effects of therapeutic agents (gastrointestinal disturbance, osteoporosis or hypertension). As such, patients with RA present with the potential for complex drug–drug and drug–patient interactions (Treharne et al. 2007).

Symptom-relieving Agents

Pain is a predominant symptom in RA and a variety of analgesics can be used. Because of the inflammatory nature of RA, non-steroidal anti-inflammatory drugs (NSAIDs), which have both analgesic and anti-inflammatory activity mediated through blocking the enzyme cyclo-oxygenase (which assists conversion of arachidonic acid to prostaglandin H_2), used to be considered 'first-line agents' for the management of RA (Upchurch and Kay 2012). Treatment with agents with a more specific effect on inflammation has altered the use of NSAIDs over time, such that NSAIDs are now frequently used on an as-needed rather than regular basis (Fries et al. 2004). NSAIDs can be subdivided into those blocking cyclo-oxygenase 1 (COX-1) and cyclo-oxygenase 2 (COX-2) enzymes (sometimes referred to as traditional NSAIDs), and those with more specific COX-2 inhibition (or COX-2 blockers). Upper gastrointestinal irritation is greater with traditional NSAIDs than with COX-2 blockers. Both agents have the potential for increasing blood pressure and worsening renal function. NSAIDs can also independently increase cardiovascular risk. The relative risk or safety of individual compounds is subject to much debate (Trelle et al. 2011).

For many patients, either because of controlled inflammatory disease or because of side effects or contraindications to NSAIDs, pure analgesics are used. Available pure analgesic agents vary greatly in both efficacy and side effects. There is a hierarchy of analgesics, starting with paracetamol/acetaminophen with modest analgesia, through partial opioid antagonists such as codeine or tramadol, to pure opioids such as morphine. Paracetamol has advantages of relative safety and low side effect profile, though a constant elimination rate increases the risk of toxicity in overdose greatly (Trescot et al. 2008). Opioid antagonists have greater analgesic effects but their use is limited by problems of constipation, CNS and respiratory depression, as well as potential for dependency and abuse.

Disease-modifying Agents

The term 'disease-modifying anti-rheumatic drugs (DMARDs)' is a collective term used to describe a diverse group of agents that can modify the long-term outcome of RA. Drugs that can inhibit the progression of erosive damage of RA as shown in controlled trials are considered members of the group of DMARDs. The group can be divided into conventional (or traditional) DMARDs, small molecules discovered through either serendipity or traditional drug discovery programmes, and biologic DMARDs, which are generally manufactured proteins that interfere with important biological functions or structures thought to be important in RA.

Conventional. The following drugs are considered traditional DMARDs: gold, D-penicillamine, sulfasalazine, azathioprine, anti-malarials, methotrexate, ciclosporin-A, and leflunomide. All traditional DMARDs have a slow onset of action, usually over several weeks to months, and a range of side effects that usually require long-term monitoring.

Methotrexate has become the most widely used conventional DMARD for use in RA. It was originally developed as a cytotoxic drug for use in the chemotherapy of cancer. In high doses in cancer chemotherapy, its mode of action is by inhibition of cell-cycle-specific folate antagonism. Its mode of action in the lower doses used in the treatment of RA is less clear (Cutolo et al. 2001). Methotrexate in RA is usually given as a single weekly dose. Supplemental folic acid is often given, primarily to reduce the incidence of GI upset, the most common side effect of methotrexate. Other potentially important side effects of methotrexate include known teratogenicity, haematological cytopenia, liver function test abnormality and rare cases of interstitial pneumonitis, liver cirrhosis, lymphoma and opportunistic infection. Despite these cautions, patients with RA taking methotrexate appear to have no clinically significant increase in hospitalization compared with RA patients not on DMARD therapy (Bernatsky et al. 2007). Indeed, the use methotrexate appears to reduce the risk of congestive heart failure (Bernatsky et al. 2005).

Because of concern regarding post-operative infection risk, some surgeons used to recommend cessation of methotrexate around the time of surgery. Following a randomized controlled trial showing that this practice did not increase the infection risk but did increase the rate of RA flares, it is now recommended to continue methotrexate over the period of surgery (Grennan et al. 2001).

Biologic Disease-Modifying Anti-Rheumatic Drugs. With an advancing understanding of the immune pathogenesis of RA, it has become increasingly possible to create proteins that interfere with specific inflammatory pathways (Otter et al. 2004). This can be conducted by a number of different methods, including 'cepts', which are protein constructs to block protein–cell or cell–cell interactions, and 'mabs', monoclonal antibodies that can block a similar set of interactions or, depending on their specificity, induce lysis of a particular cell line. Given the multiple pathways involved in RA and the various methods of producing biologic agents, the number of agents licensed for use in RA has increased dramatically in the last two decades. In 2011, the following agents were licensed for use in the UK: abatacept, adalimumab, certolizumab pegol, etanercept, golimumab, infliximab, rituximab and tocilizumab (Kiely et al. 2012).

Because biologic DMARDs are protein-based, and therefore subject to digestion if given orally, they can also be provided through subcutaneous or intravenous administration. Unlike conventional DMARDs, some biologic DMARDs have a very rapid onset of action. The risk of serious infection with biologic DMARDs appears to be increased about twofold, particularly in the first year of their administration (Dixon et al. 2006). In addition to the increased risk of common infections, the very specific mode of action of biologic DMARDs increases the risk of a very small number of very rare infections where the inflammatory pathway being blocked appears to be a critical component of host immunity. In particular, there is a risk of reactivation of latent tuberculosis in patients given monoclonal inhibitors of anti-TNF.

FOOT HEALTH MANAGEMENT

Further to early aggressive medical management, guidelines (ARMA 2004; NICE 2009) suggest that management requires an integrated co-ordinated multidisciplinary, multiprofessional approach, with care focused upon the needs of the affected person, providing access to a combination of expertise and competencies. Patients should have access to a full multidisciplinary team for assessment and intervention early in the disease process, and this includes foot health assessment (Williams et al. 2011).

The ethos of the foot health guidelines developed by Williams et al. (2011) echoes the work of Helliwell (2007) and aims to relieve pain, maintain function and improve quality of life utilizing specific interventions. These interventions include palliative treatment for the nails and skin, prescribed foot orthoses and specialist footwear and management and prevention of foot ulceration with the need for education and information in all aspects of foot health. In order to guide and inform the assessment and management process, a screening pathway has been developed by Williams et al. (2011) (Figure 2-4).

Foot Health Assessment

Through the structured assessment process, the specific foot health problems are identified, and hence a management plan can then be negotiated with the patient (Williams et al. 2011). Understanding the impact of the disease and foot problems on the patient is crucial to negotiating a suitable management plan. It may be easiest to get the patient to describe a typical day, from getting out of bed to washing, dressing, and toileting. The impact of the disease on the patient's employment will be important. Questions concerning the things a person would like to do, but is currently unable to, may pinpoint key problems. If there are problems with mobility and function then referral to physiotherapy and/or occupational therapy may be appropriate. Negotiations with the patient on balancing the risks and benefits of an intervention will be greatly affected by the patient's priorities for treatment. Patients' perceptions/knowledge and expectations in relation to their presenting symptoms also need to be ascertained in order to create appropriate dialogue and understanding and engagement with interventions and advice (Graham et al. 2012a, 2012b).

Examination for signs of the extra-articular features of RA nodules, bursa, vasculitis, tendonitis, and tenosynovitis will also determine the type of foot intervention. For example, if the disease is in remission and there is evidence of painful tendonitis or bursitis then corticosteroid injections may be warranted. A detailed assessment of foot and lower limb function and structure (static and during gait), followed by a 'feel, look and move' approach to the foot assessing the foot position, deformities, range of movement and location of painful, tender, swollen sites will determine the need for foot orthoses, specialist footwear and in some instances referral for foot surgery. A lower limb vascular assessment and neurological examination will determine any complications associated with RA or as co-morbid pathology.

Examination of patients' footwear and its suitability for both home and outdoor use is required, as changing the footwear style often helps to improve symptoms. The features of specialist therapeutic footwear have been described in relation to their appropriateness for the structure and function of the RA foot (Williams et al. 2007a; Williams and Nester 2006). However, there is currently no specific tool for evaluating the suitability of retail footwear for people with RA.

A footwear assessment tool with good face validity has been developed by Barton et al. (2009) to assist

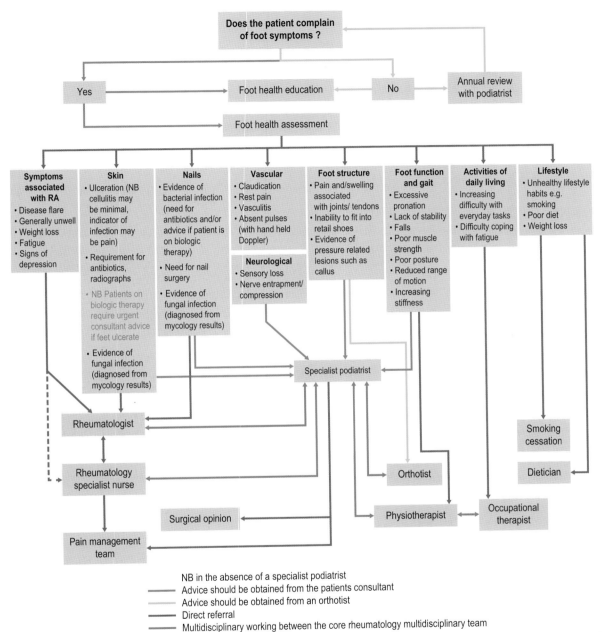

FIGURE 2-4 Foot-screening pathway. (Reprinted with permission from Williams AE, Davies S, Graham A, et al 2011. Guidelines for the management of the foot health problems associated with rheumatoid arthritis. Musculoskeletal Care 9(2):86–92. Copyright © 2011 John Wiley & Sons, Ltd.)

in footwear assessment and it generally has good internal reliability. Although also considered to be reliable for assessing footwear in relation to general foot health, it may not be comprehensive enough for patients with moderate to severe RA foot deformity. Further to an initial foot health and footwear assessment, it is recommended that an annual review should be offered to those with existing problems. Also, those with no current foot problems should be monitored and reassessed for changes in foot health status.

Management of Plantar Callus

In RA, prominent metatarsal heads are subject to excessive shear and compressive forces during gait. These stresses stimulate the stratum corneum to produce well-circumscribed painful skin lesions or callosities. A study investigating foot pain, foot function and foot impact by Siddle et al. (2013) built on earlier work by Davys et al. (2005), and concluded that the effect of sharp scalpel debridement was no greater than the sham scalpel debridement. Siddle et al. (2013) found that, at 18 months' follow-up, there were no differences between groups for the primary outcome VAS-measured forefoot plantar pain. There was little change in scores of overall function and foot impact in either group and there were no significant changes in gait parameters noted. The authors concluded that the long-term effects of sharp scalpel debridement of painful forefoot plantar callosities in people with RA, when used in conjunction with foot orthoses and footwear modification (combined intervention), produced no additional benefit over the combined intervention alone. Davys et al. (2005) and Siddle et al. (2013) reported that reduction of the plantar foot pressures that cause the callus is an alternative treatment. This can be achieved with foot orthoses and appropriate footwear (Hennessy et al. 2007). A consensus of opinion from both specialist podiatrists and academics recommend that adhesive plantar padding should not be used to provide pressure relief, especially where there are concerns regarding tissue viability (Williams et al. 2011). Additionally, they recommended a caveat to the recommendation of minimal or no debridement, and this is when infection is suspected. Overlying callus should then be debrided in order to expose the underlying infection, and in the case of existing foot ulceration it is appropriate that surrounding callus and necrotic tissue is debrided.

Footwear and Foot Orthoses

In order to negate the excessive foot pressures that lead to callus and ulcer formation, and improve foot posture and motion, guidelines recommend that specialist footwear and foot orthoses are beneficial (ARMA 2004; NICE 2009). For the purposes of clarity, foot orthoses and footwear options will be discussed separately.

Foot Orthoses. There is a broad range of orthoses that employ a variety of different approaches to modify foot and lower limb structure and function. The main groups of orthoses are: (a) simple cushioning insoles; (b) insoles to which additional padding/additions, and (c) contoured orthoses intended to change the function of leg and foot joints. However, the boundaries between the modes of action of the types are not exact and an individual device may include elements with more than one mode of action (Williams et al. 2010).

In the early stages of RA, it has been shown that early, targeted management of foot pathology with foot orthoses during a 'window of opportunity' is crucial before irreversible damage occurs (Woodburn et al. 2010). Woodburn et al. (2002b) demonstrated that foot orthoses are beneficial in reducing the pain and also in improving foot posture. This may have sustainable effects over a longer period, in dealing with an abnormal mechanical component that can predispose the patient to the development of a foot deformity.

Customized accommodative foot orthoses (also known as total contact orthoses) are designed so that the material follows the contours of the underside of the foot closely. The purpose is to redistribute the pressures applied to the foot in standing and walking more evenly. This is particularly useful where there are areas of increased pressure (e.g. under the metatarsal heads in those with established foot deformity). In this instance, the pressure is shifted to areas of the foot that do not normally bear weight, such as the arch area (Li et al. 2000). They are particularly used where there is limited or no joint mobility, such as in the established RA foot and where tissue viability is poor. These orthoses are often made from materials that also provide a cushioning effect.

In their review of the evidence for foot orthoses in an RA cohort, Clark et al. (2006) reported that there is limited evidence pertaining to the cost effectiveness of foot orthoses to reduce rearfoot and forefoot pain as well as improvements in functional ability and reduction in hallux valgus. Further, although Hennessy et al. (2012) found that custom orthoses may be beneficial in reducing pain and elevated forefoot plantar pressures, they also concluded that the evidence was inconclusive for foot function, walking speed, gait parameters, and for reducing hallux valgus angle progression.

From a biomechanical perspective, there is only limited evidence for the use of simple cushioning insoles. Two small studies indicate that prefabricated metatarsal padding (dome- and bar-shaped metatarsal pads) reduce mean peak plantar foot pressure by up to 21% with bars and 12% with domes (Jackson et al. 2004) and both equally (Hodge et al. 1999) in patients with RA. Despite the limited evidence, foot orthoses are recommended by national guidelines (NICE 2009) for the management of both early and established functional and structural foot problems (Williams et al. 2011).

Footwear. All footwear is capable of modifying elements of the structure and function of the foot. Inappropriate footwear can be a major contributing factor to foot impairment. However, it also has the potential to alleviate pain and increase mobility and hence independence (with or without foot orthoses) (Williams et al. 2007a).

Footwear can be subdivided into three main groups: (a) standard retail footwear, (b) niche retail (including comfort footwear as well as extra depth, extra width and unusual sizes), and (c) specialist therapeutic footwear. There are now many manufacturers of standard retail footwear that are appropriate for the foot health of patients. According to Williams and Nester (2006), the features of this footwear that are valuable for the RA foot are: (1) stable heel – broad enough for stability or elongated/flared to increase this effect further, (2) extended heel counter to provide support for the rearfoot, (3) padding around the top opening of the shoe – to reduce irritation to the retro-calcaneal area and the infra-malleolar areas, (4) no prominent internal seams to prevent rubbing, (5) winged 'toe puff' to ensure no pressure over the toes, (6) increased toe spring or rocker sole to reduce forefoot plantar pressures, and (7) low laces for ease of access.

Furthermore, the suitability of retail footwear can be assessed using the tool developed by Barton et al. (2009). This is crucial in relation to managing the effects of RA on the foot even during the early stages when foot deformity may be minimal but symptoms severe and compounded by ill-fitting footwear. If the foot dimensions are outside of what is available from retail suppliers or if there are pressure areas/localized pain caused by the footwear, or excessive wear to parts of the shoe, then it is recommended that patients are referred for specialist therapeutic footwear. Specialist therapeutic footwear can be either 'stock' footwear that is of standard fittings of extra depth and/or width, or bespoke that is made for the individual (NICE 2009; Williams et al. 2011).

Two systematic reviews (Egan et al. 2003; Farrow et al. 2005) indicated that specialist therapeutic footwear is likely to be beneficial in reducing pain and increasing activity for patients with RA. However, the two reviews concluded that an obstacle is the patient's agreement to wear them sufficiently to maximize the potential for these benefits to be achieved. The obstacle identified in this study was the low level of engagement in one arm of the study, owing to the participants rejecting the footwear due to its unacceptable appearance. Previous studies investigating patient experiences of wearing therapeutic footwear that the practitioners who refer patients for specialist therapeutic footwear need to be mindful of this point (Williams et al. 2007b, 2010). They should inform the patient prior to referral that this footwear often appears different in design to popular designs of retail footwear and allow the patient choice as to whether they are referred or not.

In conclusion, foot orthoses and footwear can be helpful in reducing pain and increasing activity when people with RA have established foot problems and can provide an important effect in reducing the mechanical component that contributes to the development of deformity in the first place.

SURGICAL STRATEGIES

Whilst it is recognized that advances in the medical management of RA with biologic therapies have seen a reduction in some of the major foot problems that require surgery, some patients still develop problems with their feet and ankles and may require surgical intervention. Reasons for surgical referral may include persistent pain, stiffness, synovitis in the foot or ankle joints, tenosynovitis or tendon ruptures, foot deformities causing restriction in mobility due to pain, or recurrent ulceration and osteomyelitis/septic arthritis. It is generally accepted that referrals for surgical opinion should be considered for patients with RA when optimal conservative management has failed to bring their symptoms to an acceptable level. However, clinicians should always be aware of potential exceptions, such as the requirement for earlier synovectomy in severe disease to prevent rapid joint destruction (Aho and Halonen 1991).

In a systematic review of interventions for RA foot disease, Farrow et al. (2005) found that evidence was lacking for foot surgery with an absence of RCTs but they concluded that prospective observational studies suggest that forefoot arthroplasty and first MTP joint implants are effective at improving reduction in pain and improving appearance. Through comparative retrospective analyses, these authors also suggested that some procedure variants may be better than others, and surgery may relieve pain more than foot orthoses.

A study by Canseco et al. (2012) found that surgery effectively restored alignment and weightbearing capacity in rheumatoid feet. Post-operatively the hallux position was significantly restored, forefoot abduction decreased and forefoot valgus was also decreased, although this was not significant. However, hallux range of motion significantly decreased after surgery. Although stance duration continued to be prolonged, walking speed showed slight improvement. Canseco et al. (2012) concluded that, although the purpose of the surgery was the restoration of alignment and weightbearing capacity in the rheumatoid foot, a fused MTP joint is neither mechanically nor physiologically normal and continues to produce an altered gait pattern compared with healthy individuals. The presence of altered mechanics following surgery stresses the importance of post-operative rehabilitation (such as the use of foot orthoses) and gait training.

Further to these considerations for post-operative management, the patients' expectations and evaluation of outcome needs to be considered. Patients interpret the outcome of foot surgery using a multitude of interrelated factors (Backhouse et al. 2012), particularly functional ability, appearance and surgeons' appraisal of the procedure. Although a reduction in pain was often noted by Backhouse et al. (2012), it appeared less important than appearance and functional ability in the overall outcome of the surgery.

PHYSICAL STRATEGIES

Physiotherapy is considered one of the key rehabilitative interventions for people with RA in relation to enhancing and maintaining function and mobility, and it is recommended that physiotherapists are also included in the management of lower limb and foot problems. A Cochrane review of balance interventions by Silva et al. (2010) identified 17 studies that described general exercises in rheumatoid arthritis patients. The main interventions recommended were exercises to improve muscle strength, endurance, and dynamic exercises (swimming, walking, and other physical activities). There were no studies investigating the effects of balance training, either alone or in combination with other therapies, in patients with rheumatoid arthritis.

In a review of the literature of non-pharmacological interventions, Vliet Vlieland and van den Ende (2011) found that exercise and physical activity programmes needed further development in respect to intensity, frequency, duration and mode of delivery. In a further review of tai chi as an intervention for RA (Lee et al. 2007), some positive findings on a disability index, quality of life, depression and mood were observed. Two RCTs (Wang et al. 2005; Lee 2005) assessed pain outcomes and did not show tai chi to be more effective for pain reduction than education plus stretching exercise and usual activity control. The extent of heterogeneity in these RCTs prevented a meaningful meta-analysis, with few focusing on RA, and most had low methodological quality. Hence the authors concluded that the evidence is not convincing enough to suggest that tai chi was an effective treatment for RA.

LIFESTYLE AND EDUCATION STRATEGIES

Patient education is considered to be an integral component in the management strategies, to support and facilitate self-management of the disease and long-term outcomes. Lorig et al. (2005) and Kjeken et al. (2006) demonstrated that people with RA who are actively involved in their disease management have better outcomes, improved self-efficacy, less pain and reduced incidence of depression. In relation to foot problems, it has been recommended that patient-centred education should be provided to enable patients to make informed choices about their footcare (Graham et al. 2012a, 2012b; Williams et al. 2011).

There is currently a lack of research into the effectiveness of foot-focused patient education. However, two qualitative studies have highlighted what foot-specific patient education should be and how it should be delivered from both the practitioner's and patient's perspective (Graham et al. 2012a, 2012b). These two studies suggest that patient education encompasses information about the disease and how it affects the feet, information about the effectiveness of interventions and advice on self-care. Further, education should be individually tailored as group education may not meet all the requirements of the individual.

FUTURE DIRECTIONS

The incidence of RA is falling owing to earlier detection (Emery et al. 2002), earlier targeted therapy, earlier use of biologic therapies (NICE 2009) and changes in how RA is classified (Aletaha et al. 2010). Aligned with this are improvements in diagnosis, with ultrasonography being increasingly used to visualize bursae, tendons, ligaments and other structures (Bowen et al. 2010; Wakefield 1999). Furthermore, newer, more specific laboratory investigations such as anti-cyclic citrullinated peptide antibodies are increasingly being used (Bas 2005).

The aetiology of RA remains an area of intense interest. In recent years, there have been major advances in understanding of genetic risk, aided by the genome-wide association studies (Kallberg et al. 2007). There has also been renewed interest in environmental triggers and lifestyle influences (Lahiri et al. 2012). The known lifestyle risk factors such as smoking, which can be modified, mean that there is the potential for preventative population strategies for RA akin to the well-established programmes for cardiovascular disease and cancer.

Despite advances in assessment and medical management, people are still reporting foot problems (Otter et al. 2010). This is due to foot pathology being caused by abnormal mechanics in addition to the destructive nature of inflammation (Göksel-Karatepe et al. 2010). It is known that foot problems are often overlooked, yet their assessment is vital for improved management of people with RA. Early targeted intervention for the RA foot is recommended in guidelines and by specialist teams (ARMA 2004; NICE 2009; Williams et al. 2011) and the Podiatric Rheumatic Care Association (PRCA 2008), so efforts must be made to ensure that feet are incorporated into general disease assessment tools such as the DAS (Anderson et al. 2012).

There are developments occurring in the technology utilized to produce foot orthoses and footwear (Pallari et al. 2010; Telfer and Woodburn 2010). In a review of literature on 3D scanning of the foot, it was concluded that modern 3D surface scanning systems can obtain accurate and repeatable digital representations of foot shape (Telfer and Woodburn 2010). These systems have been successfully used in medical, ergonomic and footwear development applications. The increasing affordability of these systems presents opportunities for manufacturers of footwear and foot orthoses, particularly when customization is needed.

INVITED COMMENTARY

Rheumatoid arthritis is the commonest inflammatory arthritis seen in the UK, Europe and North America. It causes inflammation and destruction of synovial joints and, in many cases, has an additional systemic component that is associated with increased morbidity and mortality. The cost of the disease, in both individual and societal terms, is considerable. Rheumatoid arthritis comprises the bulk of the work done by a general rheumatologist and is the commonest reason for referral from rheumatology to podiatry. The treatment of rheumatoid arthritis is rapidly

Continued on following page

INVITED COMMENTARY (Continued)

changing and with new treatments has come new hope of preventing the deformities seen after many years of disease.

Nevertheless, the foot remains a neglected area in rheumatology. Clinically, it is far easier to look at the hands than to look at the feet, and widespread use of the disease activity score (DAS28) reinforces this neglect. Examining the foot and ankle requires both examiner and patient to undergo activity that may incur pain and may prolong the consultation. From my experience in post-graduate education, I know that rheumatologists and podiatrists feel in need of more knowledge and skills with respect to the foot in rheumatoid arthritis. I hope this chapter helps.

Unusually in rheumatology, the specialty of orthopaedics has contributed significantly to what we know about the foot in rheumatoid arthritis, but this is changing with the emergence of academic departments of podiatry carrying out research published in the top rheumatology journals. Surgery is now seen as a failure of medical and podiatry management, but it is still a common intervention in our existing cohort of patients. Patients need to have stable disease activity if surgery is to be a success, thus demanding a combined approach to this intervention.

What are the major changes that have occurred in rheumatoid arthritis over the last 15 years? There is evidence that the disease is changing in incidence and severity and we are seeing cases earlier in the course of their disease. We now treat aggressively until the patient is in low disease activity and there is evidence that this has improved long-term outcomes. We have clearer treatment paradigms, and powerful new drugs that quickly suppress disease activity. Having said that, there is still a need for a multidisciplinary approach as patients come with complex problems that need addressing from different angles. There is also evidence that even in the low-disease-activity states that we seek; there is still continuing, grumbling disease that can cause damage. We argue that joint protection is necessary in this group but how can you 'protect' effectively the joints of the foot and ankle? I think this is one reason why it is so difficult to demonstrate the efficacy of orthoses in rheumatoid arthritis.

There are a number of challenges facing the foot specialist in rheumatology. The first is how to show the efficacy of local interventions when systemic interventions are now so powerful and effective. Somehow the added value of treatments for the foot, including mechanical, anti-inflammatory and surgical, need to have their worth demonstrated. It would be nice to think that effective systemic treatments will make local therapies obsolete, but this is unlikely given the comments above. Secondly, closer working with other disciplines, both medical and non-medical, will be necessary to meet the demands of those 'high-risk' patients who will ulcerate, fracture, become infected, and lose their jobs due to poor mobility. Most healthcare delivery is organized on a parallel model but it will be necessary to make this an integrated approach, not for everyone of course but to meet those few patients where this will prevent future problems. Thirdly, the spectre of cost must be tackled and all interventional studies should include an economic analysis. The direct costs of healthcare in rheumatoid arthritis are increasing due to the use of biologic drugs and these high-cost interventions have had to undergo extreme cost-effectiveness analysis. The same should be done for interventions in the foot, if only to demonstrate how they compare with others in an increasingly cash-strapped healthcare system.

Despite all this, times are exciting in foot and ankle research. New imaging techniques are now providing the ability to see structures both in anatomical detail and in functional configuration including their role in pathogenesis. New technology will enable better assessment of the biomechanics of the foot and provide more insights into the effect of mechanical interventions. To me, the foot still has a lot of secrets to give up in a disease that can affect all the components of the musculoskeletal system, and may provide insights into other disease processes.

Phillip S. Helliwell MA, DM, PhD, FRCP
Senior Lecturer in Rheumatology,
Leeds Institute of Molecular Medicine, Section of
Musculoskeletal Disease, University of Leeds, UK

REFERENCES

Ahmad, S., Garg, S., Dhar, M., et al., 2012. Predictors of atherosclerosis in rheumatoid arthritis. Vasa 41, 353–359.

Aho, H., Halonen, P., 1991. Synovectomy of the MTP joints in rheumatoid arthritis. Acta Orthopaedia Scandinavia 37, 243–244.

Alam, S.M., Kidwai, A.A., Jafri, S.R., et al., 2011. Epidemiology of rheumatoid arthritis in a tertiary care unit, Karachi, Pakistan. Journal of the Pakistan Medical Association 61, 123–126.

Alcalde, M., D'Agostino, M.A., Bruyn, G.A., et al., 2012. A systematic literature review of US definitions, scoring systems and validity according to the OMERACT filter for tendon lesion in RA and other inflammatory joint diseases. Rheumatology 51, 1246–1260.

Aletaha, D., Landewe, R., Karonitsch, T., et al., 2008. Reporting disease activity in clinical trials of patients with rheumatoid arthritis: EULAR/ACR collaborative recommendations. Annals of the Rheumatic Diseases 67, 1360–1364.

Aletaha, D., Neogi, T., Silman, A.J., et al., 2010. Rheumatoid arthritis classification criteria: an American College of Rheumatology/European League Against Rheumatism collaborative initiative. Arthritis and Rheumatism 62, 2569–2581.

Aletaha, D., Smolen, J., 2005. The Simplified Disease Activity Index (SDAI) and the Clinical Disease Activity Index (CDAI): a review of their usefulness and validity in rheumatoid arthritis. Clinical and Experimental Rheumatology 25, S100–S108.

Allaart, C.F, Goekoop-Ruiterman, Y.P., de Vries-Bouwstra, J.K., et al., 2006. Aiming at low disease activity in rheumatoid arthritis with initial combination therapy or initial monotherapy strategies: the BeSt study. Clinical and Experimental Rheumatology 24, S77–S82.

Anderson, J., Caplan, L., Yazdany, J., et al., 2012. Rheumatoid arthritis disease activity measures: American College of Rheumatology recommendations for use in clinical practice. Arthritis Care and Research 64, 640–647.

ARMA, 2004. Arthritis and Musculoskeletal Alliance – standards of care for people with inflammatory arthritis. Online. Available: <http://www.nras.org.uk/includes/documents/cm_docs/2012/a/arma_standards_of_care_for_ia.pdf>.

Arnett, F.C., Edworthy, S.M., Bloch, D.A., et al., 1988. The American Rheumatism Association 1987 revised criteria for the classification of rheumatoid arthritis. Arthritis and Rheumatism 31, 315–324.

Baan, H., Drossaers-Bakker, W., Dubbeldam, R., et al., 2011. We should not forget the foot: relations between signs and symptoms, damage, and function in rheumatoid arthritis. Clinics in Rheumatology 30, 1475–1479.

Baan, H., Dubbeldam, R., Nene, A.V., et al., 2012. Gait analysis of the lower limb in patients with rheumatoid arthritis: a systematic review. Seminars in Arthritis and Rheumatism 41, 768–788, e768.

Backhouse, M.R., Vinall, K.A., Redmond, A., et al., 2012. Complex reasoning determines patient's perception of outcome following foot surgery in rheumatoid arthritis. Rheumatology 51, iii52–iii92.

Backman, C.L., Kennedy, S.M., Chalmers, A., et al., 2004. Participation in paid and unpaid work by adults with rheumatoid arthritis. Journal of Rheumatology 31, 47–56.

Baka, Z., Buzas, E., Nagy, G., 2009. Rheumatoid arthritis and smoking: putting the pieces together. Arthritis Care and Therapy 11, 238.

Bakker, M.F., Jacobs, J.W., Kruize, A.A., et al., 2012. Misclassification of disease activity when assessing individual patients with early rheumatoid arthritis using disease activity indices that do not include joints of feet. Annals of the Rheumatic Diseases 71, 830–835.

Bal, A., Aydog, E., Aydog, S.T., et al., 2006. Foot deformities in rheumatoid arthritis and relevance of foot function index. Clinics in Rheumatology 25, 671–675.

Banal, F., Dougados, M., Combescure, C., et al., 2009. Sensitivity and specificity of the American College of Rheumatology 1987 criteria for the diagnosis of rheumatoid arthritis according to disease duration: a systematic literature review and meta-analysis. Annals of the Rheumatic Diseases 68, 1184–1191.

Barn, R., Rafferty, D., Turner, D.E., et al., 2012. Reliability study of tibialis posterior and selected leg muscle EMG and multi-segment foot kinematics in rheumatoid arthritis associated pes planovalgus. Gait and Posture 36, 567–571.

Barn, R., Turner, D.E., Rafferty, D., et al., 2013. Tibialis posterior tenosynovitis and associated pes plano valgus in rheumatoid arthritis: EMG, multi-segment foot kinematics and ultrasound features. Arthritis Care and Research (Hoboken) 65 (4), 495–502.

Barrett, E.M., Scott, D.G., Wiles, N.J., et al., 2000. The impact of rheumatoid arthritis on employment status in the early years of disease: a UK community-based study. Rheumatology 39, 1403–1409.

Barton, C., Bonanno, D., Menz, H., 2009. Development and evaluation of a tool for the assessment of footwear characteristics. Journal of Foot and Ankle Research 2, 10.

Bas, S., 2005. Usefulness of anti-citrullinated protein antibodies in the diagnosis and prognosis of rheumatoid arthritis. Revue Médicale Suisse 1, 674, 677–678, 680.

Bennett, P.J., Patterson, C., Wearing, S., et al., 1998. Development and validation of a questionnaire designed to measure foot-health status. Journal of the American Podiatric Medical Association 88, 419–428.

Bergsten, U., Bergman, S., Fridlund, B., et al. 2011. Patterns of background factors related to early RA patients' conceptions of the cause of their disease. Clinics in Rheumatology 30, 347–352.

Bernatsky, S., Hudson, M., Suissa, S., 2005. Anti-rheumatic drug use and risk of hospitalization for congestive heart failure in rheumatoid arthritis. Rheumatology 44, 677–680.

Bernatsky, S., Hudson, M., Suissa, S., 2007. Anti-rheumatic drug use and risk of serious infections in rheumatoid arthritis. Rheumatology 46, 1157–1160.

Bowen, C.J., Hooper, L., Culliford, D., et al., 2010. Assessment of the natural history of forefoot bursae using ultrasonography in patients with rheumatoid arthritis: a twelve-month investigation. Arthritis Care and Research 62, 1756–1762.

Bowling, A., 2001. Measuring disease: a review of disease-specific quality of life measurement scales. OUP, Buckingham.

Bruynesteyn, K., van der Heijde, D., Boers, M., et al., 2002. Determination of the minimal clinically important difference in rheumatoid arthritis joint damage of the Sharp/van der Heijde and Larsen/Scott scoring methods by clinical experts and comparison with the smallest detectable difference. Arthritis and Rheumatism 46, 913–920.

Budiman-Mak, E., Conrad, K., Stuck, R., et al., 2006. Theoretical model and Rasch analysis to develop a revised Foot Function Index. Foot and Ankle International 27, 519–527.

Budiman-Mak, E., Conrad, K.J., Roach, K.E., 1991. The Foot Function Index: a measure of foot pain and disability. Journal of Clinical Epidemiology 44, 561–570.

Canseco, K., Long, J., Smedberg, T., et al., 2012. Multisegmental foot and ankle motion analysis after hallux valgus surgery. Foot and Ankle Surgery 33, 141–147.

Clark, H., Rome, K., Plant, M., et al., 2006. A critical review of foot orthoses in the rheumatoid arthritic foot. Rheumatology 45, 139–145.

Combe, B., Landewe, R., Lukas, C., 2007. EULAR recommendations for the management of early arthritis: report of a task force of the European Standing Committee for International Clinical Studies Including Therapeutics (ESCISIT). Annals of the Rheumatic Diseases 66 (1), 34–45.

Cutolo, M., Sulli, A., Pizzorni, C., et al., 2001. Anti-inflammatory mechanisms of methotrexate in rheumatoid arthritis. Annals of the Rheumatic Diseases 60, 729–735.

Davys, H.J., Turner, D.E., Helliwell, P.S., et al., 2005. Debridement of plantar callosities in rheumatoid arthritis: a randomized controlled trial. Rheumatology 44, 207–210.

de Jong, P.H., Weel, A.E., de Man, Y.A., et al., 2012. Brief report: to squeeze or not to squeeze, that is the question! Optimizing the disease activity score in 28 joints by adding the squeeze test of metatarsophalangeal joints in early rheumatoid arthritis. Arthritis and Rheumatism 64, 3095–3101.

de P Magalhães, E., Davitt, M., Filho, D.J., et al., 2006. The effect of foot orthoses in rheumatoid arthritis. Rheumatology 45, 139–145.

Dixon, W.G., Watson, K., Lunt, M., et al., 2006. Rates of serious infection, including site-specific and bacterial intracellular infection, in rheumatoid arthritis patients receiving anti-tumor necrosis factor therapy: results from the British Society for Rheumatology Biologics Register. British Society for Rheumatology Biologics Register. Arthritis and Rheumatism 54, 2368–2376.

Egan, M., Brosseau, L., Farmer, M., et al., 2003. Splints/orthoses in the treatment of rheumatoid arthritis. Cochrane Database Systemic Reviews (1), CD004018.

Emery, P., Breedveld, F.C., Dougados, M., et al., 2002. Early referral recommendation for newly diagnosed rheumatoid arthritis: evidence based development of a clinical guide. Annals of the Rheumatic Diseases 61, 290–297.

Faguer, S., Ciroldi, M., Mariotte, E., et al., 2013. Prognostic contributions of the underlying inflammatory disease and acute organ dysfunction in critically ill patients with systemic rheumatic diseases. European Journal of Internal Medicine 24 (3), e40–e44.

Farrow, S.J., Kingsley, G.H., Scott, D.L., 2005. Interventions for foot disease in rheumatoid arthritis: a systematic review. Arthritis and Rheumatism 53, 593–602.

Felson, D.T., Anderson, J.J., Boers, M., et al., 1993. The American College of Rheumatology preliminary core set of disease activity measures for rheumatoid arthritis clinical trials. The Committee on Outcome Measures in Rheumatoid Arthritis Clinical Trials. Arthritis and Rheumatism 36, 729–740.

Firth, J., Helliwell, P., Hale, C., et al., 2008. The predictors of foot ulceration in patients with rheumatoid arthritis: a preliminary investigation. Clinics in Rheumatology 27, 1423–1428.

Fransen, M., Edmonds, J., 1997. Off-the-shelf orthopedic footwear for people with rheumatoid arthritis. Arthritis Care and Research 10, 250–256.

Fransen, M., Edmonds, J., 1999. Gait variables: appropriate objective outcome measures in rheumatoid arthritis. Rheumatology 38, 663–667.

Fries, J.F., Murtagh, K.N., Bennett, M., et al., 2004. The rise and decline of nonsteroidal antiinflammatory drug-associated gastropathy in rheumatoid arthritis. Arthritis and Rheumatism 50, 2433–2440.

Garrow, A.P., Papageorgiou, A.C., Silman, A.J., et al., 2000. Development and validation of a questionnaire to assess disabling foot pain. Pain 85, 107–113.

Göksel Karatepe, A., Günaydin, R., Adibelli, Z.H., et al., 2010. Foot deformities in patients with rheumatoid arthritis: the relationship with foot functions. International Journal of Rheumatic Diseases 13, 158–163.

Graham, A.S., Hammond, A., Williams, A.E., 2012a. Foot health education for people with rheumatoid arthritis: the practitioner's perspective. Journal of Foot and Ankle Research 5, 2.

Graham, A.S., Hammond, A., Walmsley, S., et al., 2012b. Foot health education for people with rheumatoid arthritis – some patient perspectives. Journal of Foot and Ankle Research 5, 23.

Grennan, D.M., Gray, J., Loudon, J., et al., 2001. Methotrexate and early postoperative complications in patients with rheumatoid arthritis undergoing elective orthopaedic surgery. Annals of the Rheumatic Diseases 60, 214–217.

Grigor, C., Capell, H., Stirling, A., et al., 2004. Effect of a treatment strategy of tight control for rheumatoid arthritis (the TICORA study): a single-blind randomised controlled trial. Lancet 364, 263–269.

Grondal, L., Tengstrand, B., Nordmark, B., et al., 2008. The foot: still the most important reason for walking incapacity in rheumatoid arthritis: distribution of symptomatic joints in 1,000 RA patients. Acta Orthopaedica 79, 257–261.

Hawker, G., 1997. Update on the epidemiology of the rheumatic diseases. Current Opinion in Rheumatology 9, 90–94.

Helliwell, P., Reay, N., Gilworth, G., et al., 2005. Development of a foot impact scale for rheumatoid arthritis. Arthritis and Rheumatism 53, 418–422.

Helliwell, P., Woodburn, J., Redmond, A., et al., 2007. The foot and ankle in rheumatoid arthritis. a comprehensive guide, Churchill Livingstone, Edinburgh.

Helliwell, P.S., 2003. Lessons to be learned: review of a multidisciplinary foot clinic in rheumatology. Rheumatology 42, 1426–1427.

Hennessy, K., Burns, J., Penkala, S., 2007. Reducing plantar pressure in rheumatoid arthritis: a comparison of running versus off-the-shelf orthopaedic footwear. Clinical Biomechanics 22, 917–923.

Hennessy, K., Woodburn, J., Steultjens, M.P., 2012. Custom foot orthoses for rheumatoid arthritis: A systematic review. Arthritis Care and Research 64, 311–320.

Hewlett, S., 2003. Patients and clinicians have different perspectives on outcomes in arthritis. Journal of Rheumatology 30, 877–879.

Hewlett, S., Choy, E., Kirwan, J., 2012. Furthering our understanding of fatigue in rheumatoid arthritis. Journal of Rheumatology 39, 1775–1777.

Hodge, M.C., Bach, T.M., Carter, G.M., 1999. Novel Award first prize paper. Orthotic management of plantar pressure and pain in rheumatoid arthritis. Clinical Biomechanics 14, 567–575.

Hooper, L., Bowen, C.J., Gates, L., et al., 2012. Prognostic indicators of foot-related disability in patients with rheumatoid arthritis: results of a prospective three-year study. Arthritis Care and Research 64, 1116–1124.

Hulsmans, H.M., Jacobs, J.W., van der Heijde, D.M., et al., 2000. The course of radiologic damage during the first six years of rheumatoid arthritis. Arthritis and Rheumatism 43, 1927–1940.

Isacson, J., Broström, L.A., 1988. Gait in rheumatoid arthritis: an electrogoniometric investigation. Journal of Biomechanics 21, 451–457.

Jaakkola, J.I., Mann, R.A., 2004. A review of rheumatoid arthritis affecting the foot and ankle. Foot and Ankle International 25, 866–874.

Jackson, L., Binning, J., Potter, J., 2004. Plantar pressures in rheumatoid arthritis using prefabricated metatarsal padding. Journal of the American Podiatric Medical Association 94, 239–245.

Kallberg, H., Padyukov, L., Plenge, R.M., et al., 2007. Gene–gene and gene–environment interactions involving HLA-DRB1, PTPN22, and smoking in two subsets of rheumatoid arthritis. American Journal of Human Genetics 80, 867–875.

Kane, D., Balint, P.V., Sturrock, R.D., 2003. Ultrasonography is superior to clinical examination in the detection and localization of knee joint effusion in rheumatoid arthritis. Journal of Rheumatology 30, 966–971.

Keenan, M.A., Peabody, T.D., Gronley, J.K., et al., 1991. Valgus deformities of the feet and characteristics of gait in patients who have rheumatoid arthritis. Journal of Bone and Joint Surgery, American Volume 73, 237–247.

Kiely, P.D., Deighton, C., Dixey, J., et al., 2012. Biologic agents for rheumatoid arthritis – negotiating the NICE technology appraisals.; British Society for Rheumatology Standards, Guidelines and Audit Working Group. Rheumatology 51, 24–31.

Kirwan, J.R., 1995. The effect of glucocorticoids on joint destruction in rheumatoid arthritis. The Arthritis and Rheumatism Council Low-Dose Glucocorticoid Study Group. New England Journal of Medicine 333, 142–146.

Kitas, G.D., Erb, N., 2003. Tackling ischaemic heart disease in rheumatoid arthritis. Rheumatology 42, 607–613.

Kjeken, I., Dagfinrud, H., Mowinckel, P., et al., 2006. Rheumatology care: involvement in medical decisions, received information, satisfaction with care, and unmet health care needs in patients with rheumatoid arthritis and ankylosing spondylitis. Arthritis and Rheumatism 55, 394–401.

Kwok, J.S., Hui, K.H., Lee, T.L., et al., 2005. Anti-cyclic citrullinated peptide: diagnostic and prognostic values in juvenile idiopathic arthritis and rheumatoid arthritis in a Chinese population. Scandinavian Journal of Rheumatology 34, 359–366.

Lahiri, M., Morgan, C., Symmons, D.P., et al., 2012. Modifiable risk factors for RA: prevention, better than cure? Rheumatology 51, 499–512.

Landorf, K.B., Keenan, A.M., 2002. An evaluation of two foot-specific, health-related quality-of-life measuring instruments. Foot and Ankle International 23, 538–546.

Lard, L.R., Visser, H., Speyer, I., et al., 2001. Early versus delayed treatment in patients with recent-onset rheumatoid arthritis: comparison of two cohorts who received different treatment strategies. American Journal of Medicine 111, 446–451.

Larsen, A., Dale, K., Eek, M., 1977. Radiographic evaluation of rheumatoid arthritis and related conditions by standard reference films. Acta Radiologica: Diagnosis 18, 481–491.

Lee, E.N., 2005. Effects of a tai-chi program on pain, sleep disturbance, mood and fatigue in rheumtoid arthritis patients. Journal of Rheumatology and Health 12, 57–68 (in Korean).

Lee, M.S., Pittler, M.H., Ernst, E., 2007. Tai chi for rheumatoid arthritis: systematic review. Rheumatology 46, 1648–1651.

Lempp, H., Ibrahim, F., Shaw, T., et al., 2011. Comparative quality of life in patients with depression and rheumatoid arthritis. International Review of Psychiatry 23, 118–124.

Li, C.Y., Imaishi, K., Shiba, N., et al., 2000. Biomechanical evaluation of foot pressure and loading force during gait in rheumatoid arthritic patients with and without foot orthosis. Kurume Medical Journal 47, 211–217.

Liao, K.P., Solomon, D.H., 2013. Traditional cardiovascular risk factors, inflammation and cardiovascular risk in rheumatoid arthritis. Rheumatology 52, 45–52.

Locke, M., Perry, J., Campbell, J., et al., 1984. Ankle and subtalar motion during gait in arthritic patients. Physical Therapy 64, 504–509.

Lopez-Hoyos, M., Ruiz de Alegria, C., Blanco, R., et al., 2004. Clinical utility of anti-CCP antibodies in the differential diagnosis of elderly-onset rheumatoid arthritis and polymyalgia rheumatica. Rheumatology 43, 655–657.

Lorig, K., Ritter, P.L., Plant, K., 2005. A disease-specific self-help program compared with a generalized chronic disease self-help program for arthritis patients. Arthritis and Rheumatism 53, 950–957.

MacSween, A., Brydson, G.J.H., 1999. The effects of custom moulded ethyl vinyl acetate foot orthoses of the gait of patients with rheumatoid arthritis. Foot 9, 128–133.

Maillefert, J.F., Dardel, P., Cherasse, A., et al., 2003. Magnetic resonance imaging in the assessment of synovial inflammation of the hindfoot in patients with rheumatoid arthritis and other polyarthritis. European Journal of Radiology 47, 1–5.

March, L., Lapsley, H., 2001. What are the costs to society and the potential benefits from the effective management of early rheumatoid arthritis? Best Practice and Research in Clinical Rheumatology 15, 171–185.

McDonough, A.L., Batavia, M., Chen, F.C., et al., 2001. The validity and reliability of the GAITRite system's measurements: A preliminary evaluation. Archives of Physical Medicine and Rehabilitation 82, 419–425.

Mejjad, O., Vittecoq, O., Pouplin, S., et al., 2004. Foot orthotics decrease pain but do not improve gait in rheumatoid arthritis patients. Joint, Bone, Spine: Revue Du Rhumatisme 71, 542–545.

Michelson, J., Easley, M., Wigley, F.M., et al., 1994. Foot and ankle problems in rheumatoid arthritis. Foot and Ankle International 15, 608–613.

Miller, A., Green, M., Robinson, D., 1983. Simple rule for calculating normal erythrocyte sedimentation rate. British Medical Journal 286, 266.

Mitchell, D.M., Spitz, P.W., Young, D.Y., et al., 1986. Survival, prognosis and causes of death in rheumatoid arthritis. Arthritis and Rheumatism 29, 706–714.

Mottonen, T., Hannonen, P., Leirisalo-Repo, M., et al., 1999. Comparison of combination therapy with single-drug therapy in early rheumatoid arthritis: a randomised trial. FIN-RACo trial group. Lancet 353, 1568–1573.

Nell, V.P., Machold, K.P., Eberl, G., et al., 2004. Benefit of very early referral and very early therapy with disease-modifying anti-rheumatic drugs in patients with early rheumatoid arthritis. Rheumatology 43, 906–914.

NICE, 2009. Guidance for the management of rheumatoid arthritis in adults. Online. Available: <www.nice.org.uk/nicemedia/pdf/CG79NICEGuideline.pdf>.

Nikolaisen, C., Rekvig, O.P., Nossent, H.C., 2007. Diagnostic impact of contemporary biomarker assays for rheumatoid arthritis. Scandinavian Journal of Rheumatology 36, 97–100.

Oliver, J.E., Silman, A.J., 2006. Risk factors for the development of rheumatoid arthritis. Scandinavian Journal of Rheumatology 35, 169–174.

Otter, S.J., Young, A., Cryer, J.R., 2004. Biologic agents used to treat rheumatoid arthritis and their relevance to podiatrists: a practice update. Musculoskeletal Care 2, 51–59.

Otter, S.J., Lucas, K., Springett, K., et al., 2010. Foot pain in rheumatoid arthritis prevalence, risk factors and management: an epidemiological study. Clinical Rheumatology 29, 255–271.

Otter, S.J., Lucas, K., Springett, K., et al., 2012. Identifying patient-reported outcomes in rheumatoid arthritis: the impact of foot symptoms on self-perceived quality of life. Musculoskeletal Care 10, 65–75.

Palkonyai, E., Kolarz, G., Kopp, M., et al., 2007. Depressive symptoms in early rheumatoid arthritis: a comparative longitudinal study. Clinical Rheumatology 26, 753–758.

Pallari, J.H., Dalgarno, K.W., Woodburn, J., 2010. Mass customization of foot orthoses for rheumatoid arthritis using selective laser sintering. IEEE Transactions in Biomedical Engineering 57, 1750–1756.

Platto, M.J., O'Connell, P.G., Hicks, J.E., et al., 1991. The relationship of pain and deformity of the rheumatoid foot to gait and an index of functional ambulation. Journal of Rheumatology 18, 38–43.

PRCA, 2008. Standards of care for people with musculoskeletal foot health problems. Online. Available: <www.prcassoc.org.uk/standards-project>.

Priolo, F., Bacarini, L., Cammisa, M., et al., 1997. Radiographic changes in the feet of patients with early rheumatoid arthritis. GRISAR (Gruppo Reumatologi Italiani Studio Artrite Reumatoide). Journal of Rheumatology 24, 2113–2118.

Quinn, M.A., Conaghan, P.G., Emery, P., 2001. The therapeutic approach of early intervention for rheumatoid arthritis: what is the evidence? Rheumatology 40, 1211–1220.

Quinn, M.A., Gough, A.K., Green, M.J., et al., 2006. Anti-CCP antibodies measured at disease onset help identify seronegative rheumatoid arthritis and predict radiological and functional outcome. Rheumatology 45, 478–480.

Raptopoulou, A., Sidiropoulos, P., Katsouraki, M., et al., 2007. Anti-citrulline antibodies in the diagnosis and prognosis of rheumatoid arthritis: evolving concepts. Critical Reviews in Clinical and Laboratory Sciences 44, 339–363.

Rat, A.C., Boissier, M.C., 2004. Rheumatoid arthritis: direct and indirect costs. Joint, Bone, Spine: Revue Du Rhumatisme 71, 518–524.

Ravindran, V., Rachapalli, S., 2011. An overview of commonly used radiographic scoring methods in rheumatoid arthritis clinical trials. Clinical Rheumatology 30, 1–6.

Riskowski, J.L., Hagedorn, T.J., Hannan, M.T., 2011. Measures of foot function, foot health, and foot pain: American Academy of Orthopedic Surgeons Lower Limb Outcomes Assessment: Foot and Ankle Module (AAOS-FAM), Bristol Foot Score (BFS), Revised Foot Function Index (FFI-R), Foot Health Status Questionnaire (FHSQ), Manchester Foot Pain and Disability Index (MFPDI), Podiatric Health Questionnaire (PHQ), and Rowan Foot Pain Assessment (ROFPAQ). Arthritis Care and Research 63 (S11), S229–S239.

Ritchie, D.M., Boyle, J.A., McInnes, J.M., et al., 1968. Clinical studies with an articular index for the assessment of joint tenderness in patients with rheumatoid arthritis. Quarterly Journal of Medicine 37, 393–406.

Rosenbaum, D., Schmiegel, A., Meermeier, M., et al., 2006. Plantar sensitivity, foot loading and walking pain in rheumatoid arthritis. Rheumatology 45, 212–214.

Scott, D.L., Wolfe, F., 2010. Rheumatoid arthritis. Lancet 25, 1094–1108.

Shi, K., Tomita, T., Hayashida, K., et al., 2000. Foot deformities in rheumatoid arthritis and relevance of disease severity. Journal of Rheumatology 27, 84–89.

Siddle, H.J., Hodgson, R.J., Redmond, A.C., et al., 2012a. MRI identifies plantar plate pathology in the forefoot of patients with rheumatoid arthritis. Clinical Rheumatology 31, 621–629.

Siddle, H.J., Hodgson, R.J., O'Connor, P., et al., 2012b. Magnetic resonance arthrography of lesser metatarsophalangeal joints in patients with rheumatoid arthritis: relationship to clinical, biomechanical, and radiographic variables. Journal of Rheumatology 39, 1786–1791.

Siddle, H.J., Redmond, A.C., Waxman, R., et al., 2013. Debridement of painful forefoot plantar callosities in rheumatoid arthritis: the CARROT randomised controlled trial. Clinical Rheumatology 32 (5), 567–574.

Sierakowski, S., Cutolo, M., 2011. Morning symptoms in rheumatoid arthritis: a defining characteristic and marker of active disease. Scandinavian Journal of Rheumatology 125, 1–5.

Silva, K.N., Mizusaki Imoto, A., Almeida, G.J., et al., 2010. Balance training (proprioceptive training) for patients with rheumatoid arthritis. Cochrane Database Systemic Reviews (5), CD007648.

Söderlin, M.K., Bergsten, U., Svensson, B., et al., 2011. Patient-reported events preceding the onset of rheumatoid arthritis: possible clues to aetiology. Musculoskeletal Care 9, 25–31.

Spiegel, T.M., Spiegel, J.S., 1982. Rheumatoid arthritis in the foot and ankle – diagnosis, pathology, and treatment. The relationship between foot and ankle deformity and disease duration in 50 patients. Foot and Ankle 2, 318–324.

Studenic, P., Radner, H., Smolen, J.S., et al., 2012. Discrepancies between patients and physicians in their perceptions of rheumatoid arthritis disease activity. Arthritis and Rheumatism 64, 2814–2823.

Sugiyama, D., Nishimura, K., Tamaki, K., et al., 2010. Impact of smoking as a risk factor for developing rheumatoid arthritis: a meta-analysis of observational studies. Annals of the Rheumatic Diseases 69, 70–81.

Symmons, D., 2002. Epidemiology of rheumatoid arthritis: determinants of onset, persistence and outcome. Best Practice and Research in Clinical Rheumatology 16, 707–722.

Symmons, D., 2005. Looking back: rheumatoid arthritis – aetiology, occurrence and mortality. Rheumatology 44, iv14–iv17.

Taylor, P., Gartemann, J., Hsieh, J., et al., 2011. A systematic review of serum biomarkers anti-cyclic citrullinated peptide and rheumatoid factor as tests for rheumatoid arthritis. Autoimmune Disease 2011, 815038.

Telfer, S., Woodburn, J., 2010. The use of 3D surface scanning for the measurement and assessment of the human foot. Journal of Foot and Ankle Research 3, 19.

Treharne, G.J., Douglas, K.M., Iwaszko, J., et al., 2007. Polypharmacy among people with rheumatoid arthritis: the role of age, disease duration and comorbidity. Musculoskeletal Care 5, 175–190.

Trelle, S., Reichenbach, S., Wandel, S., et al., 2011. Cardiovascular safety of non-steroidal anti-inflammatory drugs: network meta-analysis. British Medical Journal 11, 342.

Trescot, A.M., Helm, S., Hansen, H., et al., 2008. Opioids in the management of chronic non-cancer pain: an update of American Society of the Interventional Pain Physicians' (ASIPP) Guidelines. Pain Physician 11, S5–S62.

Turner, D.E., Helliwell, P.S., Emery, P., et al., 2006. The impact of rheumatoid arthritis on foot function in the early stages of disease: a clinical case series. BMC Musculoskeletal Disorders 7, 102.

Turner, D.E., Helliwell, P.S., Woodburn, J., 2007. Methodological considerations for a randomised controlled trial of podiatry care in rheumatoid arthritis: lessons from an exploratory trial. BMC Musculoskeletal Disorders 8, 109.

Turner, D.E., Woodburn, J., 2008. Characterising the clinical and biomechanical features of severely deformed feet in rheumatoid arthritis. Gait and Posture 28, 574–580.

Turner, D.E., Woodburn, J., Helliwell, P.S., et al., 2003. Pes planovalgus in RA: a descriptive and analytical study of foot function determined by gait analysis. Musculoskeletal Care 1, 21–33.

Upchurch, K.S., Kay, J., 2012. Evolution of treatment for rheumatoid arthritis. Rheumatology 51 (vi), 28–36.

van Aken, J., Lard, L.R., le Cessie, S., et al., 2004. Radiological outcome after four years of early versus delayed treatment strategy in patients with recent onset rheumatoid arthritis. Annals of the Rheumatic Diseases 63, 274–279.

van der Heijde, D., 1999. How to read radiographs according to the Sharp/van der Heijde method. Journal of Rheumatology 26, 743–745.

van der Heijde, D.M., van 't Hof, M.A., van Riel, P.L., et al., 1990. Judging disease activity in clinical practice in rheumatoid arthritis: first step in the development of a disease activity score. Annals of the Rheumatic Diseases 49, 916–920.

van der Leeden, M., Steultjens, M., Dekker, J.H., et al., 2006. Forefoot joint damage, pain and disability in rheumatoid arthritis patients with foot complaints: the role of plantar pressure and gait characteristics. Rheumatology 45, 465–469.

van der Leeden, M., Steultjens, M.P., Ursum, J., et al., 2008. Prevalence and course of forefoot impairments and walking disability in the first eight years of rheumatoid arthritis. Arthritis and Rheumatism 59, 1596–1602.

van Gestel, A.M., Prevoo, M.L., van 't Hof, M.A., et al., 1996. Development and validation of the European League Against Rheumatism response criteria for rheumatoid arthritis. Comparison with the preliminary American College of Rheumatology and the World Health Organization/International League Against Rheumatism Criteria. Arthritis and Rheumatism 39, 34–40.

Verstappen, S., Jacobs, J., van der Veen, M., et al., 2007. Intensive treatment with methotrexate in early rheumatoid arthritis: aiming for remission. Computer Assisted Management in Early Rheumatoid Arthritis (CAMERA, an open-label strategy trial). Annals of the Rheumatic Diseases 66, 1443–1449.

Vliet Vlieland, T.P., van den Ende, C.H., 2011. Non-pharmacological treatment of rheumatoid arthritis. Current Opinion in Rheumatology 23 (3), 259–264.

Wakefield, R.J., Gibbon, W.W., Emery, P., 1999. The current status of ultrasonography in rheumatology. Rheumatology 38, 195–198.

Walmsley, S., Williams, A.E., Ravey, M., et al., 2010. The rheumatoid foot: a systematic literature review of patient-reported outcome measures. Journal of Foot and Ankle Research 3, 12.

Walmsley, S., Ravey, M., Graham, A., et al., 2012. Development of a patient-reported outcome measure for the foot affected by rheumatoid arthritis. Journal of Clinical Epidemiology 65, 413–422.

Wang, C., Roubenoff, R., Lau, J., et al., 2005. Effect of Tai Chi in adults with rheumatoid arthritis. Rheumatology 44, 685–687.

Wetteland, P., Røger, M., Solberg, H.E., et al., 1996. Population-based erythrocyte sedimentation rates in 3910 subjectively healthy Norwegian adults. A statistical study based on men and women from the Oslo area. Journal of Internal Medicine 240, 125–131.

Whalley, D., McKenna, S.P., de Jong, Z., et al., 1997. Quality of life in rheumatoid arthritis. British Journal of Rheumatology 36, 884–888.

Wickman, A.M., Pinzur, M.S., Kadanoff, R., et al., 2004. Health-related quality of life for patients with rheumatoid arthritis foot involvement. Foot and Ankle International 25, 19–26.

Williams, A.E., Nester, C.J., 2006. Patient perceptions of stock footwear design features. Prosthetics and Orthotics International 30, 61–71.

Williams, A.E., Graham, A.S., 2012. 'My feet: visible, but ignored …' A qualitative study of foot care for people with rheumatoid arthritis. Clinical Rehabilitation 26, 952–959.

Williams, A.E., Rome, K., Nester, C.J., 2007a. A clinical trial of specialist footwear for patients with rheumatoid arthritis. Rheumatology 46, 302–307.

Williams, A.E., Nester, C.J., Ravey, M.I., 2007b. Rheumatoid arthritis patients' experiences of wearing therapeutic footwear – a qualitative investigation. BMC Musculoskeletal Disorders 8, 104.

Williams, A.E., Nester, C.J., Ravey, M.I., et al., 2010. Women's experiences of wearing therapeutic footwear in three European countries. Journal of Foot and Ankle Research 3, 23.

Williams, A.E., Davies, S., Graham, A., et al., 2011. Guidelines for the management of the foot health problems associated with rheumatoid arthritis. Musculoskeletal Care 9, 86–92.

Wilske, K.R., 1993. Inverting the therapeutic pyramid: observations and recommendations on new directions in rheumatoid arthritis therapy based on the author's experience. Seminars in Arthritis and Rheumatism 23, 11–18.

Wolfe, F., Michaud, K., 2007. Assessment of pain in rheumatoid arthritis: minimal clinically significant difference, predictors, and the effect of anti-tumor necrosis factor therapy. Journal of Rheumatology 34, 1674–1683.

Woodburn, J., Turner, D.E., Helliwell, P.S., et al., 1999. A preliminary study determining the feasibility of electromagnetic tracking for kinematics at the ankle joint complex. Rheumatology 38, 1260–1268.

Woodburn, J., Helliwell, P.S., Barker, S., 2002a. Three-dimensional kinematics at the ankle joint complex in rheumatoid arthritis patients with painful valgus deformity of the rearfoot. Rheumatology 41, 1406–1412.

Woodburn, J., Barker, S., Helliwell, P.S., 2002b. A randomized controlled trial of foot orthoses in rheumatoid arthritis. Journal of Rheumatology 29, 1377–1383.

Woodburn, J., Hennessy, K., Steultjens, M.P., et al., 2010. Looking through the 'window of opportunity': is there a new paradigm of podiatry care on the horizon in early rheumatoid arthritis? Journal of Foot and Ankle Research 3, 8.

World Health Organization, 2013. International classification of disease-10. Online. Available: <http://www3.who.int/icf/icftemplate.cfm>.

Yazici, Y., Pincus, T., Kautiainen, H., et al., 2004. Morning stiffness in patients with early rheumatoid arthritis is associated more strongly with functional disability than with joint swelling and erythrocyte sedimentation rate. Journal of Rheumatology 31, 1723–1726.

Young, A., Dixey, J., Kulinskaya, E., et al., 2002. Which patients stop working because of rheumatoid arthritis? Results of five years' follow up in 732 patients from the early rheumatoid Arthritis Study (ERAS). Annals of the Rheumatic Diseases 61, 335–340.

Chapter 3

Gout

Keith Rome and Mike Frecklington

Chapter Outline

INTRODUCTION

Gout, the most common form of inflammatory arthritis, has significant functional, social and financial impacts (Brook et al. 2010; Lindsay et al. 2011). Gout is a disorder that manifests itself as a spectrum of clinical and pathological features built on a foundation of an excess body burden of uric acid, manifested in part by hyperuricaemia, variably defined as a serum urate level greater than 6.8 or 7.0 mg/dL (Arromdee et al. 2002; Lawrence et al. 2008). Tissue deposition of monosodium urate (MSU) crystals in supersaturated extracellular fluids of the joint, and certain other sites, mediates most of the clinical and pathological features of gout (Khanna et al. 2012a). Typically, the disease initially presents as acute episodic arthritis. Gout also can manifest as chronic arthritis of one or more joints (Arromdee et al. 2002; Lawrence et al. 2008). Tophi, mainly found in articular, periarticular, bursal, bone, auricular, and cutaneous tissues, are a pathognomonic feature of gout (Khanna et al. 2012b).

Traditionally, the onset of gout is reported to occur during the fourth to sixth decades of life (Grahame and Scott 1970). The incidence of gout is increasing throughout the world and it is now the most common form of inflammatory arthritis affecting men (Annemans et al. 2008). Singh (2013) reported that women are protected against gout in the premenopausal period by the uricosuric effect of female sex hormones. Men outnumber women in all age groups for gout prevalence, more in the younger than older age groups by a ratio of $5:1$ to $10:1$.

The overall prevalence of gout in the US has risen over the last 20 years and it now affects 8.3 million (3.9%) American adults (Zhu et al. 2011). In New Zealand, rates of gout have also increased, with the most recent prevalence estimates of 3.2% for European adults, 6.1% for Māori adults and 7.6% for

Pacific Island adults (Winnard et al. 2012). In Australia, there has been a significant rise in the prevalence amongst the Australian Aboriginal population from 0% in 1965 to 9.7% in males and 2.9% in females in 2002 (Robinson et al. 2012). Robinson et al. (2012) also reported more than 1 in 6 elderly male Australians suffer from gout. The reasons behind an increase in the incidence and prevalence of gout are probably multifactorial, potentially related to increasing longevity, rising rates of obesity and the metabolic syndrome, as well as shifts in dietary habits and lifestyle (Richette and Bardin 2010; Richette et al. 2013).

PREVALENCE

Despite numerous studies reporting the predilection of gout in the foot, due to the variations in diagnostic criteria and study designs a comparison of the figures reported in the foot is difficult. The earliest study examining the epidemiological features of gout in the foot was a large prospective study of 760 New Zealand Māoris between 1962 and 1963 (Prior and Davidson 1966). These authors found that the prevalence of gout in the first metatarsophalangeal joint (MTPJ) was 8.8% in males and 0.8% in females. A sample from this study was followed up by Bauer and Prior (1978), who examined 531 participants who did not suffer from gout at baseline. Upon reassessment 11 years later, the incidence of gout affecting the foot was reported to be 10.3% and 4.3% in males and females respectively. Subsequent studies provide evidence that the first MTPJ is most often affected, varying between 23 and 76% (Bauer and Prior, 1978; Grahame and Scott, 1970; Puig et al. 2008; Wright et al. 2007). These data also suggest that, since the original work by Prior and Davidson (1966), the prevalence of gout in the foot has increased.

Previous studies have identified the involvement of other joints in the foot, although the data presented across studies has not always provided numbers for specific locations. For instance, Grahame and Scott (1970) noted that 50% had involvement of other foot structures including the ankle joint. Of note, Rubin et al. (2004) reported the ankle joint to be affected in 25% of cases and the proximal interphalangeal joint of the hallux in 11%. Some studies have identified the presence of tophi in the foot. Puig et al. (2008)

reported that men with tophi had 90% located in the foot compared with 40% in females. A more recent study by Kumar and Gow (2002) of 45 patients who underwent surgery for gout-related tophi reported an 18% involvement in the foot. Other foot structures affected by gout include sesamoid bones, the talus, talonavicular and ankle joints (Dalbeth et al. 2011a, 2013). Some individuals also have tophus deposits within their tendons, and there have also been cases of tendon rupture secondary to gout in the peroneal and tibialis anterior tendons reported (Jerome et al. 2008; Lagoutaris et al. 2005).

PATHOGENESIS

Mechanisms of Crystal Formation and Inflammation

In approximately 25% of those whose serum uric acid concentration exceeds its solubility (around 6.8 mg/dL, or 0.36 mmol/L), MSU crystallizes and precipitation in joints and soft tissues increases (Choi et al. 2005). MSU crystals are pro-inflammatory stimuli that can initiate, amplify and sustain an intense inflammatory response (Choi et al. 2005), seen clinically as an acute flare (Doherty 2009). However, deposited MSU crystals within cartilage and fibrous tissue are relatively protected from contact with inflammatory mediators, which explains why patients with known MSU deposits can remain clinically quiescent for years (Busso and So 2010). When crystals are shed into joint space or bursae they are quickly phagocytized by monocytes and macrophages (Schiltz et al. 2002), which activate the NALP3 inflammasome and trigger the release of interleukin-1 and other cytokines and consequently the infiltration of neutrophils (Martinon et al. 2006). The state of phagocyte differentiation determines whether the MSU crystals will trigger this inflammatory response (Yagnik et al. 2004). While monocytes are involved in stimulating such a response, differentiated macrophages have been shown to inhibit leukocyte and endothelial activation and play a central role in terminating an acute flare (Ortiz-Bravo et al. 1993). Persistent accumulation of large numbers of MSU crystals can cause pressure erosion on cartilage and bone and low-grade inflammation, seen clinically as features of chronic tophaceous gout (Dalbeth and Haskard 2005). MSU crystals have been shown to reduce the osteoblastic activity of bone, resulting in poor resolution of erosions (Bouchard et al. 2002). Even during intercritical periods, low-grade inflammation persists owing to the ongoing intra-articular phagocytosis of MSU crystals by leukocytes (Pascual et al. 1999).

Natural History

The natural history of gout is composed of four phases: asymptomatic hyperuricaemia, episodes of acute attacks of gout, interspersed with asymptomatic intercritical periods, and then a chronic phase that involves structural changes to joints and tissues (Teng et al. 2006). The time course for disease progression from asymptomatic hyperuricaemia to chronic gout varies widely from 3 to 42 years (mean 11.6 years) and is correlated with the severity and duration of hyperuricaemia (Harris et al. 1999). Figure 3-1 illustrates the four phases of gout.

Asymptomatic   Hyperuricaemia. Asymptomatic hyperuricaemia is defined as an abnormally high serum urate concentration exceeding 0.36 mmol/L in the absence of any clinical symptoms (Harris et al. 1999). The prevalence of hyperuricaemia is higher than the prevalence of gout, with an estimated prevalence of 21.4% in the US population (Zhu et al. 2011). Reflecting the gender differences in gout, hyperuricaemia is more prevalent in males, with an estimated 21.6% prevalence compared with 8.6% in females in China (Liu et al. 2011). A slightly higher prevalence

has been reported in developing countries (in males 35.1% and in women 8.7%) (Conen et al. 2004).

Acute Gout. The biochemical basis of gout is oversaturation of urate levels in the extracellular fluids, which results in precipitation of urate crystals in extra-articular tissues (Khanna et al. 2011). Acute gout is characterized by a sudden onset of severe pain, often during the night, waking the patient from sleep (Doherty 2009). This pain reaches its maximum in 6 to 24 hours and without treatment usually resolves in 7–10 days (Teng et al. 2006). The pain is accompanied by erythema, swelling, and limited motion of the affected joint. Inflammation of the peri-articular tissue is also evident and concurrent systemic features, although rare, may be present (Teng et al. 2006). As the inflammatory process begins to subside, extensive exfoliation of skin overlying the affected joint may occur (Richette and Bardin 2010). Although 90% of first attacks are monoarticular, oligoarticular and poly-articular involvement can occur in elderly patients (De Leonardis et al. 2007). Joints in the lower limb and feet, especially the first MTPJ, are the most commonly involved in an initial flare (Richette and Bardin 2010). Acute attacks of the ankle, midfoot, knee, wrist, fingers, and elbow can also occur, as well as periarticular structures including bursae and tendons (Teng et al. 2006). Compared with patients with serum urate of <6 mg/dL, the odds ratio for a gout flare is 1.33 for a serum urate level of 6–7 mg/dL and 2.15

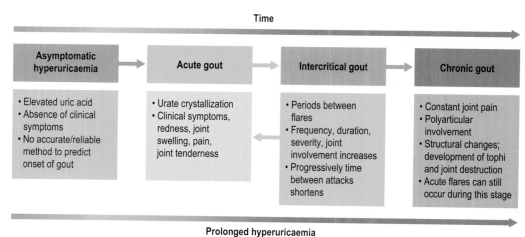

FIGURE 3-1 The four phases of gout.

for a serum urate level > 9 mg/dL (Annemans et al. 2008).

Intercritical Gout. Intercritical gout is characterized by asymptomatic periods after or between an acute flare, during which there are minimal symptoms (Brook et al. 2010). Emphasis is placed on a management programme and includes pharmacological interventions, as well as dietary and lifestyle changes, to reduce the risk of recurrent flare attacks (Hoskison and Wortmann 2006).

Chronic Gout. Chronic gout is characterized by more frequent flares with destructive polyarticular involvement, and persistent pain (Teng et al. 2006). Twelve percent of patients will develop chronic tophaceous gout after 5 years of untreated disease, and 55% after 20 years, owing to deposits of aggregated MSU crystals (Wallace and Singer 1988). Tophi comprise the characteristic needle-shaped MSU crystals surrounded by chronic mononuclear and giant cell reactions. They can form anywhere in the body and typically progress insidiously, but the rate of formation correlates with the degree and duration of hyperuricaemia (Gutman 1973). Tophi are frequently seen around the knees, over the olecranon process at the elbow, the Achilles tendon, and within and around the toe and finger joints – particularly over osteoarthritic Herbeden's or Bouchard's nodes (De Souza et al. 2005). They can also form intradermally, appearing as white or yellowish deposits beneath taut overlying skin (Chopra and Grossman 2002). Skin overlying tophi may ulcerate and extrude white, chalky material and may become infected (Harris et al. 1999). Although tophi are asymptomatic and acute symptoms during flares may be adequately controlled, tophaceous gout results in prominent joint damage and musculoskeletal disability (Alvarez-Nemegyei et al. 2005), causing functional impairment and reduced health-related quality of life (Alvarez-Hernandez et al. 2008; Dalbeth et al. 2007; Roddy et al. 2007b; Schumacher et al. 2007).

PREDISPOSING FACTORS

Co-morbidities

Increasing longevity, increasing prevalence of co-morbidities, the use of certain prescription medications, and changing dietary and lifestyle trends all have been shown to elevate risk for the development of gout (Brook et al. 2010). In a recent study conducted in the USA among individuals with gout, 74% (6.1 million) had hypertension, 71% (5.5 million) had chronic kidney disease stage ≥ 2, 53% (4.3 million) were obese, 26% (2.1 million) had diabetes, 24% (2.0 million) had nephrolithiasis, 14% (1.2 million) had myocardial infarction, 11% (0.9 million) had heart failure, and 10% (0.9 million) had suffered a stroke (Zhu et al. 2012). The authors also reported that, with increasing levels of hyperuricaemia, there were graded increases in the prevalence of the co-morbidities. In the top category (serum urate ≥ 10 mg/dL), 86% of subjects had chronic kidney disease stage ≥ 2, 66% had hypertension, 65% were obese, 33% had heart failure, 33% had diabetes, 23% had myocardial infarction, and 12% had stroke. The prevalence figures were 3–33 times higher than those in the lowest serum urate category (< 4 mg/dL). Sex-specific odds ratios tended to be larger among women than men, and the overall co-morbidity prevalence was highest among individuals with both gout and hyperuricaemia. A recent study from New Zealand reports similar findings with a high co-prevalence of gout, diabetes and cardiovascular disease (CVD) in the adult population (Winnard et al. 2013). The authors reported that one in three of the Māori, Pacific and Asian ethnic groups with gout were identified as having diabetes, with 40% of the population with gout identified as having diabetes and/or CVD, and nearly one in ten having all three conditions. Notably, women with gout had a higher co-prevalence of diabetes and/or CVD (50%) than males (Winnard et al. 2013).

Gout is a metabolic disorder associated with cardiovascular–metabolic sequelae (Choi 2010; Choi et al. 2008). Becker et al. (2009) reported that 87% of gout patients had other conditions (metabolic or cardiovascular) and 75% had more than one coexisting condition. Serum uric acid concentrations are strongly correlated with abdominal adiposity, and have been shown to predict the development of type 2 diabetes, hypertension, CVD, and renal failure (Suppiah et al. 2008). Patients with gout have high rates of metabolic syndrome and type 2 diabetes compared to individuals without gout (Liu et al. 2012). The association with the metabolic syndrome is also more common in gout compared with other forms of arthritis (Brook et al. 2010).

Lifestyle Factors

Large-scale studies have provided evidence for a number of long-suspected relations between lifestyle factors, hyperuricaemia, and gout (Choi 2010). Choi (2010) reported that increasing intake of fructose- and sugar-sweetened soft drinks was associated with increasing risk of gout. The risk was significantly increased with an intake level of 5–6 servings a week and the risk rose with increasing intake. The risk of incident gout was 85% higher among men who consumed two or more servings of sugar-sweetened soft drinks daily compared with those who consumed less than one serving monthly. In contrast, diet soft drinks were not associated with the risk of incident gout. These studies confirmed some of the long-purported dietary risk factors including meat, seafood and liquor (Choi 2010). Other putative risk factors, such as protein and purine-rich vegetables were exonerated, and a potential protective effect of dairy products, coffee and vitamin C supplements has been identified (Choi et al. 2007, 2009; Dalbeth et al. 2012a). Subsequently, several novel factors that had not been included in traditional lifestyle recommendations have been identified, including fructose- and sugar-sweetened soft drinks (Choi et al. 2007, 2009b).

Gout and Osteoarthritis

The correlation between gout and osteoarthritis (OA) has been reported in a number of studies (Roddy et al. 2007a, 2008, 2012; Muehleman et al. 2008). Roddy et al. (2007a) found a significant association between acute attacks and the presence of OA at the first MTPJ (aOR 2.06) and the midfoot (aOR 2.85). Muehleman et al. (2008) reported a strong relationship between MSU crystal deposition and cartilage degeneration in the talus, with 92% of patients with crystal involvement displaying degenerative changes in articular cartilage.

In a recent editorial by Roddy and Doherty (2012), the authors explored the reasons that the first MTPJ is often affected by gout. Simkin (1977) demonstrated that synovium is more permeable to water than urate, postulating that a synovial effusion develops in the osteoarthritic first MTPJ during the day and that, as this resolves when the joint is rested overnight, water leaves the joint more rapidly than urate leading to a localized increase in intra-articular urate concentration and predisposition to nucleation and precipitation of MSU crystals. Roddy and Doherty (2012) stated that this theory potentially explains the clinical observation that attacks of gout commonly occur overnight and following physical trauma. Roddy and Doherty (2012) also postulated that OA results in changes in tissue factors, either an increase in promoters or a reduction in inhibitors of crystal nucleation and growth, which predisposes to MSU crystal deposition. However, recent developments in understanding the mechanisms of crystal-induced inflammation have focused on MSU crystal-initiated joint damage (Dalbeth and So 2010).

Genetics

Common primary gout in men often shows a strong familial predisposition, although the genetic basis remains unknown (Doherty 2009). Twin studies have shown high heritability for both uric acid renal clearance (60%) and uric acid : creatinine ratio (87%) and several susceptibility loci for this have been reported (Roddy et al. 2007c). Genetic mutations in genes encoding for renal urate transporters may potentially be associated with poor uric acid excretion efficiency (Smith et al. 2011). Renal urate transport consists of glomerular filtration, near-complete reabsorption, secretion, and post-secretory reabsorption (Choi et al. 2005). The balance between urate reabsorption and secretion is critically linked to net uric acid elimination in the urine. Certain polymorphisms of genes encoding for renal urate transporters in proximal tubule epithelial cells may lead to reduced renal urate excretion and subsequent hyperuricaemia. Dehghan et al. (2008) reported that mutations identified in the following genes encoding for transporter proteins may potentially increase the risk of developing gout: SLC22A12 encoding for URAT-1 (regulates urate reabsorption at the apical membrane); ABCG2 and SLC17A3 (mediate urate secretion at the apical membrane); and SLC2A9 (leads to urate reabsorption into the circulation, and possibly into proximal tubule cells, at the basolateral membrane).

DIAGNOSIS AND CLASSIFICATION

A diagnosis of gout can be made by the identification of MSU crystals in synovial fluid or tophus aspirates (Pascual and Doherty 2009; Zhang et al. 2006b). Synovial aspirates are typically taken from inflamed joints but can also be present in uninflamed joints during intercritical periods even if those joints have never experienced an acute flare (Pascual and Doherty 2009). Although MSU crystals are easily observed using ordinary light microscopy, they are best seen under compensated polarized light microscopy (Wortmann 2002). MSU crystals are large (10–20 μm) long, needle-shaped crystals, showing strong light intensity and a negative sign of birefringence meaning the crystals appear yellow when parallel to the microscope compensator and blue when perpendicular (Dieppe and Swan 1999; Schumacher 1996). In many cases synovial fluid or tophus aspiration may not be possible (Chen and Schumacher 2008). Practitioner inexperience, time constraints during clinical visits, inaccessibility or inconvenience of compensated polarized light microscopy are among the reasons. Occasionally, joints are inaccessible or detectable joint effusions or visible tophaceous deposits are absent. In addition, some patients may be unwilling to undergo aspiration. In such cases a presumptive diagnosis based on clinical presentation may be reasonable (Zhang et al. 2006b).

Classification of gout for research purposes is based upon the American College of Rheumatology (ACR) criteria (Box 3-1), of which six are needed to make a diagnosis (Wallace et al. 1977). More recently, Janssens et al. (2010) generated a diagnostic tool that could discriminate patients with gout using scores for the following seven variables that are easily ascertainable in primary care: male sex (2.0), previous patient-reported arthritis attack (2.0), onset within 1 day (0.5), joint redness (1.0), one MTPJ involvement (2.5), hypertension or one or more cardiovascular diseases (angina pectoris, myocardial infarction, heart failure, cerebrovascular accident, transient ischaemic attack, or peripheral vascular diseases) (1.5), and serum uric acid level exceeding 5.88 mg/dL (3.5). A score of 4 or less ruled out gout in almost 100% of patients. Among patients with a score of 8 or higher, gout was confirmed in more than 80%.

The European League against Rheumatism (EULAR) recommendations for the diagnosis of gout confirm that a clinical composite of rapid-onset pain, tenderness, redness and swelling affecting the first MTPJ is an excellent clinical marker for gout, especially in the presence of hyperuricaemia (Box 3-2) (Zhang et al. 2006a). EULAR guidelines indicate that a definitive diagnosis of gout requires identification of MSU crystals (Figure 3-2) (Pelaez-Ballestas et al. 2010).

IMAGING

In addition to laboratory testing, various imaging techniques aid in the diagnosis of gout. Imaging may also

BOX 3-1 ACR CRITERIA FOR GOUT

DIAGNOSTIC CRITERIA
1. More than one attack of acute arthritis
2. Maximum inflammation developed within 1 day
3. Monoarthritis attack
4. Redness observed over joint(s)
5. First metatarsophalangeal joint painful or swollen
6. Unilateral first metatarsophalangeal joint attack
7. Unilateral tarsal joint attack
8. Tophus (proven or suspected)
9. Hyperuricaemia
10. Asymmetric swelling within a joint on X-ray
11. Subcortical cysts without erosion on X-ray
12. Joint fluid culture negative for organisms during attack

BOX 3-2 EULAR RECOMMENDATIONS FOR THE DIAGNOSIS OF GOUT

EULAR multidisciplinary guidelines: 10 key propositions generated by Delphi consensus approach to create a diagnostic ladder in which an increasing number of symptoms suggest an increasing likelihood of accurate diagnosis. Acute gout diagnosis likelihood ratios (LRs) of the individual findings:
- MSU crystal indemnification in joint fluid: >500
- Tophi: 40.0
- Classic podagra: 30.6
- Hyperuricaemia: 9.7
- Subcortical cysts on plain radiographs: <7

Adapted by permission from BMJ Publishing Group Limited. Zhang W, Doherty M, Pascual E, Bardin T, Barskova V, Conaghan P. EULAR evidence based recommendations for gout. Part II: Management. Report of a task force of the EULAR standing committee for international clinical studies including therapeutics (ESCISIT). Ann Rheum Dis 2006; 65:1312–1324.

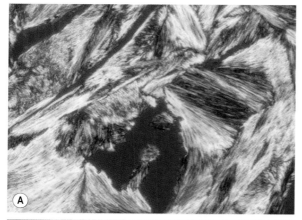

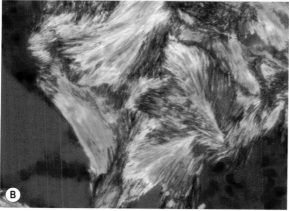

FIGURE 3-2 (A, B) Monosodium urate crystals. (This figure was first published in Pascual E, Martínez A, Ordóñez S, Gout: the mechanism of urate crystal nucleation and growth. A hypothesis based in facts. Joint Bone Spine 80(1);1–4. Copyright ©2013. Published by Elsevier Masson SAS on behalf of the Société Française de Rhumatologie. All rights reserved.)

play a role in assessment of disease complications, guiding joint aspiration, monitoring of disease progression, and understanding the mechanisms of disease (Dalbeth et al. 2012b). Imaging techniques include plain radiography, ultrasonography, conventional computed tomography (CT), dual-energy computed tomography (DECT), and magnetic resonance imaging (MRI) (Dalbeth et al. 2012b).

Radiography

Most often, X-rays do not reveal any abnormalities during the early stages of gout. Tophi can be seen on X-rays before they become apparent on physical examination. Early radiological findings in gout are limited to the soft tissues and involve asymmetrical swelling in the affected joints. In the intercritical stage of disease, gout causes subtle changes in the bony structures and these can be observed on plain-film radiographs. Dalbeth et al. (2012b) reported that plain radiography may not be optimal as the sole assessment tool of structural change in chronic gout as it has lower sensitivity and specificity for bone erosion compared with other advanced imaging methods.

Ultrasound

Although the gold standard for diagnosis of gout remains positive identification of uric acid crystals via arthrocentesis, musculoskeletal ultrasound (MSUS) can aid diagnosis, monitor disease progression and provide insights into pathological changes (Dalbeth and McQueen 2009). Advantages of MSUS include: no radiation, high-resolution, multiplane images, dynamic examinations of joints, good repeatability, relatively low cost in comparison to other advanced imaging techniques, and a patient-friendly procedure (Thiele and Schlesinger 2007). MSUS is able to detect various specific and non-specific pathological features of gout. Non-specific features include those findings that may be common amongst other inflammatory rheumatic conditions such as: joint effusion, synovitis, hypervascularization, bony erosion and proliferative new bone formation (Farrant et al. 2007). Detection of MSU crystals by MSUS allows for non-invasive assessment and a potential method of monitoring disease progression.

Magnetic Resonance Imaging (MRI)

MRI has been used to identify gout in the foot (Carter et al. 2009). There is significantly less research on the performance of MRI in identifying gout, probably because the high cost of MRI scans impedes access for patients (McQueen et al. 2011, 2012).

Computed Tomography (CT)

CT has the potential to play a role in clinical assessment of chronic gout in a number of situations; in assessing complications of gout non-invasive diagnosis of subcutaneous nodules, in identification of deep intra-articular tophi, and in evaluation of bone erosion associated with gout (Fraser et al. 2007; Perez-Ruiz et al. 2009). A recent study has reported excellent correspondence with dual-energy CT for detecting tophi and it may be that this modality has great potential in gout, although it remains expensive and difficult to access for routine clinical management (McQueen et al. 2012).

Dual-energy CT (DECT)

DECT is a recently developed technology that enables excellent visualization of soft-tissue structures, such as tendons and ligaments, and detection of MSU crystal deposits (McQueen et al. 2013). Dalbeth et al. (2013) demonstrated that MSU crystal deposition within tendons is common in patients with long-standing tophaceous gout.

IMPAIRMENTS

In this section we will discuss typical impairments, which include foot pain, joint range of motion, foot and ankle muscle strength in both acute and chronic gout stages. Joint pain and swelling during gout flares may lead to considerable morbidity and disability, having an effect on patient's work productivity and social participation (Dalbeth et al. 2011a).

Patients with gout often speak of pain, dependency and isolation (Lindsay et al. 2011). Gout is regarded as the most painful of all acute arthritic conditions with a rapid onset and build-up of pain, especially at the first MTPJ. Pain during rest and activity as well as pain intensity during and between flares has been reported specifically at the first MTPJ (Rome et al. 2012). Rome et al. (2011a) reported measuring foot pain using the pain domain of the Foot Function Index, which measures pain over the past week (Budiman-Mak et al. 1991). The results found that the patients with chronic gout experienced greater foot pain (mean: 28.2 mm on a 100 mm VAS) compared with controls (mean: 3.8 mm). These findings are similar to studies of other rheumatic diseases such as rheumatoid arthritis (RA) (Turner et al. 2006, 2009). In a subsequent study, Rome et al. (2012) reported on the clinical features of 20 patients with acute flares. Based on a 100 mm VAS foot pain scale, mean pain was 60 mm during a flare, and reduced to 16 mm at a follow-up visit after the flare had resolved, a 73% reduction. These data are in broad agreement with previous studies reporting on the severity of pain during an acute flare and indicate clearly that most patients experience considerable pain (Roddy et al. 2007b; Rubin et al. 2004). The scores further suggest that pain associated with acute flares is at least as great as that experienced by patients with RA (Turner et al. 2006, 2008). Of note, Rome et al. (2012) observed that, at the follow-up visit, pain levels did not return to minimal values, suggesting that foot-related pain may be a constant feature in patients with recurrent flares. This depiction of pain has been reported by Lindsay et al. (2011) in a qualitative study where patients with severe gout described living with constant pain.

There are a limited number of studies relating to foot impairment in gout (Rome et al. 2011a, 2012). Foot impairment has been evaluated using the two sub-scales of the Foot Impact Scale (FIS): foot impairment/footwear restriction (FISIF; range 0–21) and activity limitation/participation restriction (FISAP; range 0–29) (Helliwell et al. 2005). An elevated FISIF or FISAP score indicates greater foot impairment or activity limitation, respectively. Scores of ≤6 are considered mild, 7–13 are considered moderate, and ≥14 are considered severe for the FISIF. Scores of ≤9 are considered mild, 10–19 are considered moderate, and ≥20 are considered severe for the FISAP. A previous study suggested a change score in either the FISIF or FISAP of 3 points to be clinically relevant (Hooper et al. 2012).

Rome et al. (2011a) reported significant differences in foot impairment between 25 chronic gout cases and 25 age-matched controls. The authors demonstrated that over 30% of patients with chronic gout have moderate foot-related impairment and over 30% of patients have severe disability. This degree of foot-related impairment and disability is similar to that observed in patients with early and established RA (Turner et al. 2006, 2009). In a later study, Rome et al. (2012) reported on 20 patients with acute flares. In this study high levels of impairment (mean: 16) using the FIS were found with all patients at the time of an acute flare and a mean score of 9 after the flare had subsided.

Normal function of the first MTPJ plays an important role in efficient gait. Patients with gout have been shown to have significantly reduced peak pressure and pressure time integrals under the hallux compared with healthy individuals (Rome et al. 2011a). The authors postulated that this might be due to an attempt to offload a painful first MTPJ and thus avoid weightbearing at the toe-off phase of gait. However, the direct effect of first MTPJ gout on other biomechanical parameters such as joint range of motion remains unknown. Maccagno et al. (1991) graded range of motion at first MTPJ on a 5-point scale (1=normal, 2=mildly restricted, 3=moderately restricted, 4=severely restricted, and 5=immobilized) when evaluating the efficacy of two NSAIDs in the pharmacological management of acute gout. The results showed that etodolac was more effective than naproxen in increasing range of motion after 4 days.

FUNCTION

The research related to foot function and disability in gout is limited. This is surprising since the first MTPJ is the most affected joint in gout. Martini et al. (2012) reported those patients who experienced symptoms in their lower extremities were unable to put their shoes on or walk with ease and subsequently stayed at home. Rome et al. (2011a) identified slow walking velocity with associated step and stride length reductions in patients with chronic gout. The difference in gait speed between cases and controls may be related to reduced peak plantar pressure under the hallux. The underlying cause for the reduced peak plantar pressure under the hallux is uncertain. Reducing walking speed is a well-recognized compensatory mechanism for pain in the rheumatoid foot (Turner and Woodburn 2008).

Plantar pressures under the hallux have been shown to be higher in patients with OA of the first MTPJ (Zammit et al. 2008). In contrast, Rome et al. (2011a) reported that people with chronic gout alter their gait pattern in an attempt to reduce pain by offloading at the first MTPJ, and thus avoid weight-bearing at the toe-off phase of gait. While speculative, the strategy of gout patients decreasing load at toe-off will involve reduced plantarflexor muscle activity, and such disuse may contribute to weakness in these muscles. Rome et al. (2011a) did not undertake kinematic or kinetic analysis of the lower limb and ankle. Future studies using three-dimensional instrumented gait analysis combined with strength testing would provide a better understanding of the mechanisms associated with dysfunction in these regions.

The Lower Limb Task Questionnaire (LLTQ) focuses solely on physical tasks associated with lower limb function, more specifically the difficulty in completing tasks and the importance of the task (McNair et al. 2007). The results from a case–control trial demonstrated a significant difference in both activity of daily living and recreational sections in individuals with chronic gout. Performing activities like standing, walking, getting up from a chair and walking up and down the stairs were most difficult in patients with gout. Rome et al. (2012) reported significant differences were also found between the activity of daily living and recreational domains of the LLTQ from the time of an acute flare (mean score for daily living: 16; mean score for recreational domain: 4) and at 8-week follow-up visit (mean daily living: 28; mean recreational score: 12 ($p=<0.001$)).

Previous studies on gout have used the Health Assessment Questionnaire Disability Index (HAQ-DI) or the Short Form-36 (SF-36) physical functioning subscale (Alvarez-Hernandez et al. 2008; Singh et al. 2011). Recently, the HAQ-DI was endorsed by the Outcome Measures in Rheumatology (OMERACT) as the measure of choice for assessing disability in patients with chronic gout (Singh et al. 2011). The HAQ-DI contains 20 items measuring physical disabilities over the past week in eight categories of daily living: dressing and grooming, rising, eating, walking, hygiene, reach, grip, and activities (Bruce and Fries 2005). Each domain is scored 0–3, with the sum of all domains divided by 10 to provide a short HAQ-II score ranging from 0 (no difficulty) to 3 (unable to do) on an ordinal scale. This questionnaire has been shown to be a valid measure of musculoskeletal disability in patients with gout (Singh et al. 2011; Taylor et al. 2008; ten Klooster et al. 2011). In these patients the scale has demonstrated high internal consistency ($\alpha=0.93$), good convergent, divergent, and discriminative validity, adequate test–retest reliability (ICC=0.76), and moderate sensitivity to change (effect size=0.62) (ten Klooster et al. 2012). However, high flooring effects have been observed, with approximately 20–42% of the patients reporting no disability (Alvarez-Hernandez et al. 2008; ten Klooster et al. 2011). Van Groen et al. (2010) further reported that disability scores between RA and OA were similar, with mean HAQ-DI scores lower for patients with gout. Furthermore, the HAQ-DI questionnaire assesses general function, and hence tools that focus more specifically on the lower limb and foot would be more suitable in examining foot function.

The short 10-item HAQ-II has been used to examine gout patients (ten Klooster et al. 2011). Rome et al. (2011a) reported significant differences using the HAQ-II in patients with chronic gout (mean: 0.5) and age–sex-matched controls (mean: 0.1). Rome et al. (2012) also reported a significant difference between scores at the time of flare (mean: 1.9) and a follow-up visit after a flare (mean: 0.9). In a study of acute gout, Rome et al. (2012) reported scores of 25/31 and 18/31 using the FIS during an acute flare and subsequent visit following the flare.

QUALITY OF LIFE

Gout is an excruciatingly painful acute arthropathy; also, because of its associations with chronic disease states such as the metabolic syndrome, OA and renal and cardiovascular morbidity, it is often difficult to attribute disability or diminished lifestyle to gout (Becker et al. 2009; Khanna et al. 2008; Singh et al. 2008). This may be an explanation for the relatively sparse literature available around health-related quality of life (HRQoL) in gout patients. Most studies to date have had limitations such as small samples, cross-sectional design and the use of generic instruments (Lee et al. 2009).

Recent data suggest that gout is associated with detrimental effects on HRQoL. Patients with gout have lower scores on the medical outcomes SF-36 in physical and social scales when compared with the US general population (Khanna et al. 2008; Lee et al. 2009; Singh and Strand 2008; Roddy et al. 2007b). In chronic gout, the frequency and severity of episodic flares may have a greater impact on patients' HRQoL. These symptoms, which may affect the patient's emotional, social and physical functioning, result in significant disability. Cross-sectional observational studies have demonstrated a detrimental impact of gout on HRQOL after adjustment for multiple co-morbidities (Lee et al. 2009; Roddy et al. 2007b; Singh and Strand 2008).

In a recent qualitative study, patients with chronic gout indicated that gout had a direct impact on their ability to work, resulting in work absence and reduced productivity (Lindsay et al. 2011). This is consistent with previous quantitative studies. A large study among US employees with all types of gout showed that they had 4.6 more annual absence days than those without gout (Kleinman et al. 2007). In this study, the total number of absence days for employees with gout was 14.4 versus 9.8 days for employees without gout. In a one-year prospective study on work productivity in people with chronic gout, a mean annual work day loss for those under 65 years old was 25.1 days (Edwards et al. 2011). Martini et al. (2012) stated that the unpredictable nature of gout attacks resulted in participants having to take many days off work, because they could not operate machinery, wear the correct uniform (for example, workboots), or were unable to walk. As Māori and Pacific people experienced symptoms at a younger age, their ability to work and maintain employment was often more negatively affected. HRQoL measurements in gout are challenging, as gout is often characterized as an intermittent, progressive chronic disease. Nevertheless, the Special Interest Group for gout outcomes at the OMERACT 10 meeting recognized the importance of HRQoL measurement in gout and included it as a core domain for clinical trials for chronic gout (Singh et al. 2011).

MANAGEMENT STRATEGIES

The recent publication of the ACR guidelines for the management of gout provides a roadmap for clinicians on both non-pharmacological and pharmacological therapeutic approaches to hyperuricaemia as well as the management of acute gout arthritis (Khanna et al. 2012a, 2012b). Harrold et al. (2013) reported that the ACR recommendations encourage providers to educate patients with hyperuricaemia on dietary and lifestyle influences on gout, treatment objectives and the need for co-morbidity management.

PHARMACOLOGICAL STRATEGIES

Xanthine oxidase inhibitor (XOI) therapy with either allopurinol or febuxostat is recommended as the first-line pharmacological urate-lowering therapy (ULT) approach in gout (Khanna et al. 2012a). Serum urate level should be lowered sufficiently to durably improve signs and symptoms of gout, with the target < 6 mg/dL at a minimum, and often < 5 mg/dL. The starting dosage of allopurinol should be no greater than 100 mg/day and less than that in moderate to severe chronic kidney disease, followed by gradual upward titration of the maintenance dose, which can exceed 300 mg daily even in patients with chronic kidney disease.

An acute gouty arthritis attack should be treated with pharmacological therapy, initiated within 24 hours of onset (Khanna et al. 2012b). Established pharmacological ULT should be continued, without interruption, during an acute attack. Non-steroidal anti-inflammatory drugs (NSAIDs), corticosteroids or oral colchicine are appropriate first-line options for treatment of acute gout, and certain combinations can be employed for severe to refractory attacks (Khanna et al. 2012b). Pharmacological anti-inflammatory prophylaxis for all gout patients is recommended when pharmacological urate lowering is initiated, and should be continued if there is any clinical evidence of continuing gout disease activity and/or the serum urate target has not yet been achieved. Oral colchicine is an appropriate first-line gout attack prophylaxis therapy, including with appropriate dose adjustment in chronic kidney disease and for drug interactions, unless there is a lack of tolerance or medical contraindication. Low-dose NSAID therapy is an appropriate choice for first-line gout attack prophylaxis, unless there is a lack of tolerance or medical contraindication.

Khanna et al. (2012b) reported that complementary therapies for acute gout attack, such as topical ice application, are an appropriate adjunctive measure to one or more pharmacological therapies for acute gouty arthritis (Schlesinger 2002). In a small study of 19 patients with acute gout, Schlesinger et al. (2002) investigated the effect of ice in conjunction with other pharmacological interventions on the duration and severity of acute gout flares over a 1-week period. The results indicated a mean decrease in pain of 7.8 cm on a 10 cm VAS for those patients treated with ice therapy compared with 4.4 cm for the control group. While there was a trend for joint circumference and synovial fluid volume to decrease, the results for these variables were non-significant. However, ACR reported

as inappropriate the use of a variety of oral complementary agents for the treatment of an acute attack (cherry juice or extract, salicylate-rich willow bark extract, ginger, flaxseed, charcoal, strawberries, black currants, burdock, sour cream, olive oil, horsetail, pears, or celery root).

PHYSICAL STRATEGIES

Non-pharmacological therapies for gout have not been well documented. Anecdotal reports and pilot studies have been published, but without compelling evidence for efficacy.

Footwear and Foot Orthoses

Footwear has been developed and modified to provide protection from the environment, conform to fashion, assist function, accommodate foot deformities, and treat musculoskeletal injury. Poorly fitting shoes have also been linked to foot pain in RA (Rome et al. 2009; Silvester et al. 2010). To date, no clinical trials have addressed footwear as an intervention for patients with gout.

In a recent study Rome et al. (2011b) reported on cushioning, support, stability and motion control in the footwear of gout patients. Overall, 56% of patients wore good footwear that included walking, athletic and Oxford-type shoes, while 42% of patients were wearing shoes that were defined as 'poor'. Shoes were frequently either too long or too short. A similar finding was also found for shoe width, although shoe depth was deemed to be good in more than 62% of patients. This study also found that 24% of shoes had no fixation. More than 60% of shoes had limited cushioning and only 36% of shoes had heel/forefoot cushioning. Minimal motion control properties were found with 26% wearing shoes that had adequate heel counter stiffness, 50% of shoes had midfoot sole sagittal stability, and 42% had sufficient midfoot sole frontal stability. More than one-half of the patients wore shoes that were more than 12 months old. The factors that patients perceived as important were comfort (98%), fit (90%), support (90%), cost (60%), and weight (63%). Patients reported style (36%) and colour (33%) as being less important. Shoe width and depth did not correlate with foot pain and disability. However, patients with poor footwear reported higher foot-related impairment. Overall, the findings indicated a mismatch between perception of important attributes of a shoe and what they actually wore on a daily basis. Thus, better education to patients about good footwear is needed.

SURGICAL STRATEGIES

Surgery is considered when pharmacological strategies have failed. The treatment of tophaceous gout is aimed at preventing skin ulceration and infection (Kemp et al. 2010). Surgery for tophaceous deposits is palliative and not curative, and the reported indications are to excise the tophaceous mass, to restore or improve function, to alleviate symptomatic discomfort, to improve cosmesis, and to eradicate draining sinuses (Ou et al. 2010). At this time, only single case studies or case series are present in the literature.

Lee et al. (2010) suggested that the minimally invasive approach, to remove the tophus surgically with soft-tissue shaving, has the advantage of decreased risk of wound complications and reduces the possibility that ligaments, nerves and blood vessels might be damaged. Wang et al. (2009) reported upon a case series of 28 male patients with persistent hyperuricaemia and repeated attacks of gout at the first MTPJ. Patients were subdivided into two groups: one group underwent an arthroscopic removal of gouty crystal; patients who declined operative intervention had a pharmacological intervention. The follow-up period was a mean of 3.9 years in the surgical group and 2.4 years in the non-surgical group. After treatment, both groups showed a significant improvement in the number of acute attacks of gouty arthritis and in their functional scores on the American Orthopedic Foot and Ankle Society Ankle–Hindfoot Scale (Kitaoka et al. 1994). On both measures, the results for the surgical group were significantly better than those for the non-surgical group. The authors concluded that arthroscopic removal of gouty crystals from the first MTPJ can reduce the rate of acute repeated attacks of gouty arthritis and increase foot and ankle function. However, in a case series of 45 patients, Kumar and Gow (2002) noted that 53% of the patients experienced delayed wound healing after surgical debridement and that 7% underwent amputation for sepsis, highlighting potential problems associated with a surgical approach.

LIFESTYLE AND EDUCATION STRATEGIES

Although there is good evidence from observational studies of an association between various lifestyle risk factors and gout development, there is a paucity of high-quality evidence from randomized controlled trials to either support or refute the use of lifestyle modifications for improving outcomes in people with chronic gout (Moi et al. 2013). Only one study (120 participants), at moderate risk of bias, was included in the review (Dalbeth et al. 2012a). Patients were randomized to one of three interventions: either skimmed milk powder (SMP) enriched with glycomacropeptide (GMP) and G600, non-enriched SMP or lactose powder, over a 3-month period. The frequency of acute gout attacks, measured as the number of flares per month, decreased in all three groups over the 3-month study period. Following treatment with SMP/GMP/G600 over the 3-month period, greater improvements were also observed in pain and fractional excretion of uric acid, with trends to greater improvement in tender joint count. There were no significant between-group differences in terms of withdrawals due to adverse effects and serious adverse events resulting in hospitalization. Gastrointestinal adverse effects were the most commonly reported.

A recent randomized controlled trial found that a modest dosage of vitamin C for 8 weeks had no clinically significant lowering effects on patients with gout, despite the fact that plasma ascorbate levels increased (Stamp et al. 2013). The authors concluded that the uricosuric effect of modest-dose vitamin C appears to be small in patients with gout, when administered or in combination with allopurinol. Choi et al. (2008) recommended that gout patients should exercise daily and reduce weight. Dessein et al. (2000) stated that many patients with gout are overweight or obese, and weight reduction through gradual calorie restriction and exercise can substantially help lower uric acid levels and the risk of gout attacks. However, there is limited evidence from randomized controlled trials to demonstrate any benefits in gout patients.

General Patient Education

EULAR recommends that the optimum long-term management of gout should include patient education (Roddy et al. 2007d; Zhang et al. 2006a). Zhang et al.

(2006a) reported that there is a strong belief that patient education and information access is an important determinant of outcome, especially in relation to successful lifestyle alteration and adherence to long-term ULT. Rees et al. (2012) reported excellent clinical outcomes in patients who received intensive education and follow-up in a nurse-led gout clinic. Dalbeth (2013) suggested healthcare professionals need to be trained to ensure that patients with gout are adequately maintained with ULT. Rees et al. (2012) also reported that patient education should not only include information on dietary and other triggers of acute gout attacks, but also provide patients with instruction so that they can initiate treatment upon signs and symptoms of an acute gout attack without the need to consult their healthcare practitioner.

Harrold (2013) highlighted a key barrier to gout management for many patients and physicians, which is the perception that gout is an acute condition that requires treatment only during a painful flare. However, in patients with gout and poorly controlled hyperuricaemia, deposition of monosodium urate crystals occurs within the joint even in the absence of clinically apparent inflammation (Pascual et al. 2009). Dalbeth (2013) also reported that a barrier to effective management of gout was the complexity of the condition, with high rates of co-morbidities leading to polypharmacy and drug interactions. Dalbeth (2013) further suggested that primary care strategies should be implemented and include a multidisciplinary team approach, laboratory alerts for patients with hyperuricaemia, clinical pathways developed with the primary care practice, and the development and implementation of software packages to ensure continuous care and monitoring of patients with gout.

Robinson and Schumacher (2013) examined 10 gout information resources for readability qualitative characteristics such as figures and jargon used, and whether they included information on the major points of gout. The authors reported the information content of the resources was high. Jargon use was low and concepts were usually explained. However, important information regarding acute flare prophylaxis during ULT initiation and titration and treating serum uric acid to target was absent from 60% of the patient education resources. There was poor use of key messages at the start. Gout patient resources have a wide range of readability. Thirty percent of resources were above the average reading level of rheumatology outpatients reported in previous studies. Sixty percent of gout patient resources omit education items that could impact on patient adherence and in turn patient outcomes. The authors concluded that further investigations were needed into the literacy levels and education requirements of patients with gout.

In the UK, a recent Green Paper suggested referral to appropriate allied health professionals within the multidisciplinary team should be made, as required, for a baseline assessment, tailored education and information, advice and appropriate intervention – for example, podiatry for assessment of joint function, footwear and orthoses; dietetics for dietary and lifestyle advice; occupational therapy if the patient's work or activities of daily living are affected, and other therapies as required (Arthritis and Musculoskeletal Alliance 2012).

FUTURE DIRECTIONS

In a study of footwear characteristics, the authors concluded that footwear should be considered in the management plan of patients with gout, and future research should be focused on assessing the role of competitively priced footwear with adequate cushioning, motion control and sufficient width at the forefoot (Rome et al. 2012b). A randomized controlled trial to determine whether a specific footwear intervention can reduce foot pain and musculoskeletal disability in patients with gout would be beneficial.

The efficiency of the gait cycle is significantly influenced by the function of muscles and tendons. Yet limited research has addressed how gout can influence muscle and tendon performance. Of particular interest is the Achilles tendon, as its performance can influence the ability to perform maximally and efficiently in walking and sporting activities. The manifestations of chronic gout on the Achilles tendon structure and function, and its impact on the gait cycle, have not been investigated.

At the feet, particularly overlying areas of joint deformity and on weightbearing areas, ulcerated tophaceous gouty lesions increase the level of foot pain, impairment and disability notably (Patel et al. 2010). Data from the UK provide some insight into the presentation patterns of foot ulceration in RA (Firth et al. 2008; Siddle et al. 2012), but the clinical characteristics of wounds in affected gout patients are poorly defined and have been reported only as case reports (Falidas et al. 2011; Kemp et al. 2010; Patel et al. 2010). Future studies could be conducted to describe in depth the wound characteristics of a cohort of chronic gout patients. This will contribute to our understanding of the nature of foot ulceration in gout and the burden to patients and the health service. Furthermore, the data can be used to evaluate the multidisciplinary approach to the assessment, management and treatment of foot ulceration, improve patient outcomes and reduce recurrence rates of ulceration.

Overall, there appears to be a strong need for more research on quality of life issues in gout and for comparisons with other chronic conditions and general populations. As opposed to other rheumatic conditions, very few studies have examined quality of life in gout despite clear indications of its relevance to patients and the community. Furthermore, no validated measure of work disability is yet available for gout studies. Given that measures such as the work instability scale have shown good psychometric properties and additional value in other musculoskeletal conditions, validating and comparing these scales in patients with gout would seem a next logical step (ten Klooster et al. 2012).

Patient education is considered to be a key role for all healthcare professionals in the management of patients with rheumatic disease (Harrold 2013). Patient education has undoubtedly led to improved clinical outcomes; however, no attempts have been made to optimize its content or delivery to maximize benefits within the context of the foot affected by gout. Providing information relating to the purpose and use of clinical interventions, such as foot orthoses and specialist footwear, has the potential to improve patient adherence. However, the most appropriate content and delivery strategies for foot health patient education have not been investigated. Refining these could improve foot health outcomes. Due to the lack of specialist podiatry provision for gout patients, there is a need for foot-related management guidelines, to provide non-specialist podiatrists and other foot health providers with key information for enhancing the management of these individuals.

INVITED COMMENTARY

Gout is now the most common form of inflammatory arthritis. The central cause of gout is deposition of monosodium urate (MSU) crystals, which form in the presence of high tissue concentrations of urate. The host tissue response to these crystals leads to the clinical manifestations of gout, which include recurrent episodes of self-limiting inflammatory arthritis, chronic gouty arthritis, and tophaceous disease.

As outlined by the authors, certain joints of the foot are most frequently affected by gout. Patients typically describe rapid onset of severe joint pain in the first metatarsophalangeal joint, midfoot or ankle. The other cardinal features of inflammation – erythema, swelling and heat – are typically present.

The patient is often immobilized and unable to walk, work, or perform self-care activities. In patients with tophaceous gout, bone erosion is frequently observed in the foot, particularly at the first metatarsophalangeal joint and midfoot. Bone erosion and foot deformities related to large tophi lead to pain, difficulty finding adequate footwear, and chronic discomfort on weightbearing.

Advanced imaging studies, particularly using dual-energy computed tomography, have further emphasized the preferential involvement of certain sites of the foot, particularly the first metatarsophalangeal joint and Achilles tendon. The frequent involvement of the first metatarsophalangeal joint is of particular interest, noting that this site is also frequently affected by osteoarthritis. The predilection of both gout and osteoarthritis for certain sites raises interesting questions about local factors that promote urate deposition and, in turn, lead to the clinical manifestations of gout.

Gout is frequently associated with cardiovascular disease and type 2 diabetes. The presence of gout can further complicate management of these co-morbid conditions, particularly in the context of foot care. Recurrent flares and tophaceous disease in the feet can lead to pain on walking or running, which may restrict the lifestyle management of cardiovascular disease and diabetes. Furthermore, tophi that discharge or lead to abnormal loading can increase the risk of foot ulceration, deformity and infection in people with diabetes and peripheral vascular disease. Training of

Continued on following page

INVITED COMMENTARY (Continued)

healthcare professionals (including nurses, podiatrists, orthotists, physiotherapists and doctors) to recognize gout in the context of these other conditions is important to optimally manage these related conditions and prevent foot ulceration, infection and potentially limb amputation.

The central strategy for effective gout management is long-term urate-lowering therapy to achieve a target serum urate of below 0.36 mmol/L (6 mg/dL). Lower serum urate concentrations may be beneficial in those with tophi and bone erosion. These serum urate targets represent sub-saturation levels, and in the long term lead to dissolution of MSU crystals, suppression of acute gout flares and regression of tophi. Although such urate-lowering therapy has been shown to have clinical benefits on the frequency of gout flares, musculoskeletal disability and tophus size, the impact of long-term serum urate lowering below saturation targets on foot pain and lower limb disability scores has not been reported. Similarly, the impact of such therapy on foot function, including gait parameters, is currently unknown.

Although lifestyle risk factors are thought to play an important role in the development of gout, there are very few clinical trials that have examined the benefits of non-pharmacological interventions for this condition. Studies to date have focused on dietary interventions, with limited benefit. Interventions that specifically target the foot have not been reported to date. The recent findings that poor footwear is associated with foot-related disability in people with gout raise the possibility that footwear interventions may be of benefit to improve foot-related function in this condition. Identification of cost-effective strategies such as footwear or orthotic interventions as an adjunct to pharmacological therapy to reduce foot pain and improve foot function is required for people with gout.

Nicola Dalbeth MBChB, MD, FRACP
Consultant Rheumatologist and Associate Professor,
Department of Medicine, University of Auckland,
Auckland, New Zealand

REFERENCES

Alvarez-Hernandez, E., Pelaez-Ballestas, I., Vazquez-Mellado, J., et al., 2008. Validation of the Health Assessment Questionnaire disability index in patients with gout. Arthritis and Rheumatism 59, 665–669.

Alvarez-Nemegyei, J., Cen-Pisté, J.C., Medina-Escobedo, M., et al., 2005. Factors associated with musculoskeletal disability and chronic renal failure in clinically diagnosed primary gout. Journal of Rheumatology 32, 2189–2191.

Annemans, L., Spaepen, E., Gaskin, M., et al., 2008. Gout in the UK and Germany: prevalence, comorbidities and management in general practice 2000–2005. Annals of the Rheumatic Diseases 67, 960–966.

Arromdee, E., Michet, C.J., Crowson, C.S., et al., 2002. Epidemiology of gout: is the incidence rising? Journal of Rheumatology 29, 2403–2406.

Arthritis and Musculoskeletal Alliance, 2012. Standards of care for people with gout. Online. Available: <http://www.eguidelines.co.uk/eguidelinesmain/guidelines/summaries/musculoskeletal_joints/arma_gout_2012.php#.UpvFTr8wOfQ>.

Bauer, G.W., Prior, I., 1978. A prospective study of gout in New Zealand Maoris. Annals of the Rheumatic Diseases 37, 466–472.

Becker, M.A., Schumacher, H.R., Benjamin, K.L., et al., 2009. Quality of life and disability in patients with treatment-failure gout. Journal of Rheumatology 36, 1041–1048.

Bouchard, L., de Médicis, R., Lussier, A., et al., 2002. Inflammatory microcrystals alter the functional phenotype of human osteoblast-like cells in vitro: synergism with IL-1 to overexpress cyclooxygenase-2. Journal of Immunology 168, 5310–5317.

Brook, R., Forsythe, A., Smeeding, J., et al., 2010. Chronic gout: epidemiology, disease progression, treatment and disease burden. Current Medical Research and Opinion 26, 2813–2821.

Bruce, B., Fries, J.F., 2005. The Health Assessment Questionnaire. Clinical and Experimental Rheumatology S39, 14–18.

Budiman-Mak, E., Conrad, K.J., Roach, K.E., 1991. The foot function index: A measure of foot pain and disability. Journal of Clinical Epidemiology 44, 561–570.

Busso, N., So, A., 2010. Mechanisms of inflammation in gout. Arthritis Research and Therapy 12, 206.

Carter, J.D., Kedar, R.P., Anderson, S.R., et al., 2009. An analysis of MRI and ultrasound imaging in patients with gout who have normal plain radiographs. Rheumatology 48, 1442–1446.

Chen, L.X., Schumacher, H.R., 2008. Gout: an evidence-based review. Journal of Clinical Rheumatology 14, S55–S62.

Choi, H.K., 2010. A prescription for lifestyle change in patients with hyperuricaemia and gout. Current Opinion in Rheumatology 22, 165–172.

Choi, H.K., Mount, D.B., Reginato, A.M., 2005. Pathogenesis of gout. Annals of Internal Medicine 143, 499–516.

Choi, H.K., Willett, W., Curhan, G., 2007. Coffee consumption and risk of incident gout in men. Arthritis and Rheumatism 56, 2049–2055.

Choi, H.K., DeVera, M.A.D., Krishnan, E., 2008. Gout and the risk of type 2 diabetes among men with a high cardiovascular risk profile. Rheumatology 47, 1567–1570.

Choi, H.K., Gao, X., Curhan, G., 2009. Vitamin C intake and the risk of gout in men: a prospective study. Archives of Internal Medicine 169, 502–507.

Choi, H.K., Al-Arfaj, A., Eftekhari, A., et al., 2009a. Dual energy computed tomography in tophaceous gout. Annals of the Rheumatic Diseases 68, 1609–1612.

Choi, H.K., Gao, X., Curhan, G., 2009b. Vitamin C intake and the risk of gout in men: a prospective study. Archives of Internal Medicine 169, 502–507.

Chopra, K.F., Grossman, M., 2002. Images in clinical medicine: Finger-pad tophi. New England Journal of Medicine 346, 1714.

Conen, D., Wietlisbach, V., Bovet, P., et al., 2004. Prevalence of hyperuricaemia and relation of serum uric acid with cardiovascular risk factors in a developing country. BMC Public Health 4, 2458–2459.

Dalbeth, N., 2013. Management of gout in primary care: challenges and potential solutions. Rheumatology (Oxford, England) 52 (9), 1549–1550.

Dalbeth, N., Haskard, D., 2005. Mechanisms of inflammation in gout. Rheumatology 44, 1090–1096.

Dalbeth, N., McQueen, F.M., 2009. Use of imaging to evaluate gout and other crystal deposition disorders. Current Opinion in Rheumatology 21, 124–131.

Dalbeth, N., So, A., 2010. Hyperuricaemia and gout: state of the art and future perspectives. Annals of the Rheumatic Diseases 69, 1738–1743.

Dalbeth, N., Collis, J., Gregory, K., et al., 2007. Tophaceous joint disease strongly predicts hand function in patients with gout. Rheumatology 46, 1804–1807.

Dalbeth, N., Doyle, A., Boyer, L., et al., 2011a. Development of a computed tomography (CT) method of scoring bone erosion in the foot and ankle of patients with gout: validation and clinical implications. Rheumatology 50, 410–416.

Dalbeth, N., Petrie, K.J., House, M., et al., 2011a. Illness perceptions in patients with gout and the relationship with progression of musculoskeletal disability. Arthritis Care and Research 63, 1605–1612.

Dalbeth, N., Ames, R., Gamble, G.D., et al., 2012a. Effects of skim milk powder enriched with glycomacropeptide and G600 milk fat extract on frequency of gout flares: a proof-of-concept randomised controlled trial. Annals of the Rheumatic Diseases 71, 929–934.

Dalbeth, N., Doyle, A., McQueen, F.M., 2012b. Imaging in gout: insights into the pathological features of disease. Current Opinion in Rheumatology 24, 132–138.

Dalbeth, N., Kalluru, R., Aati, O., et al., 2013. Tendon involvement in the feet of patients with gout: a dual-energy CT study. Annals of the Rheumatic Diseases 72 (9), 1545–1548.

De Leonardis, F., Govoni, M., Colina, M., et al., 2007. Elderly-onset gout: a review. Rheumatology International 28, 1–6.

De Souza, A., Fernandes, V., Ferrari, A., 2005. Female gout: clinical and laboratory features. Journal of Rheumatology 32, 2186–2188.

Dehghan, A., Köttgen, A., Yang, Q., et al., 2008. Association of three genetic loci with uric acid concentration and risk of gout: a genome-wide association study. Lancet 372, 1953–1961.

Dessein, P.H., Shipton, E.A., Stanwix, A.E., et al., 2000. Beneficial effects of weight loss associated with moderate calorie/carbohydrate restriction, and increased proportional intake of protein and unsaturated fat on serum urate and lipoprotein levels in gout: a pilot study. Annals of the Rheumatic Diseases 59, 539–543.

Dieppe, P., Swan, A., 1999. Identification of crystals in synovial fluid. Annals of the Rheumatic Diseases 58, 261–263.

Doherty, M., 2009. New insights into the epidemiology of gout. Rheumatology 48 (S2), ii2–ii8.

Edwards, N.L., Sundy, J.S., Forsythe, A., et al., 2011. Work productivity loss due to flares in patients with chronic gout refractory to conventional therapy. Journal of Medical Economics 14, 10–15.

Falidas, E., Rallis, E., Boumia, V.K., et al., 2011. Multiarticular chronic tophaceous gout with severe and multiple ulcerations: a case report. Journal of Medical Case Reports 5, 397.

Farrant, J.M., O'Connor, P.J., Grainger, A.J., 2007. Advanced imaging in rheumatoid arthritis. Part 1: synovitis. Skeletal Radiology 36, 269–279.

Firth, J., Hale, C., Helliwell, P., et al., 2008. The prevalence of foot ulceration in patients with rheumatoid arthritis. Arthritis and Rheumatism 59, 200–205.

Fraser, J.F., Anand, V.K., Schwartz, T.H., 2007. Endoscopic biopsy sampling of tophaceous gout of the odontoid process. Journal of Neurosurgery – Spine 7, 61–64.

Grahame, R., Scott, J.T., 1970. Clinical survey of 354 patients with gout. Annals of the Rheumatic Diseases 29, 461–469.

Gutman, A.B., 1973. The past four decades of progress in the knowledge of gout, with an assessment of the present status. Arthritis and Rheumatism 16, 431–445.

Harris, M.D., Siegel, L., Alloway, J.A., 1999. Gout and hyperuricemia. American Family Physician 59, 925–934.

Harrold, L., 2013. New developments in gout. Current Opinion in Rheumatology 25, 304–309.

Harrold, L.R., Mazor, K., Negron, A., et al., 2013. Primary care providers' knowledge, beliefs and treatment practices for gout: results of a physician questionnaire. Rheumatology 52 (9), 1623–1629.

Helliwell, P., Reay, N., Gilworth, G., et al., 2005. Development of a foot impact scale for rheumatoid arthritis. Arthritis and Rheumatism 53, 418–422.

Hooper, L., Bowen, C.J., Gates, L., et al., 2012. Prognostic indicators of foot-related disability in patients with rheumatoid arthritis: results of a prospective three-year study. Arthritis Care and Research 64, 1116–1124.

Hoskison, T., Wortmann, R., 2006. Advances in the management of gout and hyperuricaemia. Scandinavian Journal of Rheumatology 35, 251–256.

Janssens, H.J., Janssen, M., van de Lisdonk, E.H., et al., 2010. Limited validity of the American College of Rheumatology criteria for classifying patients with gout in primary care. Annals of the Rheumatic Diseases 69, 1255–1256.

Jerome, J.T., Varhese, M., Sankaran, B., et al., 2008. Tibialis anterior tendon rupture in gout: case report and literature review. Foot and Ankle Surgery 14, 16–169.

Kemp, T.J., Hirsose, C.B., Coughlin, M.J., et al., 2010. Treatment of chronic tophaceous gout with a wound vacuum-assisted device. Foot and Ankle International 31, 729–731.

Khanna, D., Ahmed, M., Yontz, D., et al., 2008. The disutility of chronic gout. Quality of Life Research 17, 815–822.

Khanna, P.P., Perez-Ruiz, F., Maranian, P., et al., 2011. Long-term therapy for chronic gout results in clinically important improvements in the health-related quality of life: short form-36 is responsive to change in chronic gout. Rheumatology 50, 74074–74075.

Khanna, D., Fitzgerald, J.D., Khanna, P.P., et al., 2012a. American College of Rheumatology guidelines for management of gout. Part 1: systematic non-pharmacologic and pharmacologic therapeutic approaches to hyperuricaemia. Arthritis Care and Research 64, 1431–1446.

Khanna, D., Khanna, P.P., Fitzgerald, J.D., et al., 2012b. American College of Rheumatology guidelines for management of gout. Part 2: therapy and anti-inflammatory prophylaxis of acute gouty arthritis. Arthritis Care and Research 64, 1447–1461.

Kitaoka, H.B., Alexander, I.J., Adelaar, R.S., et al., 1994. Clinical rating systems for the ankle-hindfoot, midfoot, hallux, and lesser toes. Foot and Ankle International 15, 349–353.

Kleinman, N.L., Brook, R.A., Patel, P.A., et al., 2007. The impact of gout on work absence and productivity. Value in Health 10, 231–237.

Kumar, S., Gow, P., 2002. A survey of indications, results and complications of surgery for tophaceous gout. New Zealand Medical Journal 115, 1–4.

Lagoutaris, E.D., Adams, H.B., DiDomenico, L.A., et al., 2005. Longitudinal tears of both peroneal tendons associated with tophaceous gouty infiltration. A case report. Journal of Foot and Ankle Surgery 44, 222–224.

Lawrence, R.C., Felson, D.T., Helmick, C.G., et al., 2008. Estimates of the prevalence of arthritis and other rheumatic conditions in the United States. Part II. Arthritis and Rheumatism 58, 26–35.

Lee, J.W., Park, J.Y., Seo, J.W., et al., 2010. Surgical treatment of subcutaneous tophaceous gout. Plastic Reconstructive and Aesthetic Surgery 63, 1933–1935.

Lee, S.J., Hirsch, J.D., Terkeltaub, R., et al., 2009. Perceptions of disease and health-related quality of life among patients with gout. Rheumatology 48, 582–586.

Lindsay, K., Gow, P., Vanderpyl, J., et al., 2011. The experience and impact of living with gout: a study of men with chronic gout using a qualitative grounded theory approach. Journal of Clinical Rheumatology 17, 1–6.

Liu, B., Wang, T., Zhao, H., et al., 2011. The prevalence of hyperuricaemia in China: a meta-analysis. BMC Public Health 11, 832.

Liu, Q., Gamble, G., Pickering, K., et al., 2012. Prevalence and clinical factors associated with gout in patients with diabetes and prediabetes. Rheumatology 51, 757–759.

Maccagno, A., Di Giorgio, E., Romanowicz, A., 1991. Effectiveness of etodolac ('Lodine') compared with naproxen in patients with acute gout. Current Medical Research Opinion 12, 423–429.

Martini, N., Bryant, L., Te Karu, L., et al., 2012. Living with gout in New Zealand: an exploratory study into people's knowledge about the disease and its treatment. Journal of Clinical Rheumatology 18, 125–129.

Martinon, F., Petrilli, V., Mayor, A., et al., 2006. Gout-associated uric acid crystals activate the NALP3 inflammasome. Nature 440, 237–241.

McNair, P.J., Prapavessis, H., Collier, J., et al., 2007. The Lower-Limb Tasks Questionnaire: an assessment of validity, reliability, responsiveness, and minimal important differences. Archives of Physical Medicine and Rehabilitation 88, 993–1001.

McQueen, F.M., Doyle, A., Dalbeth, N., 2011. Imaging in gout – what can we learn from MRI, CT, DECT and US? Arthritis Research and Therapy 13, 246.

McQueen, F.M., Chhana, A., Dalbeth, N., 2012. Mechanisms of joint damage in gout: evidence from cellular and imaging studies. Nature Reviews Rheumatology 8, 173–181.

McQueen, F.M., Reeves, Q., Dalbeth, N., 2013. New insights into an old disease: advanced imaging in the diagnosis and management of gout. Postgraduate Medical Journal 89 (1048), 87–93.

Moi, J.H.Y., Sriranganathan, M.K., Edwards, C.J., et al., 2013. Lifestyle interventions for chronic gout. Cochrane Database of Systematic Reviews (5), CD010039.

Muehleman, C., Li, J., Aigner, T., et al., 2008. Association between crystals and cartilage degeneration in the ankle. Journal of Rheumatology 35, 1108–1117.

Ortiz-Bravo, E., Sieck, M.S., Schumacher, H.R. Jr., 1993. Changes in the proteins coating monosodium urate crystals during active and subsiding inflammation. Arthritis and Rheumatism 36, 1274–1285.

Ou, K.L., Tzeng, Y.S., Yu, C.C., et al., 2010. Resurfacing tophaceous gout in the foot with anterolateral thigh flap. Micosurgery 30, 79–82.

Pascual, E., Doherty, M., 2009. Aspiration of normal or asymptomatic pathological joints for diagnosis and research: indications, technique and success rate. Annals of the Rheumatic Diseases 68, 3–7.

Pascual, E., Batlle-Gualda, E., Martínez, A., et al., 1999. Synovial fluid analysis for diagnosis of intercritical gout. Annals of Internal Medicine 131, 756–759.

Pascual, E., Martínez, A., Ordóñez, S., 2013. Gout: the mechanism of urate crystal nucleation and growth. A hypothesis based in facts. Joint, Bone, Spine: Revue Du Rhumatisme 80 (1), 1–4.

Patel, G.K., Davies, W.L., Price, P.P., et al., 2010. Ulcerated tophaceous gout. International Wound Journal 7, 423–427.

Pelaez-Ballestas, I., Hernandez-Cuevas, C., Burgos-Vargas, R., et al., 2010. Diagnosis of chronic gout: evaluating the American College of Rheumatology proposal, European League Against Rheumatism recommendations, and clinical judgment. Journal of Rheumatology 37, 1743–1748.

Perez-Ruiz, F., Dalbeth, N., Urresola, A., et al., 2009. Imaging of gout: findings and utility. Arthritis Research and Therapy 11, 232.

Prior, I.A., Davidson, F., 1966. The epidemiology of diabetes in Polynesians and Europeans in New Zealand and the Pacific. New Zealand Medical Journal 65, 375–383.

Puig, J.G., de Miguel, E., Castillo, M.C., et al., 2008. Asymptomatic hyperuricemia: impact of ultrasonography. Nucleosides, Nucleotides and Nucleic Acids 27, 592–595.

Rees, F., Jenkins, W., Doherty, M., 2012. Patients with gout adhere to curative treatment if informed appropriately; proof-of-concept observational study. Annals of the Rheumatic Diseases 72, 826–830.

Richette, P., Bardin, T., 2010. Gout. Lancet 375, 318–328.

Richette, P., Clerson, P., Périssin, L., et al., 2013. Revisiting comorbidities in gout: a cluster analysis. Annals of the Rheumatic Diseases (in press).

Robinson, P.C., Taylor, W.J., Merriman, T.R., 2012. A systematic review of the prevalence of gout and hyperuricaemia in Australia. Internal Medicine 42, 997–1007.

Robinson, P.C., Schumacher, H.R., 2013. A qualitative and quantitative analysis of the characteristics of gout patient education resources. Clinics in Rheumatic Diseases 32, 771–778.

Roddy, E., Doherty, M., 2012. Gout and osteoarthritis: a pathogenetic link? Joint, Bone, Spine: Revue Du Rhumatisme 29, 499–503.

Roddy, E., Zhang, W., Doherty, M., 2007a. Are joints affected by gout also affected by osteoarthritis? Annals of the Rheumatic Diseases 66, 1374–1377.

Roddy, E., Zhang, W., Doherty, M., 2007b. Is gout associated with reduced quality of life? A case–control study. Rheumatology 46, 1441–1444.

Roddy, E., Zhang, W., Doherty, M., 2007c. The changing epidemiology of gout. Nature Clinical Practice. Rheumatology 3, 443–449.

Roddy, E., Zhang, W., Doherty, M., 2007d. Concordance of the management of chronic gout in a UK primary-care population with the EULAR gout recommendations. Annals of the Rheumatic Diseases 66, 1311–1315.

Roddy, E., Zhang, W., Doherty, M., 2008. Gout and nodal osteoarthritis: a case–control study. Rheumatology 47, 732–733.

Rome, K., Gow, P., Dalbeth, N., et al., 2009. Clinical audit of foot problems in patients with RA treated at Counties Manukau District Health Board, Auckland. Journal of Foot and Ankle Research 2, 16.

Rome, K., Supervalli, D., Sander, S., et al., 2011a. Functional and biomechanical characteristics of foot disease in chronic gout: a case–control study. Clinical Biomechanics 26, 90–94.

Rome, K., Frecklington, M., McNair, P.J., et al., 2011b. Footwear characteristics and factors influencing footwear choice in patients with gout. Arthritis Care and Research 63, 1599–1604.

Rome, K., Frecklington, M., McNair, P.J., et al., 2012. Foot pain, impairment and disability in patients with acute gout flares; a prospective observational study. Arthritis Care and Research 64, 384–388.

Rubin, B.R., Burton, R., Navarra, S., et al., 2004. Efficacy and safety profile of treatment with etoricoxib 120 mg once daily compared with indomethacin 50 mg three times daily in acute gout: a randomized controlled trial. Arthritis and Rheumatism 50, 598–606.

Schiltz, C., Lioté, F., Prudhommeaux, F., et al., 2002. Monosodium urate monohydrate crystal-induced inflammation in vivo: quantitative histomorphometric analysis of cellular events. Arthritis and Rheumatism 46, 1643–1650.

Schlesinger, N., Detry, M.A., Holland, B.K., et al., 2002. Local ice therapy during bouts of acute gouty arthritis. Journal of Rheumatology 29, 331–334.

Schumacher, H., Taylor, W., Joseph-Ridge, N., et al., 2007. Outcome evaluations in gout. Journal of Rheumatology 34, 1381–1385.

Schumacher, H.R., 1996. Crystal-induced arthritis: an overview. American Journal of Medicine 100, 46S–52S.

Siddle, H.J., Firth, J., Waxman, R., et al., 2012. A case series to describe the clinical characteristics of foot ulceration in patients with rheumatoid arthritis. Clinical Rheumatology 31, 541–545.

Silvester, R.N., Rome, K., Williams, A.E., et al., 2010. Choosing shoes': the challenges for clinicians in assessing rheumatoid footwear: a preliminary study. Journal of Foot and Ankle Research 3, 24.

Simkin, P.A., 1977. The pathogenesis of podagra. Annals of Internal Medicine 86, 230–233.

Singh, J.A., 2013. Racial and gender disparities among patients with gout. Current Rheumatology Reports 15, 307.

Singh, J.A., Strand, V., 2008. Gout is associated with more comorbidities, poorer health related quality of life and higher health care utilization in US veterans. Annals of the Rheumatic Diseases 67, 1310–1316.

Singh, J.A., Taylor, W.J., Simon, L.S., et al., 2011. Patient-reported outcomes in chronic gout: a report from OMERACT 10. Journal of Rheumatology 38, 1452–1457.

Smith, H.S., Bracken, D., Smith, J.M., 2011. Gout: current insights and future perspectives. Journal of Pain 12, 1113–1129.

Stamp, L.K., O'Donnell, J.L., Frampton, C., et al., 2013. Clinically insignificant effect of supplemental vitamin C on serum urate in patients with gout: a pilot randomized controlled trial. Arthritis and Rheumatism 65, 1636–1642.

Suppiah, R., Dissanayake, A., Dalbeth, N., 2008. High prevalence of gout in patients with type 2 diabetes: male sex, renal impairment, and diuretic use are major risk factors. New Zealand Medical Journal 121, 43–50.

Taylor, W.J., Colvine, K., Gregory, K., et al., 2008. The Health Assessment Questionnaire Disability Index is a valid measure of physical function in gout. Clinical and Experimental Rheumatology 26, 620–626.

ten Klooster, P.M., Oude Voshaar, M.A., Taal, E., et al., 2011. Comparison of measures of functional disability in patients with gout. Rheumatology 50, 709–713.

ten Klooster, P.M., Vonkeman, H.E., van de Laar, M.A., 2012. Disability due to gouty arthritis. Current Opinion in Rheumatology 24, 139–144.

Teng, G., Nair, R., Saag, K., 2006. Pathophysiology, clinical presentation and treatment of gout. Drugs 66, 1547–1563.

Thiele, R.G., Schlesinger, N., 2007. Diagnosis of gout by ultrasound. Rheumatology 46, 1116–1121.

Turner, D.E., Woodburn, J., 2008. Characterizing the clinical and biomechanical features of severely deformed feet in rheumatoid arthritis. Gait and Posture 28, 574–580.

Turner, D.E., Helliwell, P.S., Emery, P., et al., 2006. The impact of rheumatoid arthritis on foot function in the early stages of disease: a clinical case series. BMC Musculoskeletal Disorders 21, 102–107.

Turner, D.E., Helliwell, P.S., Siegel, K.L., 2009. Biomechanics of the foot in rheumatoid arthritis: Identifying abnormal function and the factors associated with localised disease 'impact. Clinical Biomechanics 23, 93–100.

Van Groen, M.M., ten Klooster, P.M., Taal, E., et al., 2010. Application of the health assessment questionnaire disability index to various rheumatic diseases. Quality of Life Research 19, 1255–1263.

Wallace, S., Singer, J., 1988. Therapy in gout. Rheumatic Disease Clinics of North America 14, 441–457.

Wallace, S.L., Robinson, H., Masi, A.T., et al., 1977. Preliminary criteria for the classification of the acute arthritis of primary gout. Arthritis and Rheumatism 20, 895–900.

Wang, C.C., Lien, S.B., Huang, G.S., et al., 2009. Arthroscopic elimination of monosodium urate deposition of the first metatarsophalangeal joint reduces the recurrence of gout. Arthroscopy: The Journal of Arthroscopic and Related Surgery 25, 153–159.

Winnard, D., Wright, C., Taylor, W.J., et al., 2012. National prevalence of gout derived from administrative health data in Aotearoa New Zealand. Rheumatology 51, 901–909.

Winnard, D., Wright, C., Jackson, G., et al., 2013. Gout, diabetes and cardiovascular disease in the Aotearoa New Zealand adult population: co-prevalence and implications for clinical practice. New Zealand Medical Journal 1368, 1–12.

Wortmann, R.L., 2002. Gout and hyperuricemia. Current Opinion in Rheumatology 14 (3), 281–286.

Wright, S.A., Filippucci, E., McVeigh, C., et al., 2007. High-resolution ultrasonography of the first metatarsophalangeal joint in gout: a controlled study. Annals of the Rheumatic Diseases 66, 859–864.

Yagnik, D.R., Evans, B.J., Florey, O., et al., 2004. Macrophage release of transforming growth factor beta1 during resolution of monosodium urate monohydrate crystal-induced inflammation. Arthritis and Rheumatism 50, 2273–2280.

Zammit, G.V., Menz, H.B., Munteanu, S.E., et al., 2008. Plantar pressure distribution in older people with osteoarthritis of the first metatarsophalangeal joint (hallux limitus/rigidus). Journal of Orthopaedic Research 26, 1665–1669.

Zhang, W., Doherty, M., Pascual, E., et al., 2006a. EULAR evidence based recommendations for gout. Part II: Management. Report of a task force of the EULAR standing committee for international clinical studies including therapeutics (ESCISIT). Annals of the Rheumatic Diseases 65, 1312–1324.

Zhang, W., Lioté, F., McCarthy, G., et al., 2006b. EULAR evidence based recommendations for gout. Part I: Diagnosis. Report of a task force of the standing committee for international clinical studies including therapeutics (ESCISIT). Annals of the Rheumatic Diseases 65, 1301–1311.

Zhu, Y., Pandya, B.J., Choi, H.K., 2011. Prevalence of gout and hyperuricaemia in the US general population: the National Health and Nutrition Examination Survey 2007–2008. Arthritis and Rheumatism 63, 3136–3141.

Zhu, Y., Pandya, B.J., Choi, H.K., 2012. Comorbidities of gout and hyperuricaemia in the US general population: NHANES 2007–2008. American Journal of Medicine 125, 679–687.

Chapter 4

Forefoot Entities

Fiona Hawke and Vivienne Chuter

Chapter Outline

HALLUX LIMITUS AND HALLUX RIGIDUS

INTRODUCTION

Hallux limitus and hallux rigidus describe the progressive structural restriction of the sagittal plane range of motion at the first metatarsophalangeal joint (MTPJ), particularly in the direction of dorsiflexion as a result of degenerative joint changes associated with osteoarthritis (Coughlin and Shurnas 2003a; Horton et al. 1999; Lichniak 1997). Although hallux limitus and hallux rigidus are used interchangeably and there is no consensus on the diagnostic threshold separating hallux limitus and rigidus (Munuera et al. 2007), it is generally accepted that hallux limitus refers to the preliminary restriction of dorsiflexion of the hallux on the first metatarsal to less than the 65° required for normal gait (Botek and Anderson 2011; Camasta 1996; Grady et al. 2002; Van Saase et al. 1989). Progressive loss of joint range of motion develops as a result of the presence of periarticular osteophytes and alterations to the dorsal aspect of the joint, including the development of an exostosis, which creates a mechanical impingement of the proximal phalanx on the base of the first metatarsal (Zgonis et al. 2005). Hallux rigidus occurs when the degenerative joint changes progress to the point of complete loss of joint movement and subsequent joint ankylosis (Camasta 1996), with a suggested definition of no more than 10° of available hallux dorsiflexion (Stuck et al. 1988).

Hallux limitus and rigidus are reported to be the second most common pathology to affect the first MTPJ after hallux valgus (Munuera et al. 2008). Initial observations of hallux limitus were first reported in adolescents (Davies-Colley 1887); however, the incidence of osteoarthritic changes at the first MTPJ increases with older age. The condition most frequently affects those from middle age onwards, with increases in prevalence from 10% of people aged

20–34 years to between 35% and 60% of people over the age of 65 years (Taranto et al. 2007).

In addition to osteoarthritic changes at the first MTPJ, functional restrictions occurring in an otherwise normal joint have been proposed as a cause of altered gait mechanics and subsequent pathology (Dananberg 1986). Functional hallux limitus was first defined as a restriction at the first MTPJ, proposed to originate from mechanical restrictions rather than structural abnormalities, with range of motion at the first MTPJ within normal limits when non-weightbearing but restricted when weightbearing (Dananberg 1986; Laird 1972).

An initial description of functional hallux limitus provided diagnostic criteria of greater than 50° of dorsiflexion available at the first MTPJ during non-weightbearing but less than 14° during weightbearing (Laird 1972). However, more recent kinematic investigation of normal first-MTPJ motion suggests functional restriction occurs where there is less than 60° to 65° of dorsiflexion in dynamic weightbearing (Hopson et al. 1995; Nawoczenski et al. 1999). During gait, a functional hallux limitus is proposed to occur at a point following forefoot loading, when the upper body moves in front of the stance limb (Dananberg 1986). Limitation of hallux dorsiflexion at this time is suggested to disrupt the balance of forward motion, preventing both propulsion through a fulcrum for rotation about the first MTPJ and raising of the medial longitudinal arch via the windlass mechanism (Dananberg 1993; Payne and Dananberg 1997). First described by Hicks (1954), the windlass mechanism involves dorsiflexion of the hallux shortening the distance between the origin and insertion of the plantar fascia, causing the medial longitudinal arch to raise and creating a rigid foot structure for propulsion (Hicks 1954). Lack of instigation of the windlass mechanism is suggested to result in an unstable arch structure and assumed gait compensation via more proximal joints in the foot and leg (Dananberg 1993). These include excessive midtarsal or subtalar joint pronation, prolonged forefoot inversion, lack of knee extension during propulsion, propulsive instability, and postural perturbations (Dananberg 1993, 1999). Clinically functional hallux limitus usually presents not as pain in the first MTPJ but rather as pathologies thought to occur as a result of gait compensations for first-MTPJ dysfunction (Dananberg 1993).

Despite theories on the potential effects of a functional hallux limitus on gait and its role in the development of pathology, there is limited independent research evidence investigating the prevalence of the condition or its proposed compensations. The lack of research relating to prevalence of functional hallux limitus in the general population may be explained by the diagnostic challenge that faces clinicians when trying to evaluate function at the first MTPJ. As there are generally no symptoms at the joint, a diagnosis must be made via clinical assessment of joint function and/or the presence of assumed compensatory gait changes (Dananberg 1993; Durrant and Chockalingam 2009). Preliminary investigation of prevalence of functional hallux limitus determined by non-weightbearing assessment in a population of 43 asymptomatic participants (86 feet) reported the condition was present in 62% of limbs (Payne et al. 2002). Fifty-two percent demonstrated evidence of a functional hallux limitus determined via non-weightbearing assessment and an assumed gait compensation (classified as abnormal motion at the midtarsal joint on visual gait analysis). However, findings assume both the validity of the non-weightbearing and gait assessment techniques and assessed only for the presence of one of many proposed gait compensations.

PREDISPOSING FACTORS

Hallux limitus and rigidus commonly occur secondary to existing disease processes, particularly systemic arthropathies such as rheumatoid arthritis, ankylosing spondylitis, and Reiter's syndrome (Grady et al. 2002). In its primary form, the aetiology of the condition is widely considered multifactorial and a large number of risk factors have been suggested. Radiographic evidence of first-MTPJ osteoarthritis (OA) is reported to be present in up to 35% of people over the age of 35 years (Van Saase et al. 1989) with prevalence rising further in older age groups (Beeson et al. 2009; Coughlin and Shurnas 2003b). The disease presents bilaterally in up to 79% of people with 95% of those having a familial history of the disease (Coughlin and Shurnas 2003b). Previous studies on gender predilection are inconclusive. Cross-sectional data indicate higher incidence in association with female gender

(Beeson et al. 2009) with radiographic first-MTP joint OA occurring in approximately 45% of women and 30% of men at 60 years of age (Van Saase et al. 1989); however, this has not been consistently demonstrated in the literature (Trivedi et al. 2010).

Trauma, either as a single incident or due to ongoing microtrauma to the joint, is considered a common cause of first-MTPJ OA. Histological evidence of a traumatic aetiology including damage to the articular cartilage and changes to subchondral bone is present in 64% of cases (Beeson et al. 2009; McMaster 1978). Single episodes of trauma are typically associated with a unilateral presentation and younger age of onset of the disease process, frequently involving a hyperextension or hyperflexion injury of the hallux causing increased joint compression or shearing (Goodfellow 1966; Hanft et al. 1993; McMaster 1978). In contrast, ongoing microtrauma to the joint resulting in osteoarthritic change has been suggested to be associated with a number of anatomical factors including (1) foot posture and first-metatarsal function (Nilsonne 1930; Root et al. 1977), (2) radiological findings including length and position of the first metatarsal (Nilsonne 1930; Root et al. 1977), and (3) morphology of the first metatarsal and proximal phalanx of the hallux.

Foot Posture and First-Metatarsal Function

A hypermobile first metatarsal either in isolation or as a result of an excessively pronating foot has been proposed to allow dorsiflexion of the first metatarsal during the mid-stance and propulsive phases of gait, preventing normal plantarflexion of the first metatarsal (Root et al. 1977). Lack of first-metatarsal plantarflexion is suggested to block the arc of dorsiflexion of the proximal phalanx on the head of the first metatarsal, resulting in a functional hallux limitus (Dananberg 1993; Root et al. 1977). Chronic impingement then results in joint degeneration and osteoarthritic changes associated with hallux limitus and rigidus (Botek and Anderson 2011; Root et al. 1977). However, there is limited evidence to support this theory, with several radiographic investigations of medial arch angle in people with and without hallux limitus/rigidus, finding no significant association between the presence of the pathology and radiographic measures of medial arch height (Beeson et al. 2009; Coughlin 2003b). Additional investigation of the relationship

between passive weightbearing hallux dorsiflexion and frontal plane motion of the rearfoot complex (used as an indicator of excessive subtalar joint pronation) has also failed to demonstrate a relationship between increased rearfoot eversion and restricted hallux dorsiflexion (Halstead et al. 2005).

First-Metatarsal Length and Position

Excessive length of the first metatarsal has historically been considered a primary cause of hallux limitus and rigidus (Coughlin and Shurnas 2003a). A long first metatarsal was proposed to prevent the plantarflexion required to allow normal hallux dorsiflexion during gait, causing increased joint compressive forces at the first MTPJ resulting in osteoarthritic change (Nilsonne 1930; Root et al. 1977). A number of cross-sectional studies of radiographic risk factors for hallux limitus and rigidus have failed to confirm such a relationship. Coughlin and Shurnas (2003a) used radiographs to assess first-metatarsal length in 114 patients undergoing surgery for hallux rigidus and concluded 'a long first metatarsal was no more common in patients with hallux rigidus than in the general population' (Coughlin and Shurnas 2003a). Similarly, in a study of radiographs of 180 instances of hallux rigidus, Beeson et al. (2009) reported a longer first metatarsal than second metatarsal was present in only 37% of cases whereas 73% of cases had a longer first than third metatarsal – leading the authors to suggest that it was this relationship that may be more strongly associated with the development of hallux limitus and rigidus (Beeson et al. 2009).

Findings of case–control studies are less conclusive. Several studies have supported a lack of relationship between a long first metatarsal and hallux limitus or rigidus (Bryant et al. 2000; Taranto et al. 2007; Zgonis et al. 2005), with results of one such study finding the first metatarsal was actually significantly shorter in those with hallux rigidus than in the control group (Zgonis et al. 2005). However, a similar study performed on a younger cohort with hallux limitus reported contradictory findings, demonstrating a significantly longer first metatarsal in cases (mean 68.6 mm) compared with controls (mean=65.2 mm) (Munuera et al. 2007). The focus of this study was on an earlier stage of disease progression, with all cases diagnosed with hallux limitus only (between 30° and

50° of first-MTPJ dorsiflexion remaining) and in a younger cohort (mean age 23 years). Due to the early stage of the disease process in this cohort these findings have been suggested to be more likely to represent true joint changes rather than long-term consequences of joint degeneration (Munuera et al. 2007; Zammit et al. 2009; Zgonis et al. 2005).

Metatarsus primus elevatus (dorsiflexion of the first metatarsal relative to the second metatarsal) has been proposed as a common cause of hallux limitus and rigidus (Jack 1940; Root et al. 1977). Similar to the theory behind the role of excessive foot pronation and a hypermobile first metatarsal, the fixed position of the first metatarsal is proposed to prevent the amount of first metatarsal plantarflexion required to allow a normal range of dorsiflexion of the proximal phalanx of the hallux on the head of the first metatarsal during gait (Root et al. 1977). Research has generally failed to support such a relationship, with approximately 90% of cases of hallux rigidus reported to have a radiographically measured first-metatarsal elevation within normal limits (8 mm of elevation) (Beeson et al. 2009), and no evidence of differences in mean first-metatarsal elevation angle between those with and those without hallux rigidus (Horton et al. 1999). Furthermore, several case–control studies have also reported an opposite relationship, demonstrating an increase in radiographically assessed declination angle of the first metatarsal, indicating plantarflexion of the rearfoot on the forefoot (Bryant et al. 2000, 2001; Horton et al. 1999).

Despite lack of evidence supporting the role of metatarsus primus elevatus in the development of hallux limitus and rigidus, research does suggest that a first metatarsal that is dorsiflexed relative to the position of the second metatarsal may be a contributing factor (Bryant et al. 2000; Horton et al. 1999). Several studies have demonstrated radiographic evidence indicative of a relatively dorsiflexed metatarsal including a greater difference in first- and second-metatarsal declination angle (Horton et al. 1999) and higher lateral intermetatarsal angle (Bryant et al. 2000) in the presence of diagnosed hallux limitus and rigidus. These findings suggest that an altered relationship between the positions of the first and second metatarsals may be of greater importance than elevation of the first metatarsal alone.

Hallux and First-Metatarsal Morphology

Numerous other radiographic findings have been associated with the development of hallux limitus and rigidus. Munuera et al. (2007) used dorsoplantar radiographs to evaluate the size of the first metatarsodigital segment in 144 feet (94 controls and 50 cases) with and without hallux limitus (Munuera et al. 2007). In the presence of hallux limitus there was a significant increase in the length of the proximal and distal phalanges of the hallux, increased length of the medial and lateral sesamoids, and increased width of the first metatarsal and proximal phalanx (Munuera et al. 2007). Increased hallux length is proposed to increase compressive forces at the first MTPJ when wearing footwear (Zammit et al. 2009) causing high joint compression forces at the first MTPJ. The increased length of the sesamoids is suggested to impede first metatarsal plantarflexion and posterior movement of the first metatarsal during gait (Durrant and Siepert 1993), preventing the required amount of dorsiflexion of the hallux on the first metatarsal.

First metatarsal head morphology, specifically a flat or chevron shape, is suggested to place the joint at greater risk of injury through severe joint compression (or jamming) and increase the likelihood of related degenerative changes. In a cross-sectional study of radiographs of 180 feet with hallux rigidus Beeson et al. (2009) demonstrated that 131 feet (73%) had either a flat or chevron-shaped metatarsal head. Similar findings were demonstrated in a study of patients undergoing joint fusion due to painful hallux rigidus, with 93 of 127 feet (73%) found to have chevron or flat metatarsal head (Coughlin and Shurnas 2003b). These findings are consistent with the increased proximal phalanx and first-metatarsal width reported by Munuera et al. (2007). However, it is difficult to determine true incidence as flattening of the metatarsal head also occurs with progression of the disease process; therefore a high incidence in patients with long-standing hallux limitus and rigidus is to be expected (Zammit et al. 2009).

Functional Hallux Limitus

Abnormal first-metatarsal dorsiflexion and high plantar fascial tension associated with prolonged foot pronation have been suggested as possible theoretical causes of a functional hallux limitus (Fuller 2000; Scherer et al. 2006). During normal gait, plantarflexion of the ankle joint at heel-off shifts body weight to the forefoot, with dorsiflexion of the MTPJs providing a fulcrum of rotation facilitating forward progression (Dananberg 1993). Peroneus longus activity assists in stabilizing the first metatarsal (Donatelli 1985). Hallux dorsiflexion then instigates the windlass mechanism, tightening the plantar aponeurosis, raising the medial longitudinal arch, and ensuring a rigid foot structure for propulsion (Hicks 1954). Raising of the longitudinal arch has been demonstrated to produce relative plantarflexion of the first metatarsal (Hicks 1954). Adequate first-metatarsal plantarflexion is also required to allow hallux dorsiflexion to occur with dorsiflexion beyond 20° requiring 1° of relative first-metatarsal plantarflexion for every 3° of additional hallux dorsiflexion (Phillips et al. 1996). A hypermobile first metatarsal is suggested to elevate during stance with the dorsiflexed position limiting first-MTPJ dorsiflexion, resulting in a functional hallux limitus (Scherer et al. 2006).

Excessive tension on the plantar fascia through lowering of the medial longitudinal arch as may occur with prolonged foot pronation is also suggested to prevent normal hallux dorsiflexion during gait (Fuller 2000). During normal gait, tension on the plantar fascia increases as the foot is loaded during stance producing a plantarflexion moment at the hallux. This force is overcome by an external dorsiflexing moment created by extension of the hallux on the first MTPJ as the body moves forward over the fixed foot (Fuller 2000; Hicks 1954). Foot pronation into the propulsive phase is proposed to cause increased tension on the plantar fascia owing to flattening of the medial longitudinal arch, resulting in a greater magnitude of the plantarflexing moment produced by the plantar fascia at the first MTPJ. A plantarflexing moment from increased plantar fascial tension that exceeds the dorsiflexion moment produced by the hallux is suggested to prevent normal function of the windlass mechanism, resulting in a functional hallux limitus (Fuller 2000). Evidence of delayed onset of the windlass mechanism induced by passive hallux dorsiflexion in association with increased rearfoot eversion suggests that a relationship between excessive foot pronation and functional hallux limitus may exist (Kappel-Bargas

et al. 1998). However, the proposed kinetic imbalance around the first MTPJ during gait requires further investigation.

DIAGNOSIS

Diagnosis and grading of hallux limitus and rigidus are made via a combination of presenting symptoms and clinical and radiographic assessment (Vanore et al. 2003a). Clinical practice guidelines require a significant patient history including pain or joint stiffness localized to the first MTPJ with either an insidious onset, post trauma, or with a history of relevant systemic disease (Vanore et al. 2003a). Onset of symptoms is often associated with physical activity and footwear and may present with secondary pathology such as lateral forefoot pain due to gait compensation. Clinically the condition should present with a prominent dorsal exostosis, which creates a mechanical block at the first MTPJ and joint movement associated with pain and possibly crepitus (Vanore et al. 2003a). Other clinical findings may include evidence of gait compensation such as forefoot pain or associated plantar hyperkeratosis lesions at the interphalangeal joint (IPJ) of the hallux or lateral forefoot (Vanore et al. 2003a). Radiographic findings will vary according to the stage of the disease process but should be consistent with osteoarthritic changes including the presence of dorsal, lateral, and medial osteophytes, joint space narrowing, and sclerosis with possible periarticular cystic changes (Coughlin and Shurnas 2003b; Vanore et al. 2003a).

Numerous classification systems exist to determine the progression of the disease. These are based on radiographic criteria only or combine clinical and radiographic findings to classify the disease in either three or four stages (Coughlin and Shurnas 2003a; Drago et al. 1984; Geldwert et al. 1992; Hanft et al. 1993). Clinical–radiographic grading systems classify the severity of the pathology via a combination of clinical findings such as range of motion available at the joint and presenting symptoms such as joint pain and stiffness in addition to radiographic findings of osteoarthritis (Table 4-1) (Coughlin and Shurnas 2003a; Easley et al. 1999). However, a review of the classification systems available has questioned their clinical utility owing to lack of consistency in classification criteria and assessment methodology (Beeson

TABLE 4-1 Clinical-Radiographic System for Grading Hallux Rigidus

Grade	Dorsiflexion	Radiographic Findings*	Clinical Findings
0	40° to 60° and/or 10% to 20% loss compared with normal side	Normal	No pain; only stiffness and loss of motion on examination
1	30° to 40° and/or 20% to 50% loss compared with normal side	Dorsal osteophyte is main finding, minimal joint space narrowing, minimal periarticular sclerosis, minimal flattening of metatarsal head	Mild or occasional pain and stiffness, pain at extremes of dorsiflexion and/or plantar flexion on examination
2	10° to 30° and/or 50% to 75% loss compared with normal side	Dorsal, lateral and possible medial osteophytes giving flattened appearance to metatarsal head, no more than ¼ of dorsal joint space involved on lateral radiograph, mild to moderate joint space narrowing and sclerosis, sesamoids not usually involved	Moderate to severe pain and stiffness that may be constant; pain occurs just before maximum dorsiflexion and maximum plantar flexion on examination
3	≤10° and/or 75% to 100% loss compared with normal side. There is notable loss of metatarsophalangeal plantar flexion as well (often ≤10° of plantar flexion)	Same as in Grade 2 but with substantial narrowing, possibly periarticular cystic changes, more than ¼ of dorsal joint space involved on lateral radiograph, sesamoids enlarged and/or cystic and/or irregular	Nearly constant pain and substantial stiffness at extremes of range of motion but not at mid range
4	Same as in Grade 3	Same as in Grade 3	Same criteria as Grade 3 BUT there is definite pain at mid range of passive motion

*Weight bearing and anterior–posterior and lateral radiographs are used.
Adapted from Coughlin and Shurnas.
Coughlin MJ, Shurnas PS. Hallux rigidus. Grading and long-term results of operative treatment. J Bone Joint Surg Am 2003;85-A(11):2072–2088.

et al. 2008). Furthermore, diagnostic parameters for grading were found to be based on clinical experience rather than scientific evidence and the authors identified a lack of research assessing the reliability and validity of any of the classification systems (Beeson et al. 2008).

As a clinically based alternative to the variety of classification systems relying in part or completely on radiographic evaluation, Zammit et al. (2011) developed a clinical diagnostic rule for identification of osteoarthritis at the first MTPJ without use of radiographs (Zammit et al. 2011). The rule uses a combination of subjective history, clinical observation, and assessment including: reporting a pain duration >25 months, observation of a dorsal exostosis, hard-end feel to the joint, presence of joint crepitus, and first-MTPJ dorsiflexion <64° (Zammit et al. 2011). All these factors have been found to be independently

associated with radiographically identified OA. In combination, the presence of all variables demonstrated 88% sensitivity, 71% specificity, and a diagnostic accuracy of 84% for osteoarthritis of the first MTPJ (Zammit et al. 2011).

Diagnosis of functional hallux limitus is challenging in the clinical environment. Motion analysis systems can provide measurement of first-MTPJ dorsiflexion during gait, but may not be available in clinical practice and accuracy of measurement will vary according to the type of system used. Clinical testing for functional hallux limitus may include either non-weightbearing or weightbearing examination of the range of hallux dorsiflexion (Dananberg 1999; Enklaar 1956; Jack 1940). In a non-weightbearing examination the range of motion of the first metatarsophalangeal joint is determined while the first-metatarsal head is prevented from plantarflexing (Dananberg 1999).

Presence of a functional hallux limitus is indicated by loss of hallux dorsiflexion from this position. This form of clinical testing has demonstrated moderate sensitivity and specificity (72% and 66% respectively) for abnormal midtarsal joint function (presumed to be a gait compensation for functional hallux limitus) determined by visual gait analysis (Payne et al. 2002). However, the usefulness of this data is limited as the proportion of cases of functional hallux limitus presenting with abnormal midtarsal function is unknown, as is the validity of using visual gait analysis to determine its presence.

Weightbearing static assessment of first-MTPJ function is conducted using the Jack's test or the Hubscher manoeuvre, where the proximal phalanx of the hallux is manually dorsiflexed by a clinician with the patient in relaxed bilateral stance (Enklaar 1956; Jack 1953). Resistance to hallux dorsiflexion and lack of, or delayed, tightening and raising of the medial longitudinal arch is considered an indicator of the presence of a functional hallux limitus. Use of this test is based on an assumption that restriction during the static manoeuvre is predictive of functional limitation at this joint during gait (Halstead and Redmond 2006). However, investigations of the relationship between passive and dynamic hallux dorsiflexion in people with and without weightbearing restriction of first-MTPJ range of motion have reported only weak (Jack 1953) to moderate (Nawoczenski et al. 1999) correlations between the two measurements, suggesting this test may have limited clinical utility.

IMPAIRMENTS

Progressive loss of joint motion and joint pain are hallmarks of hallux limitus and rigidus. Assessment of passive non-weightbearing dorsiflexion is normally used to determine the extent of degenerative joint changes. In the early stages of hallux limitus, loss of range of motion is relatively small and may be measured as a reduction from normal range of motion on the symptomatic side (5–20°), or a reduction in range of motion on the symptomatic side compared to the unaffected side (10–20%) (Coughlin and Shurnas 2003a). Range of motion losses become progressively worse as the joint deteriorates, with end-stage hallux rigidus typically associated with less than 10° available range of dorsiflexion or significant loss compared with the affected side (e.g. more than 75%) (Coughlin and Shurnas 2003a).

Previous research investigating levels of pain associated with the condition is focused on outcomes following surgical interventions. Early stages of hallux limitus present with subjective reports of joint stiffness with absence of or minimal or occasional pain. In more severe cases, joint pain is constant with stiffness at the mid- and end-ranges of motion (Coughlin and Shurnas 2003a). Generally people seeking surgical intervention have high levels of pain, typically between 6 and 10 points on a visual analogue pain scale (Coughlin and Shurnas 2003a).

Impairments associated with functional hallux limitus are not possible to quantify. The large range of proposed gait compensations is suggested to result in a number of pathologies (Coughlin and Shurnas 2003a; Dananberg 1993, 1999) that presumably result in pain either localized to the point of compensation or secondary to altered gait patterns. The magnitude of pain reported is likely to be affected by activity level and site of compensation; however, this point has not been a focus of investigation.

FUNCTION

Patients with structural or functional hallux limitus and hallux rigidus have significant compensatory gait adaptations including changes to dynamic plantar pressures and lower limb kinematics (Bryant et al. 1999; Canseco et al. 2008; Van Gheluwe et al. 2006; Zammit et al. 2008). Case–control studies of plantar pressure change suggest that functional or structural hallux limitus/rigidus is associated with increased lateral forefoot loading (Bryant et al. 1999) and resistance at the first MTPJ during dynamic function (Van Gheluwe et al. 2006). Evidence of higher peak pressures, force, and loading rates under the hallux (Bryant et al. 1999; Van Gheluwe et al. 2006; Zammit et al. 2008) has been suggested to result from blockade of first-MTPJ dorsiflexion, and when coupled with a relative shift in forefoot pressure from medial to lateral supports alteration to propulsive gait mechanics (Van Gheluwe et al. 2006).

Several kinematic studies of the effect of hallux limitus and rigidus on gait have also demonstrated changes consistent with an altered propulsive phase and possible failure of the windlass mechanism as predicted by the sagittal plane facilitation model proposed by Dananberg (1993, 1999). Reduced first-MTPJ dorsiflexion due to hallux rigidus has been linked to altered midfoot motion, with plantarflexion of the forefoot on the rearfoot during propulsion indicating flattening of the medial longitudinal arch (Canseco et al. 2008). Artificially induced hallux limitus has been shown to increase ankle dorsiflexion during late mid-stance, the point at which restriction at the first MTPJ would prevent forward progression of the body and more proximal sagittal plane compensation would be required, and reduce peak ankle joint plantarflexion during propulsion (Hall and Nester 2004).

Investigation of changes in kinematic and kinetic parameters post-arthrodesis of the first MTPJ supports these findings (DeFrino et al. 2002). Following fusion of the first MTPJ, ankle joint plantarflexion has been demonstrated to reduce with an associated reduction in power production during propulsion (DeFrino et al. 2002). Consistent with this, surgical intervention with cheilectomy (to improve joint range of motion) for hallux rigidus has been found to have the opposite effect (Smith et al. 2012). Comparison of pre- and post-surgical gait kinetics demonstrated cheilectomy produced increased first-MTPJ dorsiflexion accompanied by significant increases in power produced at the ankle joint, indicating improved propulsive efficiency and supporting the integral role of the first MTPJ in maintenance of efficient propulsive mechanics (Smith et al. 2012).

QUALITY OF LIFE

Limited evidence exists that evaluates the impact of hallux limitus and rigidus on general quality of life measures with existing studies assessing the impact of structural hallux limitus and rigidus. In a case–control study, Bergin et al. (2012) evaluated the impact of first-MTPJ OA on health-related quality of life outcomes. Assessment of general quality of life was conducted with the Short Form-36 (SF-36), a generic questionnaire used to assess the physical, psychological, and social health and wellbeing of individuals suffering from a chronic disease (Ware Jr and Sherbourne 1992). Foot-specific quality of life was measured using the Foot Health Status Questionnaire (FHSQ), a validated, reliable self-rated questionnaire

assessing the domains of foot pain, foot function, shoe fit (footwear), and general foot health (Bennett et al. 1998). Forty-three cases with radiographic evidence of first-MTPJ OA accompanied by joint pain were compared with an age-, sex-, and BMI-matched control group (Bergin et al. 2012). Mean score for physical function in the SF-36 was found to be significantly lower in the cases compared with the controls (82.8 versus 95.2 respectively), indicating first-MTPJ OA causes considerable impairment of a wide range of physical activities. Interestingly, the severity of radiographically measured joint degeneration was not associated with the degree of self-reported impact on physical impairment. Results of the FHSQ supported the SF-36 findings of physical impairment. Participants with first-MTPJ OA reported lower scores (indicating greater impairment) across all domains of the FHSQ having more foot pain, poorer foot function, greater difficulty finding appropriate footwear, and had poorer perceived general foot health. However, as with the SF-36, lower scores indicating poorer outcomes were not dependent on the severity of joint OA.

Results of other investigations of foot-specific quality of life using the FHSQ in people with symptomatic hallux limitus and rigidus demonstrate that the condition is associated with consistent reductions across all domains of the questionnaire. Maher and Metcalfe (2008) used the FHSQ pre- and post-surgery in 29 patients undergoing first-MTPJ arthrodesis. Pre-intervention scores (out of 100) for all domains of the FHSQ demonstrated high levels of foot pain (mean score 29) poor function (mean score 46.7), difficulty with finding footwear (mean score 19.7), and poor perceptions of general foot health (mean score 28.2) (Maher and Metcalfe 2008). Gilheany et al. (2008) compared the impact of hallux rigidus and hallux valgus in a cohort of 122 patients presenting for first-MTPJ pain or deformity; for patients with hallux rigidus, mean scores were reduced across all domains: 46.9 for pain, 59.7 for function, 24.8 for footwear/shoe fit, and 36.7 for general foot health. Furthermore, scores in the domains of function and pain were significantly lower for patients presenting with hallux rigidus than for patients with hallux valgus (mean scores: 60.6 for pain, 74.7 for function), suggesting that, of the two conditions, hallux limitus is associated with poorer foot-related health-related quality of life outcomes.

MANAGEMENT STRATEGIES

Pharmacological Strategies

Pharmacological management of hallux limitus typically involves the use of anti-inflammatory agents such as corticosteroids and hyaluronic acids, often in combination with local anaesthetics delivered as peri- or intra-articular injection (Solan et al. 2001). Corticosteroids are administered to provide long-lasting pain relief (weeks to months) through the removal of the inflammatory feedback loop; however, they do not slow the course of articular cartilage degeneration causing osteoarthritis progression (Schurman and Smith 2004). Retrospective data of successful interventions used in symptomatic hallux limitus suggest treatment with corticosteroid injection is used in only a small proportion (6%) of cases treated with conservative means and there is limited research investigating its efficacy (Pons et al. 2007).

Existing research indicates the usefulness of corticosteroid injections is dependent on the severity of the presenting condition (Solan et al. 2001). Solan et al. (2001) investigated the duration of pain relief achieved following the use of a combination of corticosteroid injection with anaesthetic and joint manipulation in 29 patients with hallux rigidus. Severity of radiological changes in hallux was found to be associated with the duration of symptomatic relief experienced by patients post-treatment. Patents with early joint changes experienced the most benefit from the therapy, averaging 6 months of symptomatic relief with only one-third of patients progressing to surgery. Symptomatic relief for patients with moderate disease lasted an average of 3 months with two-thirds of patients having surgery. For those with end-stage joint changes the treatment was unsuccessful, with no reported period of symptom reduction and all patients having surgical procedures (Solan et al. 2001).

Comparative investigation of the benefits of hyaluronic acid and corticosteroid injections for symptomatic early-stage hallux limitus has demonstrated that the treatments have similar therapeutic effects (Pons et al. 2007). In a randomized controlled trial comparing the benefits of a single hyaluronic acid injection compared with a single corticosteroid injection, both agents produced similar significant reductions in pain during range of motion and walking

assessment at 84 days post-administration (Pons et al. 2007). Hallux evaluation measured using the American Orthopedic Foot and Ankle Society (AOFAS) score with subscores for pain (40 points), function (45 points), and alignment (15 points) demonstrated significant reductions in pain and improvements in function for both hyaluronic acid and corticosteroid injection; however, there was significantly greater improvement on the pain subscale for those receiving hyaluronic acid. Regardless of therapy type, approximately half of all patients receiving treatment in this trial subsequently had surgical intervention, suggesting injection therapy only delays more invasive treatment (Pons et al. 2007).

Physical Strategies

There is a broad range of physical therapies used for the treatment of hallux limitus and rigidus; however, there is limited evidence of their efficacy. Physical therapy interventions cited in the literature include whirlpool, ultrasound, first-MTPJ mobilizations, calf and hamstring stretching, marble pick-up exercise, cold packs, electrical stimulation, continuous passive motion, splinting, and chiropractic treatment (Brantingham et al. 2007; John et al. 2011; Shamus et al. 2004). Despite the variety of treatment options available there is a paucity of research investigating their outcomes. Several studies have shown success for treatment of iatrogenic (post-surgery) hallux limitus using continuous passive motion therapy and dynamic splinting to reduce post-surgical pain and stiffness at the first MTPJ and increase range of motion (Connor and Berk 1994; John et al. 2011). In cases of hallux limitus of mixed aetiology, three times weekly mobilization of the sesamoids, flexor hallucis longus strengthening, and gait retraining in addition to therapeutic modalities has been demonstrated to significantly decrease pain, increase first-MTPJ range of dorsiflexion, and increase flexor hallucis longus strength compared with the therapeutic modalities alone (Shamus et al. 2004). However, the above interventions are intensive and time-consuming, limiting their practicality in a clinical setting and increasing the risk of patient non-compliance. Further research is required to determine the efficacy of individual physical therapies as a method of conservative therapy for the treatment of this condition.

Footwear. Difficulty with footwear fitting due to pain and irritation from impingement of dorsal osteophytes is common for patients with hallux limitus and rigidus. Footwear recommendations include a low heel and deep toe box to allow for accommodation of a dorsal exostosis and increased stiffness through the shank of the shoe or a rocker-sole shoe to reduce stress on the first MTPJ during the propulsive phase of gait (Grady et al. 2002; Shereff and Baumhauer 1998). Changes in footwear alone have been demonstrated to significantly reduce pain and allow for a return to normal activities in a small proportion of patients with hallux limitus and rigidus (Grady et al. 2002); however, they are frequently used in conjunction with other forms of therapy such as foot orthoses or post-operatively.

Foot Orthoses. Foot orthoses are used in the treatment of hallux limitus and rigidus and functional hallux limitus (Camasta 1996; Cohn and Kanat 1984; Dananberg 1993; Grady et al. 2002). Orthotic therapy for earlier stages of hallux limitus and functional hallux limitus is aimed at preserving or improving first-MTPJ range of motion with the use of functional foot orthoses. In the later or more severe stages of the condition, accommodative devices are used to stabilize the joint and reduce pain (Shereff and Baumhauer 1998). These devices are designed to actively prevent movement at the first MTPJ using rigid orthotic additions extending under the medial column of the foot (such as a Morton's extension), and to reduce the dorsiflexing stress applied to the joint during propulsion and the associated joint pain (Shereff and Baumhauer 1998).

In contrast, functional foot orthoses prescribed for hallux limitus and functional hallux limitus frequently use medial rearfoot posting and device modifications such as a first-ray cut-out or forefoot posting (Nawoczenski et al. 1999; Welsh et al. 2010). Functional foot orthoses are designed to reduce the extent and alter the timing of foot pronation to achieve a stable plantarflexed position of the first metatarsal, facilitate first-MTPJ dorsiflexion for propulsion, and reduce any joint pain. However, despite widespread use of such devices, the premise behind them is largely theoretical (Welsh et al. 2010), and existing research does not support increases in dynamic first-MTPJ dorsiflexion with foot orthotic use (Deland and Williams 2012; Nawoczenski and Ludewig 2004; Welsh et al. 2010).

There is limited research assessing the outcomes of foot orthotic therapy for hallux limitus, hallux rigidus, or functional hallux limitus; however, existing data support their use as a potentially effective long-term conservative intervention to reduce pain and allow a return to previous activity in patients with first-MTPJ symptoms (Grady et al. 2002). In a review of 772 patients with symptomatic hallux limitus, 47% were considered to be treated successfully with either accommodative or functional foot orthoses when, following 12 weeks of therapy, patients reported significant reductions in pain, were able to go back to previous activities, and did not go on to have surgical intervention (Grady et al. 2002). Similarly intervention with prefabricated functional foot orthoses in people with first-MTPJ OA has been shown to significantly reduce pain measured following an 8-week intervention (Welsh et al. 2010). Pain reductions were subsequently sustained or continued to improve over a 24-week period, suggesting orthotic therapy can be used as an effective long-term intervention (Welsh et al. 2010).

Surgical Strategies

Surgical intervention for painful hallux limitus and rigidus is common, with more than 50% of symptomatic cases reported to undergo some form of surgical procedure (Grady et al. 2002). Generally surgical intervention is recommended for symptomatic patients where conservative intervention has been unsuccessful (Deland and Williams 2012). The type of surgical procedure used depends on the extent of osteoarthritic changes. In earlier stages of hallux limitus, joint-sparing procedures including cheilectomy and metatarsal and phalangeal osteotomies are recommended (Beeson 2004; DeCarbo et al. 2011). In more advanced disease, joint-destructive procedures are favoured including implant arthroplasties and arthrodesis (DeCarbo et al. 2011).

Cheilectomy. Of the joint-sparing procedures cheilectomy, usually involving resection of the dorsal third of the metatarsal head together with any peripheral osteophytes, is one of the most common (Seibert and Kadakia 2009). Indications for use of this type of procedure vary in the literature but are generally recommended in patients with early stages of osteoarthritic changes (Beeson 2004). Removal of the impingement at the first MTPJ has been demonstrated to make additional dorsiflexion possible with improvements reported of approximately 20° of dorsiflexion post-operatively (Coughlin and Shurnas 2003a). The procedure is consistently reported to provide long-term pain relief with satisfaction rates of up to, 95% reported; however, better results are seen in patients with a less advanced stage of the condition, and continued degeneration of the joint generally occurs following the procedure (Coughlin and Shurnas 2003a; DeCarbo et al. 2011; Mulier et al. 1999; Seibert and Kadakia 2009).

Phalangeal   Osteotomy. Phalangeal   osteotomy, usually involving a dorsal wedge osteotomy, is used to place the hallux in a more dorsiflexed position relative to the first metatarsal (Seibert and Kadakia 2009). Phalangeal osteotomy is normally used in conjunction with other surgical procedures and is rarely a sole intervention for hallux limitus (Seibert and Kadakia 2009). Originally believed to create additional dorsiflexion capacity, this type of procedure is now suggested to decompress the joint via positioning of the articular surface away from the diseased portion of the metatarsal head and is a successful technique for reducing joint pain (Bonney and Macnab 1952; Thomas and Smith 1999). Long-term follow-up of patient satisfaction following a combination dorsal wedge osteotomy of the proximal phalanx in conjunction with a cheilectomy has been demonstrated to be more successful that a cheilectomy alone, with 96% of patients reporting they would undergo the combined procedure again versus only 73% of patients receiving a cheilectomy (Thomas and Smith 1999).

Proximal and Distal Metatarsal Osteotomies. Proximal and distal metatarsal osteotomies used in the treatment of hallux rigidus are suggested to provide pain relief through correction of excessive first-metatarsal length or elevation or through altering the position of the articular surface of the proximal phalanx on the first metatarsal, allowing greater movement (Coughlin and Shurnas 2003a; Seibert and Kadakia 2009). A large number of different procedures

and techniques for metatarsal osteotomies exist, making comparison of surgical outcomes difficult. Retrospective and prospective evaluation of various distal metatarsal osteotomies has demonstrated high levels of patient satisfaction between 85% and 95% (Roukis et al. 2002). Long-term follow-up (an average of 5.7 years post-surgery) has reported sustained improvement in self-reported levels of pain and satisfaction with the procedure (Oloff and Jhala-Patel 2008). However, metatarsal osteotomies have been linked to high rates of secondary complications including sesamoiditis, lateral forefoot pain, and first-ray instability, which are suggested to reduce long-term efficacy of this procedure (Seibert and Kadakia 2009).

Implant Arthroplasty. Implant arthroplasty involves partial or complete joint replacement at the first MTPJ and is an alternative procedure for end-stage hallux rigidus that is aimed at restoration of function at the first MTPJ rather than joint fusion (DeCarbo et al. 2011). There are a wide variety of types of implant available, resulting in a range of surgical procedures being used and making comparison with other surgical interventions challenging. Success rates following implant surgery are varied, with outcomes relating to pain and function generally found to be inconsistent (DeCarbo et al. 2011; Gibson and Thomson 2005). Earlier studies demonstrated up to 30% of patients experience moderate to severe post-operative pain and high frequency of implant failure (Granberry et al. 1991) and other post-operative complications including pain, osteolysis, and reaction to a foreign body (DeCarbo et al. 2011; Granberry et al. 1991; Pulavarti et al. 2005). Reported improvements in joint function were tempered by evidence of 50% loss of flexion power at the first MTPJ (Vanore et al. 1984) and evidence of iatrogenic hallux limitus and excessive loading of the lesser metatarsals (Freed 1993).

More recent studies are inconclusive. A meta-analysis of patent satisfaction levels following arthroplasty demonstrated 87.5% of patients are satisfied with the surgery (Cook et al. 2009). Similarly a systematic review of pain and function following total joint arthroplasty or arthrodesis measured using the American Orthopedic Foot and Ankle Society-Hallux Metatarsophalangeal-Interphalangeal   (AOFAS-HMI) score demonstrated equivalent improvements for both types of surgeries (Brewster 2010). However, outcomes of a randomized controlled trial comparing pain measured with a VAS following arthrodesis or arthroplasty have demonstrated significantly greater improvements in pain for patients receiving arthrodesis (Gibson and Thomson 2005). These conflicting findings highlight a lack of data relating to long-term outcomes for implant arthroplasty and suggest that currently results of this form of surgery are far less predictable than more widely used procedures such as arthrodesis (Beeson 2004).

Arthrodesis. Arthrodesis is considered the gold standard for end-stage osteoarthritis of the first MTPJ causing hallux rigidus and following failed surgical procedures. The procedure is generally reported to have good outcomes, with successful joint fusion more than 90% of the time, long-term (up to 12 years) post-operative decreases in pain, and long-term improvements in pain (Coughlin and Shurnas 2003a), function (Goucher and Coughlin 2006), and quality of life (Flavin and Stephens 2004). A randomized controlled trial investigating outcomes following arthrodesis or total joint replacement arthroplasty for end-stage hallux rigidus supports joint fusion over preservation of joint movement (Gibson and Thomson 2005). Arthrodesis provided greater reductions in joint pain, fewer surgical complications, lower likelihood of revision, and incurred fewer costs compared with arthroplasty. However, although the available high-level evidence supports use of arthrodesis in favour of arthroplasty for hallux rigidus, further larger-scale investigations over longer timeframes are required before the most effective intervention can be identified with confidence.

HALLUX VALGUS

INTRODUCTION

Hallux valgus is a common, progressive deformity of the forefoot characterized by medial deviation of the first-metatarsal plus lateral deviation and rotation of the hallux (Roddy et al. 2008; Thomas and Barrington 2003). Development of hallux valgus is associated with loss of ligamentous stabilization of the medial aspect of the first MTPJ, and medial drift of the metatarsal head over the medial sesamoid placing the lateral sesamoid in the increased intermetatarsal space (Alvarez et al. 1984; Perera et al. 2011; Suzuki et al. 2004; Uchiyama et al. 2005). As a result there is articular degeneration, erosion of the crista, inflammation of the bursa over the medial aspect of the metatarsal head, and the appearance of lateral displacement of the long flexor and extensor hallucis tendons (Perera et al., 2011; Wheeler and McDougall 1954). Ligamentous and muscular attachments of the proximal phalanx including the adductor hallucis tendon and the deep transverse ligament cause valgus rotation of the proximal phalanx (Perera et al. 2011). Loss of sesamoid stabilization encourages pronation and dorsiflexion of the first metatarsal moving the medial and plantar attachments of abductor hallucis muscle inferiorly, preventing normal resistance to valgus movement of the proximal phalanx and increasing lateral forefoot plantar pressures (Perera et al. 2011).

Hallux valgus is reported as the most common pathology affecting the first MTPJ (Munuera et al. 2008). Prevalence varies widely in the literature and is reported to be up to 70% (Leveille et al. 1998), with differences attributed to differing populations surveyed and the diagnostic criteria for hallux valgus used (Roddy et al. 2008). A meta-analysis of 76 population-based surveys of hallux valgus prevalence involving 496 957 participants reported that the condition affects 23% of adults aged 18–65 and 40% of those over 65, with the incidence is higher in females (Nix et al. 2010). The impact of hallux valgus in the general population is significant with the condition associated with a high incidence of foot pain (Benvenuti et al. 1995), loss of balance and disability (Menz and Lord 2001; Menz et al. 2011), increased risk of falls (Menz and Lord 2001), and reduced quality of life (Menz et al. 2011).

PREDISPOSING FACTORS

Footwear, standing occupations, and excessive weight-bearing are all suggested as possible aetiologies of hallux valgus (Coughlin and Jones 2007). Comparison of shod and unshod populations support the relationship between wearing shoes and hallux valgus (Lazarides et al. 2005; Shine 1965). Long-term use of footwear (60 years) has been shown to be associated with an incidence of hallux valgus of 16% in males and 48% in females, compared with only 2% of people who had not worn shoes (Shine 1965). However, there remains conjecture over the role footwear plays in development of the condition (Coughlin 1995b; Perera et al. 2011). Increased forefoot loading, foot pronation, and compression of the first MTPJ associated with high heels have been proposed to contribute to increased risk of hallux valgus (Corrigan et al. 1993; Perera et al. 2011). Women regularly using high heels between the ages of 20 and 64 years have also been shown to be at increased risk of the condition [risk ratio (RR) 1.2] (Nguyen et al. 2010). However, a lack of consistent occurrence in association with history of high-heel use suggests other contributing factors may be required for the condition to develop (Nix et al. 2010). Similarly, although microtrauma from prolonged weightbearing associated with occupation or recreational activities has been implicated in the development of hallux valgus, there is little research to support the relationship (Cho et al. 2009; Mann and Coughlin 1981).

A large number of intrinsic factors have been proposed as risk factors for the development of hallux valgus. Female gender is associated with a 2.3-fold increase in risk of the condition compared with males, with an incidence in the general population of 30% in females and only 13% in males (Nguyen et al. 2010). There is increased prevalence in older age with an odds ratio (OR) of 1.61 per decade (Nguyen et al. 2010). However, joint changes have been demonstrated in children and adolescents, with juvenile-onset hallux valgus affecting approximately 8% of the population (Nix et al. 2010). Genetic predisposition has been linked to the incidence of hallux valgus in both juvenile and adult populations (Coughlin 1995b; Pique-Vidal et al. 2007). Maternal transmission has been identified in up to 94% of cases of hallux valgus in children and young adults; 90% of white adults have also been shown to have at least one relative affected by the condition, with autosomal dominance with incomplete penetrance identified as the most common pattern of inheritance (Pique-Vidal et al. 2007). Genetic links have been made to inheritable foot type (Bonney and Macnab 1952), and morphology- and gender-based differences in metatarsal articular morphology, including a more adducted first-metatarsal position (Ferrari et al. 2004) and a more rounded

smaller metatarsal head (Ferrari and Malone-Lee 2002) in females, have also been suggested to increase joint instability and account for a higher prevalence of the condition (OR 2.64) (Nguyen et al. 2010).

Foot structure and function have widely been implicated as risk factors for the development of hallux valgus. Specific foot morphologies including metatarsus primus varus (Bryant et al. 2000) and a long or short first metatarsal have all been theoretically linked to the condition; however, definitive relationships have not been identified (Mancuso et al. 2003). Metatarsus primus varus has been suggested to move the insertion of abductor hallucis inferiorly preventing resistance to valgus positioning of the hallux (Humbert et al. 1979). High incidence of metatarsus primus varus has been demonstrated in cases of juvenile hallux valgus (Banks et al. 1994), but is less common in association with hallux valgus in adults (Coughlin and Jones 2007) and it remains unknown whether the condition precedes or follows the development of hallux valgus.

Both a short and a long first metatarsal have been suggested as possible aetiologies for hallux valgus. A short first metatarsal has been suggested to encourage first-ray pronation and hypermobility creating an unstable medial column of the foot (Root et al. 1977). There is little evidence to support such an association (Coughlin and Jones 2007); however, high incidence of a long first metatarsal in people with hallux valgus has been reported (Mancuso et al. 2003). A long first metatarsal relative to the second metatarsal has been suggested to create a buckle point and an associated high intermetatarsal angle (Heden and Sorto Jr 1981). This contributes to joint instability and strain on medial ligamentous structures whilst the increased length is proposed to prevent normal first-metatarsal plantarflexion, causing jamming at the first MTPJ and encouraging joint subluxation (Root et al. 1977). It has been proposed that restriction of dorsiflexion at the first MTPJ from an excessively long first metatarsal, metatarsus primus elevates, or hypermobility of the first ray is likely to encourage lateral deviation of the hallux. This will be exacerbated when associated with a rounded first-metatarsal head due to inherent joint instability associated with this articular morphology (Okuda et al. 2007).

Theoretical links have been made between the function of the first ray, foot pronation, and functional restriction of the first MTPJ and the development of hallux valgus (Greenberg 1979). First-ray hypermobility has been proposed to occur as a result of tarsometatarsal joint instability (David et al. 1989). In turn, instability at the tarsometatarsal joint has been associated with a number of factors including an excessively long or short metatarsal and, perhaps most frequently, excessive foot pronation (Dananberg 1986). Regardless of the cause, tarsometatarsal joint instability is theorized to allow movement of the first ray during loading, causing a dorsiflexed position of the first metatarsal, and limiting first-MTPJ dorsiflexion creating a functional hallux limitus (Dananberg 1986; Roukis et al. 1996). The resistance to sagittal plane movement at the first MTPJ during propulsion is suggested to produce compensatory joint motion in other planes (Dananberg 1986). The presence of hypermobility of the first ray is proposed to allow more compensatory movement of the head of the first metatarsal and increase the risk of hallux valgus (Scherer et al. 2006). The dorsiflexed position of the first metatarsal also produces medial column instability and subsequent first-ray pronation, which increases load medially on the hallux, creating a valgus force (Dananberg 1986). The altered position of the first metatarsal prevents stabilization of the first ray by peroneus longus and weightbearing under the first MTPJ is reduced (Donatelli 1985).

In the case of an excessively pronated rearfoot, pronation moves the forefoot in an abducted position relative to the line of weightbearing, increasing force on the medial aspect of the first MTPJ and hallux during propulsion (Perera et al. 2011). Excessive firing of abductor and adductor hallucis in conjunction with an altered line of pull due to the abnormal position of the first metatarsal creates a valgus moment at the hallux (Iida and Basmajian 1974). The altered propulsive mechanics (Shereff et al. 1986) result in an increased strain on medial ligamentous structures at the first MTPJ.

Excessive foot pronation has also been suggested to contribute to the development of hallux valgus via increased tension on the plantar fascia caused by flattening of the medial longitudinal arch (Perera et al. 2011). As with its proposed role in the development of a functional hallux limitus, flattening of the medial longitudinal arch during propulsion is proposed to increase tension on the fascia, increasing the plantarflexing moment the fascia produces at the first MTPJ. The increased plantarflexing moment opposes the dorsiflexing moment produced by ground reaction forces acting on the hallux, preventing instigation of the windlass mechanism and reducing stability of the medial column of the foot during propulsion, with the hallux suggested to then move along a 'path of least resistance' into a valgus position (Perera et al. 2011).

Currently, research investigating the relationship between excessive foot pronation and hallux valgus is inconclusive. Foot pronation has been associated with pronation of the first ray, which may alter the relative position of the sesamoids causing overloading of the medial sesamoid and increasing the strain on ligamentous structures on the medial aspect of the joint (Eustace et al. 1993). Furthermore, first-metatarsal pronation has been demonstrated to occur in conjunction with medial longitudinal arch flattening and to be associated with a higher intermetatarsal angle and hallux valgus (Eustace et al. 1993). However, there is yet to be any direct link established in the literature between foot pronation and increased risk of hallux valgus.

DIAGNOSIS

Clinical practice guidelines for diagnosis of hallux valgus suggest using a combination of patient history, clinical assessment, and radiographic findings (Vanore et al. 2003b). Patient history typically involves a familial history of hallux valgus, with onset generally in older age and presence of pain associated with the medial subcutaneous bursa (Coughlin 1995b; Hardy and Clapham 1951; Vanore et al. 2003b). Clinical findings include varying degrees of first-MTPJ deformity characterized by lateral deviation of the hallux, which may be accompanied by valgus rotation, a bony prominence on the medial aspect of the joint, and medial subcutaneous bursitis and/or neuritis of the medial dorsal cutaneous nerve due to footwear irritation (Eustace et al. 1993; Perera et al. 2011; Wheeler and McDougall 1954). Common secondary findings include hammer-toe deformity of the second digit with possible plantar plate rupture, second-MTPJ subluxation, and over- or under-riding of the hallux (Coughlin 1987). Altered first-MTPJ loading is also associated with weight transfer to the lesser MTPJs, which commonly manifests as second-MTPJ pain or more generalized lateral forefoot pain with accompanying plantar hyperkeratosis (Gibbs and Boxer 1982; Raymakers and Waugh 1971). Proposed biomechanical risk factors, including an excessively pronated foot type or ankle equinus, may also be present on gait analysis (Shaw 1974; Yu et al. 1987).

Radiographical evaluation is used to assess presence and severity of the deformity (Vanore et al. 2003b). Generally a hallux abductus angle (the angle formed between the longitudinal bisections of the first metatarsal and the proximal phalanx of the hallux) of more than 15° is considered diagnostic of hallux valgus (Hardy and Clapham 1951; Piggott 1960). However, other radiographic measurements are used for detailed pre-surgical classification of the extent of the deformity (Smith et al. 1984). These most commonly assess relative position of the first metatarsal to the second metatarsal (intermetatarsal angle) and the hallux abductus interphalangeus angle (the angle formed by the longitudinal bisections of the hallucal proximal and distal phalanges), with angles greater than 10° considered abnormal in both cases (Judge et al. 1999; Menz and Munteanu 2005; Piggott 1960; Vanore et al. 2003b; Wheeler and McDougall 1954). Excellent intra- and inter-tester reliability has been reported for the hallux abductus angle (ICC: 0.87) and intermetatarsal angle (ICC: 0.96), and very good for the hallux abductus interphalangeus angle (ICC: 0.77). However, variations in measurement techniques have been suggested to potentially affect reliability (Kilmartin et al. 1992).

Non-radiographic classification of hallux valgus staging may be performed using the Manchester Scale, a clinical tool using photographs of feet with a separate picture representing four classifications: no deformity, mild deformity, moderate deformity, and severe deformity (Garrow et al. 2001) (Figure 4-1A–D). The Manchester Scale has been demonstrated to have excellent inter- and intra-tester reliability (Garrow et al. 2001; Menz et al. 2003). Good validity of the scale has also been determined with high correlation between visually determined categories and radiographical measures of the hallux abductus angle (Spearman's $\rho=0.73$) and moderate correlation with the intermetatarsal angle ($\rho=0.49$), suggesting the

scale is a useful tool for non-invasive grading of hallux valgus for clinical purposes (Menz and Munteanu 2005).

IMPAIRMENTS

Hallux valgus is associated with pain causing restricted function and loss of range of motion. Early states of hallux valgus are characterized by intermittent appearance of symptoms and no restriction of normal activities (Bonney and Macnab 1952). Range of motion is reduced at the first MTPJ but may be in only one direction. In later stages of the condition symptoms become more constant with loss of dorsiflexion and plantarflexion, progressing to joint ankylosis (Bonney and Macnab 1952). Primary concerns of patients with the condition relate to impairment of walking, joint pain, and difficulty with footwear fitting (Tai et al. 2008).

FUNCTION

Hallux valgus is associated with a reduction in physical function on measures of health-related quality of life (Cho et al. 2009; Lazarides et al. 2005; Menz et al. 2011), and gait changes as a result of the condition have been suggested to contribute to increased risk of falls in elderly populations (Pavol et al. 1999). Evidence of shorter step length and slower walking speed over irregular surfaces in an older population with hallux valgus support this proposal (Menz and Lord 2005). However, these changes have been shown only in relation to uneven terrain and have not been demonstrated in investigations on flat surfaces in cohorts, older or otherwise (Deschamps et al. 2010; Mickle et al. 2011).

There is limited research assessing kinematic changes related to the condition. Existing research suggests hallux valgus is associated with changes to propulsive phase of gait, with three-dimensional motion analysis demonstrating reduced hallux range of motion (Canseco et al. 2010; Deschamps et al. 2010) and less internal rotation of the rearfoot relative to the tibia during propulsion (Deschamps et al. 2010). Reduced hallux motion is consistent with loss of range of motion due to osteoarthritic change associated with the condition and, potentially, subsequent failure of the windlass mechanism to raise the medial longitudinal arch and create a rigid lever for

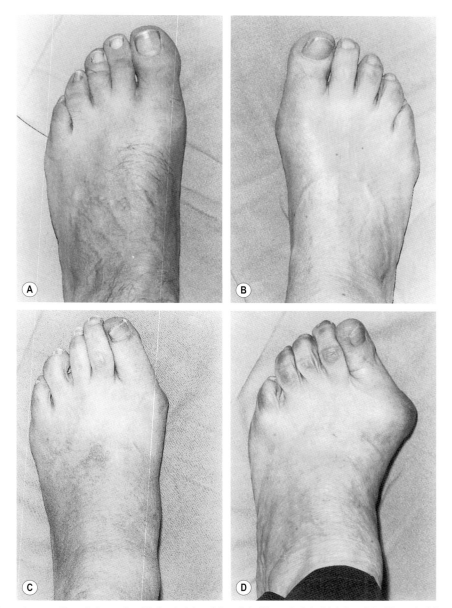

FIGURE 4-1 Hallux valgus grading photographs. (A) Grade 1 (no deformity); (B) grade 2 (mild deformity); (C) grade 3 (moderate deformity); (D) grade 4 (severe deformity).

propulsion. Furthermore, the lack of resupination suggested by the reduction in internal rotation of the rearfoot suggests prolonged foot pronation and supports a link between excessive pronation and first-ray hypermobility contributing to the development of hallux valgus.

A number of studies have investigated the effect of hallux valgus on plantar pressures; however, reported changes are inconsistent. Peak pressure under the first MTPJ has been variously reported to be significantly increased (Bryant et al. 1999; Mickle et al. 2011), significantly decreased (Komeda et al. 2001), and no different in people with hallux valgus (Martinez-Nova et al. 2010). Similarly, findings of changes under the lesser metatarsal heads are inconsistent. There is evidence of higher peak pressures under the lesser metatarsal heads (Bryant et al. 1999) and a centre of pressure pathway indicating lateral forefoot pressure during propulsion (Tokita et al. 1991), and equally studies demonstrating no differences in lesser metatarsal pressures (Komeda et al. 2001; Mickle et al. 2011). These inconclusive results have been suggested to be due to lack of heterogeneity in severity of hallux valgus with plantar pressures potentially altering according to the severity of the condition, inconsistent avoidance strategies used in the presence of associated foot pain, anatomical differences between individuals such as metatarsal morphology affecting pressure distribution, and differing plantar pressure measurement systems used for data collection (Nix et al. 2013). Based on current evidence, it is not possible to determine any changes in plantar pressures that occur consistently with the condition.

QUALITY OF LIFE

Research investigating the impact of hallux valgus on quality of life has demonstrated the condition is associated with poorer general and health-related quality of life outcomes independent of other factors including age, sex, body mass index, and other bodily pain. Several studies have assessed the impact of hallux valgus on general quality of life using the Short Form 36 (SF-36) (Lazarides et al. 2005; Menz et al. 2011). Increases in severity of hallux valgus determined by radiographic evaluation is associated with worsening quality of life outcomes, with higher hallux abductus angle significantly affecting scores for general health, and higher intermetatarsal angle associated with measures of poorer role-physical, role-emotional, and mental health subscale scores (Lazarides et al. 2005).

In a survey of 2831 people aged 56 years or over, the presence of hallux valgus was associated with significantly lower scores across all subscales of the SF-36, with poorer outcomes for hallux valgus sufferers for general health, physical function, bodily pain, mental health, vitality, social function, and role-physical and role-emotional subscales (Menz et al. 2011). Severity of hallux valgus was determined using

a validated self-assessment tool where participants compare the severity of their own hallux valgus to five line drawings depicting increasing severity of the condition, choosing the picture most closely resembling their own foot (Roddy et al. 2007). Significant decreases in scores for all subscales of the SF-36 apart from the role-physical and role-emotional subscales were demonstrated with increasing severity of the condition (Menz et al. 2011). Differences between scores for physical function, bodily pain, and general health were consistently approximately 5 points higher (indicating less severe impairment) in sufferers in the earliest stage of the condition (physical function 63.7, bodily pain 58.2, and general health 61.2) compared with those with the most severe deformity (physical function 58.4, bodily pain 52.0, and general health 55.5). Concurrent investigation of foot-specific quality of life was performed using the Manchester Foot Pain and Disability Index (Menz et al. 2011). The Manchester Foot Pain and Disability Index consists of questions relating to the pain intensity, functional limitation, and appearance. Consistent with the findings of the SF-36, participants with more severe hallux valgus deformity demonstrated poorer scores for pain and function, leading the authors to suggest that interventions that could halt or slow progression of the condition could have more extensive benefits than localized joint pain reduction (Menz et al. 2011).

MANAGEMENT STRATEGIES
Physical Strategies

There is currently no accepted protocol for the provision of conservative care for hallux valgus (du Plessis et al. 2011). Treatment options including manual therapy, manipulation, splinting, shoe modifications, interdigital wedges, and padding are suggested to help alleviate symptoms (du Plessis et al. 2011; Hart et al. 2008; Tehraninasr et al. 2008; Torkki et al. 2003). However, there have been few trials investigating the efficacy of such interventions. Juriansz (1996) assessed the effect of night splints (plastic splints used to pull the hallux into the correct position) worn for 6 months versus no treatment on hallux valgus angle and pain. Neither outcome was significantly different from the no-treatment group following completion. Outcomes of a small trial investigating the effect of 4 weeks of mobilization versus night splints suggests mobilization may provide more sustained improvement in foot function and pain, with night splints associated with regression to baseline levels of pain and loss of function (du Plessis et al. 2011). However, more extensive research is required to determine benefits of mobilization and night splints as well as other physical therapy interventions.

Footwear and Foot Orthoses. Management of hallux valgus with accommodative footwear requires extra-depth and extra-width shoes (Robinson and Limbers 2005). High heels and narrow toe boxes are suggested to force the toe into further valgus and exacerbate symptoms (Hart et al. 2008). Conservative care with footwear is recommended in cases of neurological or vascular compromise, in children with open physes, and where surgical intervention is contraindicated, for example due to old age or poor healing (Hart et al. 2008; Robinson and Limbers 2005).

Several trials have assessed the effect of foot orthoses on the prevention and progression of hallux valgus deformity and pain associated with the condition (Budiman-Mak et al. 1995; Kilmartin et al. 1994). Theoretical links between excessive foot pronation and the development of hallux valgus suggest that foot orthoses may have a role in preventing development and progression of the deformity. Current research is conflicting and limited to specific populations (Budiman-Mak et al. 1995; Kilmartin et al. 1994). Long-term intervention of foot orthoses in cases of active rheumatoid arthritis has shown foot orthoses to be associated with a lower risk of developing the condition compared with a control group (adjusted OR 0.27) (Budiman-Mak et al. 1995). However, the use of foot orthoses in cases of juvenile hallux valgus has been demonstrated to be of no benefit in preventing its progression (Kilmartin et al. 1994). Kilmartin et al. (1994) investigated the effect of foot orthoses on hallux abductus angle over a 3-year period in children aged 10–14 years. Over the course of the study the condition deteriorated at a similar rate in children treated with foot orthoses as in those not treated. Furthermore, children initially presenting with unilateral deformity developed the condition bilaterally regardless of whether they wore orthoses or not (Kilmartin et al. 1994).

High-quality investigations of the effects of foot orthoses on levels of pain from hallux valgus are similarly scarce. Pain pre- and post-intervention has been measured in several randomized controlled trials but outcomes do not support the use of orthoses as a long-term intervention for pain reduction (Kilmartin et al. 1994; Torkki et al. 2001). Compared with no treatment, pain associated with mild or moderate hallux valgus has been shown to reduce temporarily with foot orthoses but return to pre-intervention levels by 12 months (Torkki et al. 2001). Based on current research, foot orthoses intended specifically to reduce pain from this condition have limited value.

Surgical Strategies

Indications for surgical correction of hallux valgus include painful progressive deformity and limitation of activity (Hart et al. 2008). Approximately 150 different surgical procedures have been developed to reduce the severity of the deformity and restore joint function (Ferrari et al. 2009). Surgical correction usually involves a combination of soft-tissue and osseous procedures (Hart et al. 2008). Surgical procedures are aimed at increasing first-MTPJ congruency, reducing the radiographic changes associated with the condition, including the hallux valgus angle and intermetatarsal angle, and correcting sesamoid position (Hart et al. 2008; Robinson and Limbers 2005). Generally this requires a combination of procedures that may include soft-tissue realignment to alter the action of muscles and ligamentous structures, proximal phalanx resection to decompress the joint (Keller's procedure), first-metatarsal osteotomy, and arthrodesis of the first tarsometatarsal joint (Lapidus procedure) or the first MTPJ (Hart et al. 2008; Robinson and Limbers 2005).

Osteotomy may be performed on any part of the metatarsal. Distal osteotomies are more commonly used in earlier stages of the deformity, with intermediate diaphyseal and proximal osteotomies allowing greater correction of the intermetatarsal angle but, as more invasive procedures, requiring increased healing time (Robinson and Limbers 2005). Joint range of motion is increased or may be removed in the presence of extensive joint degeneration (arthrodesis), when associated with a neuromuscular disorder, systemic arthritis, or following a failed surgical procedure

TABLE 4-2   Operative Techniques for Hallux Valgus Surgery

Techniques	Sub-types	Description
Akin osteotomy (Akin 1925)		A medial closing wedge osteotomy of the proximal phalanx of the hallux with excision of protruding medial condylar eminence
Distal soft-tissue procedure (McBride 1928; Silver 1923)		The adductor hallucis and lateral joint capsule are released with the excision of the medial eminence of first metatarsal and plication of the medial joint capsule
Keller's (1904) procedure		Approximately ⅓ of proximal phalanx is resected to correct the deformity
Proximal (basal) osteotomies of the first metatarsal (allows a greater degree of correction for more severe deformities)	Proximal wedge osteotomy	Opening wedge: a single transverse cut allows opening of the wedge, lengthens the metatarsal and can require a bone graft (Threthowan 1923) Closing wedge: a V-shaped cut allows removal of a wedge of bone and leads to shortening of the metatarsal (Resch et al. 1989; Trnka et al. 1999)
	Crescentic osteotomy (Mann et al. 1992)	A crescentic cut, distal to the metatarsocuneiform joint, with the concavity proximal, allows the distal metatarsal shaft to be rotated laterally
	Proximal chevron osteotomy (Sammarco et al. 1993)	A V-shaped cut at the medial proximal metatarsal allows the shaft to be rotated laterally
Distal osteotomies of the first metatarsal (mild or moderate deformities)	Wilson procedure (Helal et al. 1974; Wilson 1963)	An oblique metaphyseal osteotomy from distal medial to proximal lateral allows displacement of the metatarsal head laterally and proximally to correct IMA and HVA
	Mitchell osteotomy (Mitchell et al. 1958)	A double step cut osteotomy through the metatarsal neck, displacing the head fragment laterally and plantarwards
	Distal chevron osteotomy (Corless 1976)	A V-shaped cut at the metatarsal neck allows lateral displacement of the metatarsal head
Intermediate diaphyseal osteotomies (if IMA between 14° and 20°)	Scarf procedure (Barouk 2000; Meyer 1926; Weil and Borelli 1991)	A Z-shaped step cut along the diaphysis followed by lateral translation of the distal metatarsal fragment to correct the IMA
	Modified Ludloff procedure (Chiodo et al. 2004; Ludloff 1918)	Longitudinal oblique osteotomy at 30° to the long axis of the diaphysis allows lateral rotation of the distal fragment to correct the IMA
Arthrodeses	First-MTPJ arthrodesis (Coughlin et al. 2005)	Surgical fixation by varied techniques (screws, wires, staples, plates)
	First tarsometatarsal joint arthrodesis – modified Lapidus (1934)	Surgical fixation of first tarsometatarsal joint with closing wedge osteotomy of medial cuneiform

HVA=hallux abducto valgus; IMA=intermetatarsal angle.

(Hart et al. 2008). A more detailed overview of common surgical procedures is provided in Table 4-2.

The expectations of patients seeking surgical intervention for hallux valgus are primarily to improve walking, have their pain alleviated, and return to normal footwear (Tai et al. 2008). Outcomes of surgical interventions are highly variable owing to the wide range of procedures used; however, patient dissatisfaction rates are approximately 25% regardless of the type of procedure used (Ferrari et al. 2009), and only

60% of patients are unrestricted in their footwear choice post-surgery (Mann and Pfeffinger 1991). Furthermore, review of comparative studies of different types of osteotomy procedures indicates that, based on current literature, there is no significant benefit in terms of pain reduction or deformity correction associated with any one technique (Ferrari et al. 2009). However, there is some evidence to suggest surgical intervention is superior to conservative care (Torkki et al. 2001); investigation of hallux valgus surgery using a chevron osteotomy procedure versus functional foot orthoses or no treatment in people with mild to moderate hallux valgus has demonstrated that surgery provides a significant reduction in pain 12 months post-intervention, whereas foot orthoses are no better than no treatment for the same time period.

Risk of post-surgical complications from hallux valgus surgery has been reported to occur in more than 35% of cases (Coetzee 2003) and is an important consideration prior to undergoing any type of procedure (Sammarco and Idusuyi 2001). Common complications include infection, recurrence of the deformity, avascular necrosis of the head of the first metatarsal in association with distal osteotomy procedures, overcorrection causing hallux varus, first-metatarsal shortening, increased pain, sensory loss, and metatarsal malunion or non-union (Coetzee 2003; Coughlin 1997; Hart et al. 2008; Robinson and Limbers 2005; Sammarco and Idusuyi 2001). Therefore, although surgery for hallux valgus has been demonstrated to be more beneficial than conservative care (Torkki et al. 2001), adequate patient counselling in relation to patient expectations and possible surgical outcomes is required prior to this form of intervention (Hart et al. 2008; Tai et al. 2008).

PLANTAR INTERMETATARSAL NERVE COMPRESSION (MORTON'S NEUROMA)

INTRODUCTION

Metatarsalgia encompasses a diverse range of pathologies that present with pain in the plantar region of the metatarsal heads, particularly the second to fourth metatarsal heads (Espinosa et al. 2010; Fuhrmann et al. 2005). Underlying pathologies include plantar intermetatarsal nerve compression (Morton's

neuroma), synovitis, capsulitis, bursitis, tendinosis of the digit flexors or forefoot, and intrinsic, stress, or acute fracture, Freiberg infarction, or one of many types of arthritis (Gregg et al. 2008). The first step towards clinical success when addressing cases of metatarsalgia is to identify the principal pathology so that a precise diagnosis can be made and treatment tailored accordingly. The following section provides a detailed review of plantar intermetatarsal nerve entrapment, a common underlying cause of chronic metatarsalgia.

Symptoms characteristically present unilaterally and in isolation, though bilateral cases and the occurrence of more than one lesion in one foot have been reported (Lee et al. 2009; Thomson et al. 2004). Case series reports consistently identify the third intermetatarsal space (between the third and fourth metatarsals) as being the most commonly affected, accounting for between 64% and 91% of cases (Addante et al. 1986; Bartolomei and Wertheimer 1983; Bennett et al. 1995; Friscia et al. 1991; Pastides et al. 2012). The second interspace is also commonly affected (18–29% of cases reported), yet rarely is the fourth interspace (3–6%) or the first interspace (0–2.5%) (Clinical Practice Guideline Forefoot Disorders et al. 2009b; Pastides et al. 2012). The predominance of the third interspace may be due to the presence of a communicating branch between the third and fourth plantar intermetatarsal nerves, which was identified by Govsa et al. (2005) in 28% of 50 adult male cadaveric feet.

PREVALENCE

No large and recent epidemiological study has been conducted to determine the prevalence or incidence of plantar intermetatarsal nerve compression in a randomly selected sample. Though it is regarded in the literature as a 'common' diagnosis (Adams 2010), there is insufficient evidence to determine the prevalence of the condition. A recent Cochrane Collaboration systematic review of interventions for Morton's neuroma included a hospital activity analysis to estimate prevalence of Morton's neuroma in Scotland (population approximately 5 200 000). In the year 1999/2000 there were 139 inpatient and day-case discharges following operations for Morton's neuroma (Thomson et al. 2004). Obviously, this figure does not include people who did not seek treatments, who received non-surgical intervention only, and who were imprecisely recorded in hospital data sets.

Iagnocco et al. (2001) performed diagnostic ultrasound on 112 people with metatarsalgia to determine the underlying pathologies. Signs of 'Morton's neuroma' were present in 15% of cases. Other common pathologies included intermetatarsophalangeal joint bursitis (21% of cases) and MTPJ effusion (12% of cases) (Iagnocco et al. 2001). Although this study is of some value in determining the relative contribution of plantar intermetatarsal nerve compression to cases of metatarsalgia, it cannot be used to estimate the prevalence of plantar intermetatarsal nerve compression in the general population as the prevalence of metatarsalgia is unknown. Retrospective audits of clinical records reveal that more females seek treatment for plantar intermetatarsal nerve compression than males (Bartolomei and Wertheimer 1983; Park et al. 2011; Rout et al. 2009). The condition almost exclusively occurs in adults, and is reported to be most prevalent between ages 45 and 65 years (Clinical Practice Guideline Forefoot Disorders et al. 2009b; Rout et al. 2009).

PREDISPOSING FACTORS

There is a paucity of evidence regarding factors that predispose individuals to developing plantar intermetatarsal nerve compression. Evidence is limited to observational studies of case series and anecdotal reports. Factors suggested to be associated with plantar intermetatarsal nerve compression include wearing narrow, high-heeled shoes (Summers 2010), equinus deformity (Barrett and Jarvis 2005), obesity (Bartolomei and Wertheimer 1983), trauma (Barrett and Walsh 2006), increased forefoot plantar pressure associated with diabetes (Adams 2010), abnormal forefoot alignment (e.g. forefoot varus or valgus) (Bartolomei and Wertheimer 1983), and subtalar joint pronation (Root et al. 1977). None of these factors has been adequately investigated to determine their contribution to plantar intermetatarsal nerve compression.

IMPAIRMENT AND FUNCTION

There is no dependable evidence of the impact of plantar intermetatarsal nerve compression. There are anecdotal reports of affected persons stopping activity to remove footwear and manipulate the forefoot or toes (Rout et al. 2009; Thomson et al. 2004) and of becoming apprehensive about walking or even putting their foot to the ground (Thomson et al. 2004).

QUALITY OF LIFE

The wider impact of plantar intermetatarsal nerve compression on important health outcomes such as health-related quality of life and participation in activities of daily living is unknown.

DIAGNOSIS

Diagnosis of plantar intermetatarsal nerve compression is typically made clinically based on history and physical examination (Adams 2010; Lallemand et al. 2003). Diagnostic imaging can be used to exclude differential diagnoses and to confirm plantar intermetatarsal nerve compression when results of clinical assessment are unclear (Pastides et al. 2012).

Physical Examination

Pain is typically reproduced on direct palpation of the intermetatarsal space (Clinical Practice Guideline Forefoot Disorders et al. 2009b). In a retrospective case series (Pastides et al. 2012) of 43 instances of plantar intermetatarsal nerve compression surgically excised from 36 patients over 68 months, direct palpation reproduced tenderness in all cases. The authors reported that care should be taken to palpate in the intermetatarsal space, not directly over the MTPJ (Clinical Practice Guideline Forefoot Disorders et al. 2009b). Direct palpation of the nerve may also invoke Tinel's sign or Valleix phenomenon (Clinical Practice Guideline Forefoot Disorders et al. 2009b). Sensory deficit is rarely noted on neurological assessment and little or no oedema is usually apparent (Clinical Practice Guideline Forefoot Disorders et al. 2009b). The adjacent digits may be splayed (Clinical Practice Guideline Forefoot Disorders et al. 2009b), yet this may be obvious only when the affected foot is weightbearing.

Various physical manoeuvres can be used to help diagnose plantar intermetatarsal nerve compression. These include the web space compression test, Mulder's click, and Bratkowski's sign (Bratkowski 1978; Clinical Practice Guideline Forefoot Disorders et al. 2009b; Mulder 1951).

The web space compression test, also called Gauthier's test, is performed by squeezing together the first to fifth metatarsal heads with one hand while pinching the involved web-space between the thumb and forefinger of the contralateral hand. A positive web space compression test produces severe pain and is suggestive of Morton's neuroma (Clinical Practice Guideline Forefoot Disorders et al. 2009b; Rout et al. 2009). This may also produce pain and paraesthesia in the adjacent toes. Upon performing the web space compression test, an audible or palpable click or pop may be noticed (Adams 2010). This phenomenon was first described by Jacob Mulder in 1951 and now bears his name (Mulder 1951). The click or clunk is suggested to occur with plantar displacement of the nerve between the metatarsal heads (Adams 2010; Rosenberg and Sferra 1998). In an ultrasonographic study of people with plantar intermetatarsal nerve compression and asymptomatic controls, Mulder's click was associated with intermetatarsal nerve width greater than 5 mm (Symeonidis et al. 2012). Bratkowski (1978) described the technique of extending the affected metatarsophalangeal joints to their end ranges and palpating the symptomatic intermetatarsal space. In cases of plantar intermetatarsal nerve compression, a tender, thickened, longitudinal mass may be palpable.

There is a lack of high-quality data on the sensitivity or specificity of these physical manoeuvres to diagnose plantar intermetatarsal nerve compression. In a retrospective case series (Owens et al. 2011) of 76 feet that underwent surgery for plantar intermetatarsal nerve compression, physical examination revealed web space tenderness in 95% of cases, pain on lateral compression of the metatarsal heads in 88% of cases, positive response to plantar percussion in 61% of cases, and sensation deficit when on tip toe in 67% of cases.

Diagnostic Imaging

Ultrasound. Ultrasonography is used widely for assisting the diagnosis of plantar intermetatarsal nerve compression (Fazal et al. 2012) and is recommended as the imaging modality of choice (Pastides et al. 2012). In many regions, ultrasonography is readily accessible and much less expensive than other soft-tissue imaging modalities [e.g. magnetic resonance imaging (MRI)]. Plantar intermetatarsal nerve compression is best observed on the coronal view (Kankanala and Jain 2007) and appears as an ovoid, hypoechoic mass parallel to, but not abutting, adjacent metatarsals (Beggs 1999; Park et al. 2011). Clarity of mass margination is inconsistent between cases (Park et al. 2011). The interdigital nerve may appear thickened (>5 mm) though this is in itself not diagnostic as nerve thickening has been identified in asymptomatic controls, particularly among elderly people (Symeonidis et al. 2012). 'Gingko leaf sign' (the appearance of a biconcave shape of the mass due to compression from adjacent structures) may also be apparent. In Park et al's (2011) ultrasonographic study of 14 cases of plantar intermetatarsal nerve compression, 10 of the cases demonstrated gingko leaf sign; this sign was not seen in any other forefoot pathology investigated and the authors suggested that this sign might be specific to plantar intermetatarsal nerve compression. Plantar intermetatarsal nerve compression may also be visualized using dynamic ultrasound, in which the mass is imaged as the metatarsal heads are squeezed together by the sonographer (Perini et al. 2006). The American Journal of Roentgenology provides an excellent online video outlining the use of ultrasonography in diagnosing plantar intermetatarsal nerve compression (Lee 2009).

There are few reports of the diagnostic accuracy of ultrasonography for plantar intermetatarsal nerve compression. Some authors have retrospectively analysed case series to establish the accuracy of initial ultrasonography in patients who eventually underwent surgical intervention. Kankanala and Jain (2007) reported a retrospective analysis of 48 cases of plantar intermetatarsal nerve compression to explore the diagnostic accuracy of ultrasound findings when compared with post-operative histopathology findings (Kankanala and Jain 2007). There was 91% sensitivity, 100% specificity, 100% positive predictive value, and 20% negative predictive value. In similar retrospective studies of surgically confirmed cases of plantar intermetatarsal nerve compression, Fazal et al. (2012) identified 24 of 25 cases on ultrasound (sensitivity 96%) and Pastides et al. (2012) identified 28 of 31 cases on ultrasound (90% sensitivity); in this study, ultrasound was reported to be of slightly higher sensitivity than MRI, particularly for nerves less than

5 mm diameter. Although ultrasound is sensitive, Sharp et al. (2003) reported that ultrasound had poor specificity for lesions <6 mm diameter and therefore carried a risk of false positives, particularly when used as a single modality for diagnosis.

Magnetic Resonance Imaging. MRI is generally less accessible and more expensive than ultrasound and has been recommended for atypical presentations and to rule out multiple nerve lesions (Clinical Practice Guideline Forefoot Disorders et al. 2009b). Plantar intermetatarsal nerve compression appears as a well-demarcated mass of low signal intensity on T1- and T2-weighted images (Mendicino and Rockett 1997). The low signal intensity results from the fibrous content and differentiates plantar intermetatarsal nerve compression from nerve neoplasm (e.g. schwannoma) or bursitis, which have high signal intensity (Timins 2000). In Pastides and colleagues' retrospective case series review of 16 surgically confirmed cases of plantar intermetatarsal nerve compression that were imaged with MRI, MRI had a sensitivity of 88% (Pastides et al. 2012).

Plain Film Radiographs. The visibility of plantar intermetatarsal nerve compression on X-ray is disputed and at best inconsistent. In cases of plantar intermetatarsal nerve compression, X-ray may detect no obvious pathology (Clinical Practice Guideline Forefoot Disorders et al. 2009b; Grace et al. 1993) or a faint radiopaque shadow (Wu 1996). Splaying of the digits may also be apparent on images taken while weightbearing (Sullivan 1967). X-ray can be used to investigate potential aetiology (e.g. close proximity of adjacent metatarsal heads) (Clinical Practice Guideline Forefoot Disorders et al. 2009b).

Histomorphological Examination

Although histomorphological examination is considered by many to be the gold standard diagnostic test for plantar intermetatarsal nerve compression, there are no diagnostic criteria, histopathological findings are inconsistent and histomorphology is rarely referred for unless the nerve is surgically resected (Thomson et al. 2004). Cases of plantar intermetatarsal nerve compression may present with endoneural, epineural, and perineural fibrosis, demyelination, and densely packed whorls of collagen called Renaut bodies (Rosenberg and Sferra 1998; Valente et al. 2008), yet these abnormalities are not isolated to plantar intermetatarsal nerve compression and in one study there was no consistent histopathological difference between symptomatic cases and asymptomatic controls (Bourke et al. 1994).

Neurodiagnostics

Regional block with local anaesthetic can provide useful diagnostic information (Clinical Practice Guideline Forefoot Disorders et al. 2009b), though is not routinely performed. Electromyography and nerve conduction testing have been recommended when symptoms of plantar intermetatarsal nerve compression are suspected to arise from a proximal nerve lesion or regional/systemic nerve dysfunction (Rosenberg and Sferra 1998). Uludag et al. (2010) reported a new electrodiagnostic test for plantar intermetatarsal nerve compression; in four cases of plantar intermetatarsal nerve compression and 20 asymptomatic controls, they demonstrated that interlatency differences between branches of the common plantar interdigital nerves were abnormal in all patients. A larger study is required to establish the sensitivity and specificity of this diagnostic test.

MANAGEMENT STRATEGIES

There is no consensus on the best approach to managing plantar intermetatarsal nerve compression (Adams 2010; Rout et al. 2009; Schreiber et al. 2011). The evidence base is starkly incomplete and treatment practices differ greatly among health practitioners. Individualized treatment regimens are encouraged to account for differences in aetiologies, activities of daily living, and resources (Espinosa et al. 2010). A protocol of stepped care is generally accepted, in which treatment begins with the most conservative options and escalates incrementally if treatment response is insufficient (Clinical Practice Guideline Forefoot Disorders et al.; Kunze and Wulker 2011; Rout et al. 2009). In a recent review of the literature, Schreiber et al. (2011) concluded that the strongest evidence supported a stepped care protocol of: (step 1) patient education and footwear or insole changes, (step 2) corticosteroid changes, and (step 3) surgery. Conservative treatments are reported anecdotally to be effective in most cases (Lallemand et al. 2003), though empirical evidence is lacking.

A systematic review of all randomized controlled trials evaluating surgical and non-surgical interventions for Morton's neuroma in adults was published in 2004 (Thomson et al. 2004). Only three randomized controlled trials that included a total of 121 participants were eligible for inclusion (Colgrove et al. 2000; Kilmartin and Wallace 1994; Nashi et al. 1997). Participants were predominantly female and the mean age of participants in each study ranged from 43 to 53 years, which reflects what is known of plantar intermetatarsal nerve compression prevalence in the general population. In the two studies that reported diagnostic criteria, diagnosis was made on patient history and physical examination, and was not supported by diagnostic imaging or histomorphology. Interventions evaluated were 'supinatory and pronatory insoles' (foot orthoses) (Kilmartin and Wallace 1994), excision of the nerve through dorsal or plantar incision (Nashi et al. 1997), and transaction and transposition of the nerve (Colgrove et al. 2000). The primary outcome of the review was pain relief, defined as the proportion of patients reporting at least 50% pain relief after 3 months. All three studies included pain as an outcome, though the description of how pain was assessed was not always clear. Kilmartin and Wallace (1994) used a 100-mm visual analogue scale for pain, Colgrove et al. (2000) used a 100-point scale administered by telephone interview, and the method of pain assessment by Nashi et al. (1997) was not reported. Other outcomes measured included length of hospital stay following surgery (Nashi et al. 1997), time taken to return to work and activity (Nashi et al. 1997), and the McMaster-Toronto Arthritis patient function preference questionnaire patient specific measure of maximal function (Kilmartin and Wallace 1994). Due to differences in study interventions, no meta-analysis was performed. The findings of individual studies are presented in the following sections. Overall, the reviewers reported a distinct lack of quality research to support any treatment for plantar intermetatarsal nerve compression. In the randomized controlled trials that had been completed, the reviewers highlighted deficiencies in study design that exposed the studies to a high risk of bias, inadequate outcome assessment, and incomplete reporting.

Non-invasive Therapies

Non-invasive therapies aim to reduce compression of the plantar intermetatarsal nerve (Adams 2010).

Patients should be encouraged to avoid all factors, where possible, that exacerbate symptoms. Patients should also be encouraged to wear shoes with wide and deep toe boxes with secure, but not tight, fastening and to avoid high-heeled shoes (Adams 2010; Clinical Practice Guideline Forefoot Disorders et al. 2009b). Plantar metatarsal pads or domes may be used to alter plantar pressure distribution and alleviate symptoms (Clinical Practice Guideline Forefoot Disorders et al. 2009b). Hsi et al. (2005) evaluated optimum position of a metatarsal pad for plantar pressure reduction in 10 people with metatarsalgia. They found that peak pressure at the metatarsal head was most reduced when the metatarsal pad was placed just proximal to the metatarsal head. The effect of metatarsal pads or domes for symptom reduction in plantar intermetatarsal nerve compression has not been evaluated in a randomized trial.

Use of foot orthoses is a component of routine conservative therapy for plantar intermetatarsal nerve compression in some regions (Thomson et al. 2004). One randomized controlled trial has compared 'supinatory' and 'pronatory' insoles in 23 participants diagnosed with Morton's neuroma (Kilmartin and Wallace 1994). In that trial, 50% of participants in the supinatory insole group and 45% of participants in the pronatory insole group reported a decrease in pain of greater than 50% (RR 1.10) at the 12 months endpoint (Thomson et al. 2004). This difference was not statistically or clinically significant.

Other non-surgical interventions include manipulation (Cashley 2000), massage (Nunan and Giesy 1997), oral non-steroidal anti-inflammatory drugs (Schreiber et al. 2011), ultrasound (Nunan and Giesy 1997), whirlpool (Nunan and Giesy 1997), and percutaneous electrocoagulation (Finney et al. 1989). None of these has been evaluated in randomized controlled trials.

Extracorporeal Shockwave Therapy

Fridman et al. (2009) evaluated extracorporeal shockwave therapy in a small, randomized controlled trial. Twenty-five participants with plantar intermetatarsal nerve compression were randomly assigned to receive extracorporeal shockwave ($n=13$) or sham therapy ($n=12$). Shockwave therapy was performed under intravenous sedation and local anesthesia (5 mL of bupivacaine hydrochloride) and was directed inferiorly to the site of plantar intermetatarsal nerve compression. The sham group received local anaesthesia under intravenous sedation. Two patients in the sham group did not complete the study. Unfortunately, the authors did not report important baseline characteristics of the two groups or the statistical significance of differences between groups in final pain scores. After 12 weeks, nine people in the treatment group (69%) and four people in the sham group (40%) reported an improvement in pain severity of greater than 50% and a final pain score $\leq 3/10$ on a visual analogue scale. One participant in the active group (8%) and three people in the sham group ($n=3$) did not experience a reduction in pain. There were no adverse effects in either group. Due to the small size of the study and substantial flaws in reporting and statistical analyses, this study's findings should be viewed with caution (Landorf 2009). Adverse effects of extracorporeal shockwave therapy reported elsewhere in the literature include local soft-tissue damage and haemorrhage (Delius 1994) and nerve damage (Coombs et al. 2000). Extracorporeal shockwave therapy is contraindicated at sites close to open epiphyseal plates as it can cause premature union (Coombs et al. 2000).

Emerging Therapies

Radio-frequency ablation has also been described for plantar intermetatarsal nerve compression (Genon et al. 2010). Moore et al. (2012) reported a series of cases in which 29 patients underwent radiofrequency thermoneurolysis therapy for plantar intermetatarsal nerve compression. Recovery time was 2 days. Twenty-four patients (83%) reported complete relief of symptoms and five (17%) reported no to minimal relief. One patient experienced foot cellulitis, which was treated by oral antibiotics. Average follow-up was 13 months. Over this time, three patients pursued further therapy and two patients were lost to follow-up. Radiofrequency ablation should be evaluated for plantar intermetatarsal nerve compression in a randomized controlled trial to establish its effectiveness.

Injection Therapies

Injection therapies are widely described and used for plantar intermetatarsal nerve compression (Clinical Practice Guideline Forefoot Disorders et al. 2009b) and are the first-line therapy in some centres (Rout et al. 2009). Most commonly, either corticosteroid or alcohol is administered, though injection with phenol (Magnan et al. 2005), homeopathic remedies (Drury 2011), and vitamin B_{12} (cyanocobalamin) (Steinberg 1955) have been described. Users of alternative injection therapies that utilize alcohol as a preserving agent should take care to avoid misattributing the potentially beneficial sclerosing effect of the alcohol to the alternative therapy (Adams 2010; Clinical Practice Guideline Forefoot Disorders et al. 2009b).

Corticosteroid Injection. Corticosteroid for plantar intermetatarsal nerve compression is typically mixed with local anaesthetic and administered perineurally via the intermetatarsal web-space under ultrasound guidance (Adams 2010; Markovic et al. 2008; Rout et al. 2009). Yap and McNally (2012) measured pain severity using a 100-mm visual analogue scale during ultrasound-guided corticosteroid injection in 68 patients with Morton's neuroma. Injections were perceived as being less painful if administered from a dorsal approach [mean (SD): 2.9 (2.0) mm] than a plantar approach [4.4 (2.3) mm]. Preliminary subcutaneous local anaesthetic did not confer any statistically significant benefit for pain severity during skin puncture or needle advancement when either the dorsal or plantar approaches were used (Yap and McNally 2012).

One randomized controlled trial has compared corticosteroid injection with footwear modifications in 82 people with clinically diagnosed Morton's neuroma (Saygi et al. 2005). Participants were randomly assigned to receive either: (1) metatarsal pads and shoes with wide toe boxes and low heels, or (2) two injections given 3 weeks apart of prilocaine hydrochloride and methylprednisolone acetate to the site of maximal interspace tenderness. The only outcome of participant-perceived satisfaction was measured after 1, 6, and 12 months. After 6 months participants in the footwear group who were not completely satisfied were offered the injection therapy, so 12-month data are not presented in this summary. Satisfaction was rated as being: complete satisfaction (complete pain relief), satisfaction with some discomfort (partial pain relief) and dissatisfaction. Sixty-nine participants with 71 instances of Morton's neuroma completed the study. After 1 and 6 months, participants in the corticosteroid group were more than twice as likely to rate their level of satisfaction as complete and were less than half as likely to be dissatisfied.

Other reports in the literature suggest that corticosteroid injection may provide greater and longer pain relief for lesions smaller than 5 mm (Makki et al. 2012), though results are conflicting (Markovic et al. 2008). As a single injection may offer only short-term relief (Markovic et al. 2008) patients may require periodic injection (Adams 2010). Care should be taken to avoid administering more than the maximum safe dose over a 12-month period as adverse effects including skin and plantar fat pad atrophy, altered pigmentation, metatarsophalangeal joint subluxation, and steroid flare have been reported (Basadonna et al. 1999; Greenfield et al. 1984; Reddy et al. 1995).

Alcohol Injection. For over a decade dilute alcohol (4–20%) has been used for its sclerosing effects in treating plantar intermetatarsal nerve compression (Dockery 1999). Alcohol (with or without local anaesthetic) is administered percutaneously to the affected web-space, with or without ultrasound guidance (Dockery 1999; Espinosa et al. 2011). Repeat injections are performed at 5- to 14-day intervals (Dockery 1999; Espinosa et al. 2011). In one report of 101 cases of alcohol injection for plantar intermetatarsal nerve compression, the average number of injections per patient was 4.1 (Hughes et al. 2007), though up to seven injections per patient has been reported (Dockery 1999). Results of case series reports are conflicting, with 32% to 84% of patients reporting complete relief of symptoms (Espinosa et al. 2011; Hughes et al. 2007; Musson et al. 2012). Alcohol injection therapy is suggested to be more effective in younger patients with solitary lesions, though this is untested (Musson et al. 2012). Alcohol injection therapy should be evaluated in a randomized controlled trial to properly determine its effectiveness for plantar intermetatarsal nerve compression.

Surgical Strategies

Complete resection of the affected nerve is the most common procedure performed (Adams 2010;

Thomson et al. 2004). The resected nerve may be left in situ or implanted (transpositioned) into a tendon or intermuscular space to reduce risk of stump cord neuroma (Thomson et al. 2004). Colgrove et al. (2000) conducted a quasi-randomized controlled trial with 46 participants to compare standard resection versus resection and transposition for plantar intermetatarsal nerve compression. At the 36- to 48-month end-point, 100% of patients in the transposition group and 86% of patients in the resection group reported a decrease in pain of greater than 50% (relative risk (RR) 1.79) (Thomson et al. 2004). A separate quasi-randomized controlled trial including 42 participants has evaluated nerve resection by dorsal versus plantar incision (Nashi et al. 1997). Plantar incision is a more straightforward procedure but has longer recovery time and carries a risk of troublesome plantar scarring (Thomson et al. 2004). After 3 months, 80% of participants in the dorsal incision group and 65% of participants in the plantar incision group reported a decrease in pain of greater than 50% (RR 1.26). In each group, 2 of 26 participants had a subsequent infection and 1 of 26 participants had recurrence of neuroma. Painful postoperative scars were reported by two participants in the dorsal incision group and five participants in the plantar incision group (Thomson et al. 2004).

Although nerve resection is reportedly the most commonly performed procedure, there is call in the literature for it to be reserved for cases in which macroscopic thickening or pseudoneuroma is present (Villas et al. 2008) or when surgical decompression has failed (Clinical Practice Guideline Forefoot Disorders et al. 2009a). Decompression aims to reduce irritation of the affected nerve by transecting the deep transverse metatarsal ligament (Barrett and Walsh 2006). This has been performed as an open procedure, a minimally invasive procedure, or endoscopically (Barret and Pignetti 1994; Dellon 1992; Zelent et al. 2007). The transected ligament may be left in situ or transpositioned inferiorly to the affected nerve (Vito and Talarico 2003). The effectiveness of surgical decompression for plantar intermetatarsal nerve entrapment has not been evaluated in a randomized trial.

Another surgical option for plantar intermetatarsal nerve compression is cryogenic neuroablation. It is used to provoke Wallerian degeneration of the axons and myelin (Caporusso et al. 2002; Hodor et al. 1997). The risk of stump neuroma formation is purported to be low, as the epineurium and perineurium remain intact (Clinical Practice Guideline Forefoot Disorders et al. 2009a). The clinical effect is not permanent, however, and may be reduced in large lesions and in the presence of fibrosis (Clinical Practice Guideline Forefoot Disorders et al. 2009a). Again, the effectiveness of cryogenic neuroablation for plantar intermetatarsal nerve entrapment has not been evaluated in a randomized trial.

Adverse Effects of Surgery. The potential benefits of surgical intervention must preoperatively be weighed against potential adverse effects by both the health practitioner and patient. Potential adverse effects include infection (Schreiber et al. 2011), haematoma (Clinical Practice Guideline Forefoot Disorders et al. 2009a), scar sensitivity (Schreiber et al. 2011), scar hyperkeratosis, particularly if plantar (Richardson et al. 1993), keloid scar (Adams 2010), residual pain (Schreiber et al. 2011), sensory deficits (Schreiber et al. 2011), stump neuroma (which may be caused by resecting the nerve too distally, incomplete excision, or tethering of the nerve to local structures) (Adams 2010; Barret and Pignetti 1994), complex regional pain syndrome (Adams 2010), adhesive neuritis (Fridman et al. 2009), and post-operative hammer toe due to inadvertent resection of the lumbrical tendon (Adams 2010).

LESSER DIGIT DEFORMITIES

INTRODUCTION

A lesser digit deformity may occur as an isolated pathology or as a component of a more complex foot deformity. The second digit is most commonly involved (particularly for hammer or mallet toe), though any lesser digit may be affected (American College of Foot and Ankle Surgeons Preferred Practice Guidelines Committee 1999; Atinga et al. 2011; Coughlin 1995a). Lesser digit deformities tend to develop insidiously and become rigid over time, and may not be noticed until a secondary pathology arises (Ellington 2011). Perhaps the most common secondary pathology is painful callosity at the digit apex, dorsal to the interphalangeal joints, interdigitally, or

plantar to the MTPJ (American College of Foot and Ankle Surgeons Preferred Practice Guidelines Committee 1999). These tend to develop at sites of irritation from footwear or adjacent digits and are at risk of ulcerating in people with neuropathy or vascular compromise (Molloy and Shariff 2011). Other secondary pathologies include nail deformities due to damage to the nail germinal matrix or plate (Molloy and Shariff 2011), ingrown toenail, adventitious bursae over bony prominences (American College of Foot and Ankle Surgeons Preferred Practice Guidelines Committee 1999), interdigital maceration (American College of Foot and Ankle Surgeons Preferred Practice Guidelines Committee 1999), interdigital fungal or bacterial infection, and medial tibial pain associated with overuse of the flexor digitorum longus (FDL) (Garth and Miller 1989). Patients may also report difficulty with footwear fitting and dissatisfaction with the appearance of affected digit/s. As the deformity progresses, patients may experience pain of the MTPJ as part of a 'pre-subluxation syndrome' (Clinical Practice Guideline Forefoot Disorders et al. 2009a).

PREVALENCE

There is a paucity of epidemiological data describing the prevalence or incidence of lesser digit deformities (American College of Foot and Ankle Surgeons Preferred Practice Guidelines Committee 1999). In one study of 1691 Americans aged over 50 years (Golightly et al. 2012), the prevalence of hammer toes was 35%. Similar rates of claw or hammer toes have been reported in people with diabetes (Holewski et al. 1989; Smith et al. 1997). Mallet toe is much less common and has been reported to account for just 5% of lesser digit deformities (Molloy and Shariff 2011). Peak incidence is reported to be at 30 to 60 years of age (Good and Fiala 2010). The deformity is typically observed to worsen over time, which may be due to secondary muscle imbalance, degeneration of affected joints, fat pad migration, and soft-tissue changes, including failure of the plantar plate (Chadwick and Saxby 2011; Good and Fiala 2010; Molloy and Shariff 2011). The incidence is reportedly greater among females than males, though high-quality data are lacking (Clinical Practice Guideline Forefoot Disorders et al. 2009a).

PREDISPOSING FACTORS

Knowledge of the pathogenesis of lesser digit deformity is incomplete. A plethora of factors have been suggested to contribute to development of deformity. Loss of MTPJ stability is perhaps the most popularly accepted theory. MTPJ instability may result from malfunction of any of the active and/or passive MTPJ stabilizers, including the extensor digitorum longus (EDL), extensor digitorum brevis (EDB), flexor digitorum longus (FDL), flexor digitorum brevis (FDB), lumbricals, interrossei, plantar plate, MTPJ collaterals, and transverse intermetatarsal ligament. Potential causes include intrinsic muscle atrophy due to motor neuropathy (Boulton 1996; Delbridge et al. 1985), plantar fat pad displacement (Schrier et al. 2009), muscle contracture in neuromuscular disease, which may present with cavus foot type (Molloy and Shariff 2011), hyperextension of the MTPJ (e.g. with high-heel use) (Chadwick and Saxby 2011), constrictive footwear (Coughlin 1984), deforming force from adjacent digits (American College of Foot and Ankle Surgeons Preferred Practice Guidelines Committee 1999), acute trauma (Clinic Clinical Practice Guideline Forefoot Disorders et al. 2009a), overactivity of EDL due to weak tibialis anterior (Hansen Jr 2000; Sahrmann 2002), overactivity of EDL due to tight calf muscles (Kwon et al. 2009), inflammatory and non-inflammatory arthritides (Clinical Practice Guideline Forefoot Disorders et al. 2009a) abnormal metatarsal and/or digit length (Coughlin 1995a; Ellington 2011), pes planus (Oliver et al. 1996), and as a potential complication of harvesting vascularized fibular grafts, though the hallux is more likely to be affected than lesser digits (Arai et al. 2002; Minami et al. 2000; Takakura et al. 2000).

In one small case–control study of 10 participants with idiopathic claw toe deformity and 10 matched patients with normally aligned toes (all participants had diabetic neuropathy), differences between groups in mean intrinsic foot muscle atrophy scores rated using MRI were not statistically significant (Bus et al. 2009), and intrinsic muscle atrophy scores were not correlated with degree of toe deformity ($r=-0.18$). EDL was atrophic in six cases and four controls. FDL was atrophic in three cases and four controls. There was no evidence of EDL or FDL fibrosis (a marker of contracture) in either group. Despite the small size of this study, the authors concluded that other factors, including plantar aponeurosis discontinuity and MTPJ capsule pathology, may be more important than intrinsic muscle atrophy in the pathogenesis of claw toe deformity (Bus et al. 2009).

In a study of 27 feet with hammer toe and 31 age-matched feet without hammer toe (Kwon et al. 2009), mean extensor/flexor muscle strength ratios for digits two to four were higher in cases than controls (second digit: 2.4 versus 0.8; third digit: 1.9 versus 0.8; fourth digit: 1.6 versus 0.7; all $p<0.001$). Cases had less mean (SD) ankle dorsiflexion range of motion (4.7 versus 10.3°, $p<0.01$) and less mean (SD) calcaneal eversion range of motion (7.1 versus 9.9°, $p<0.01$) than controls. The ratio of toe extensor/flexor muscle strength accounted for 48–64% of the variance in MTPJ angle. Calcaneal eversion range of motion added a unique additional 6–11% of the variance in MTPJ angle in toes 2–4 to explain a total of 59–73% of the total variance in MTPJ angle in toes 2–4. Ankle dorsiflexion range of motion did not account for a unique amount of the variance in MTPJ angle once ratio of extensor/flexor muscle strength had been added.

DIAGNOSIS

Physical Examination

The affected digit is inspected visually to identify the joints involved and the extent of the deformity (American College of Foot and Ankle Surgeons Preferred Practice Guidelines Committee 1999). Common sites of hyperkeratosis in claw and hammer toe are plantar to the MTPJ and dorsal to the proximal interphalangeal joint (Ellington 2011). Common sites of hyperkeratosis in mallet toe are the digit apex and dorsal to the distal interphalangeal joint (Clinical Practice Guideline Forefoot Disorders et al. 2009a; Ellington 2011). In all three toe deformities, interdigital hyperkeratosis at points of irritation is common (Clinical Practice Guideline Forefoot Disorders et al. 2009a). Areas of hyperkeratosis are at risk of present and future ulceration (Molloy and Shariff 2011). Careful debridement of hyperkeratosis may reveal underlying ulceration, particularly if the hyperkeratosis was haemorrhagic (American College of Foot and Ankle Surgeons Preferred Practice Guidelines Committee 1999). The interdigital space should also be examined for signs of maceration, tinea pedis, and intertrigo (American College of Foot and Ankle Surgeons Preferred Practice Guidelines Committee 1999). Bulbous subcutaneous lesions overlying bony prominences (potential adventitious bursa) should be noted and palpated (American College of Foot and Ankle Surgeons Preferred Practice Guidelines Committee 1999; Clinical Practice Guideline Forefoot Disorders et al. 2009a).

Range of motion testing of the interphalangeal and metatarsophalangeal joints will reveal whether the deformity is flexible (reducible), semi-rigid (partially reducible), or rigid (non-reducible) (American College of Foot and Ankle Surgeons Preferred Practice Guidelines Committee 1999; Chadwick and Saxby 2011; Ellington 2011). Range of motion tests may be conducted non-weightbearing with the ankle in neutral position, dorsiflexed, and plantarflexed, and while weightbearing (Ellington 2011). This will help to determine the contribution of the EDL and FDL to the deformity and guide intervention selection (Good and Fiala 2010). During weightbearing assessment, the digits should also be checked for ground contact and splay. Gait assessment may also be of use in characterizing the deformity; for example, excessive extension of the lesser digits in swing phase may identify tibialis anterior weakness or gastric soleal tightness and might contribute to footwear irritation and subsequent hyperkeratosis/ulceration dorsal to an interphalangeal joint (Clinical Practice Guideline Forefoot Disorders et al. 2009a). Plantar pressure studies may be useful (e.g. in determining MTPJ involvement), though this modality is not readily accessible to many practitioners (American College of Foot and Ankle Surgeons Preferred Practice Guidelines Committee 1999).

The MTPJ should be assessed for stability using the vertical drawer test, in which the examiner stabilizes the metatarsal and moves the proximal phalanx vertically (Ellington 2011). Pain, subluxation, and/or dislocation should be noted (Good and Fiala 2010). Results should be compared with adjacent and contralateral MTPJs.

Strength and flexibility of the digit flexors and extensors, and ankle dorsiflexors and plantarflexors, can be assessed to help establish potential aetiologies of the deformity. Footwear should be assessed for shape and fit, particularly in respect to toe box depth and width, adequacy of fixation, heel elevation, and forefoot flex point (Chadwick and Saxby 2011). Hallux position and any foot deformities should be assessed for their possible contribution. A neurological assessment should be conducted in cases where an underlying neurological pathology is suspected (Ellington 2011). If routine neurological assessment does not satisfy concerns, the patient should be referred for neurological consultation (American College of Foot and Ankle Surgeons Preferred Practice Guidelines Committee 1999). A vascular assessment is warranted in cases of ulceration, notable risk of ulceration, or where surgical intervention is considered (Ellington 2011).

Diagnostic Imaging and Other Modalities

Diagnostic imaging is not required to diagnose lesser digit deformities though it may help to identify the underlying cause and to guide intervention selection, particularly if surgical intervention is considered. Blood biochemical studies are not indicated unless underlying inflammatory or metabolic diseases are suspected.

Plain film radiographic assessment may include weightbearing anterior–posterior, lateral and lateral–oblique projections, stress projections, and isolated digit projections (Clinical Practice Guideline Forefoot Disorders et al. 2009a; Good and Fiala 2010). X-rays have been used to assess abnormalities of soft tissue, joint space, and bone dimension, quality, and alignment (Ellington 2011). Radiographic superimposition of phalanges due to subluxation or dislocation should not be confused with arthritic degeneration (Good and Fiala 2010; Kwon and De Asla 2011). In a severe deformity where a phalanx is flexed or extended to 90°, a 'gun-barrel' sign may be seen, in which the phalanx base is superimposed over its head (Ellington 2011; Good and Fiala 2010). X-rays have also been used to identify possible contributors to the deformity, including abnormal metatarsal length or inclination and metatarsus adductus (Ellington 2011).

Sung et al. (2012) recently evaluated the diagnostic accuracy of MRI for plantar plate injury with reference to intraoperative findings. In 45 feet of 42 participants, MRI showed high accuracy (96%), sensitivity (95%), specificity (100%), positive predictive value (100%), and negative predictive value (67%). The authors concluded that, as clinical diagnosis was also highly accurate (91%), MRI should be reserved for cases in which surgical intervention is not clearly indicated by clinical assessment results.

IMPAIRMENT AND FUNCTION

The impact of lesser digit deformities has not been explored. There are anecdotal reports of detrimental effects on participation in activities of daily living and on quality of life (Angirasa et al. 2011; Ellington 2011), though these have not been validated. Commonly, patients report frustration with difficulty in footwear fitting and dissatisfaction with digit appearance. Certain populations have increased risk of complications of lesser digit deformities. For example, claw and hammer toe deformities are associated with increased peak plantar pressure at the affected MTPJ and may dangerously increase risk of ulceration in people with neuropathy or other risk factors for ulceration (Bus et al. 2005).

MANAGEMENT STRATEGIES

Management of digital deformities is guided principally by each patient's treatment goals. Treatment goals may include reduced pain, improved function, improved footwear options, reduced toe deformity, and prevention of progression.

There is a plethora of treatment options for digital deformities (American College of Foot and Ankle Surgeons Preferred Practice Guidelines Committee 1999). Where possible, treatment should address the cause of the deformity, including underlying systemic disease (American College of Foot and Ankle Surgeons Preferred Practice Guidelines Committee 1999; Clinical Practice Guideline Forefoot Disorders et al. 2009a). Interventions for lesser digit deformities can be broadly divided into non-surgical and surgical treatments. Selection of any particular treatment is informed by the degree of deformity, severity of symptoms, and impact on daily living, previous treatments and responses, presence of other medical conditions, availability of resources, and patient preference (Clinical Practice Guideline Forefoot Disorders et al. 2009a).

Typically, non-surgical intervention is first-line therapy (Ellington 2011; Molloy and Shariff 2011) and surgical intervention is reserved for cases in which non-surgical therapy does not adequately achieve patient goals (Good and Fiala 2010; Kernbach 2012; Kwon and De Asla 2011). Surgery may be considered a first-line therapy when the MTPJ is subluxed or dislocated, when the risks and impacts of uncorrected deformity are great, and when requested by the patient (American College of Foot and Ankle Surgeons Preferred Practice Guidelines Committee 1999; Chadwick and Saxby 2011; Kwon and De Asla 2011). Any intervention should be preceded by an appropriate education regarding the diagnosis and treatment options.

Non-surgical Strategies

For many people with lesser digit deformities, footwear is a source of discomfort and provides a sensible starting point for non-surgical intervention (Clinical Practice Guideline Forefoot Disorders et al. 2009a). General features of footwear appropriate for lesser digit deformities include: adequate shoe length, wide and deep toe box, soft upper material, cushioned inner sole, and low heel height (Chadwick and Saxby 2011). Footwear may also be modified through stretching and patching to allow more room for deformed digits (Molloy and Shariff 2011).

If changes in footwear alone do not provide adequate relief of symptoms or if a patient is unwilling to wear the footwear recommended, then splinting, taping, and/or padding can be used to reduce irritation of the digit/s (Clinical Practice Guideline Forefoot Disorders et al. 2009a). Splinting and taping are reserved for flexible deformities. Padding may be applied directly to the digit to cushion or deflect, or can be applied proximally to affect digit position; for example, a metatarsal bar may be applied proximal to the metatarsal head to reduce extension of the flexible MTPJ. Other commonly used products include toe sleeves, toe separators, and toe props, each of which can be made of a wide variety of materials (Angirasa et al. 2011). None of these interventions has been evaluated in a randomized controlled trial for lesser digit deformities, though there is evidence suggesting that toe props for claw toes reduce plantar pressure at the digit apex and MTPJ (Claisse et al. 2004).

Painful or otherwise troublesome hyperkeratosis should be addressed in first-line treatment plans. Treatment typically involves sharp debridement but may include application of topical keratolytics under careful medical supervision. If a putty toe separator or prop is to be made to deflect pressure from a corn, the prop might be best made before debridement to increase deflective capability of the device. Toe separators and props for digital deformities have not been evaluated in randomized trials.

Although muscle imbalance has long been suggested as a potential cause of lesser digit deformities, there is limited evidence supporting muscle strengthening and/or stretching for intrinsic muscles of the foot (Angirasa et al. 2011; Kwon et al. 2009; Molloy and Shariff 2011). In the absence of research evidence supporting an alternative intervention, a trial of muscle stretching and strengthening with clear goals and careful monitoring may be deemed appropriate.

Injection of corticosteroids may be of use for MTPJ swelling and synovitis, and bursitis (Chadwick and Saxby 2011; Clinical Practice Guideline Forefoot Disorders et al. 2009a). Botox injection may emerge as a treatment option, though the single published report is limited to use for hallux claw toe in cadavers (Lee et al. 2012).

Surgical Strategies

Many surgical techniques have been described for lesser digit deformities. No single procedure is appropriate for all digit deformities and there is no consensus on the best technique for each type of digit deformity (Atinga et al. 2011; Kernbach 2012; Molloy and Shariff 2011). Not surprisingly, variation in procedure selection and conduct between surgeons is marked (Angirasa et al. 2011).

Surgery plans should be patient-centred and may involve a stepwise progression of soft-tissue or bone procedure/s, or a combination of both (Chadwick and Saxby 2011). Procedure selection is guided by the flexibility of the deformity and associated pathology (Clinical Practice Guideline Forefoot Disorders et al. 2009a). Soft-tissue procedures alone are reserved for flexible deformities but may be combined with one or more bone procedures for semi-rigid or rigid deformities. Commonly employed soft-tissue procedures include flexor tenotomy (Tamir et al. 2008) or tendon lengthening (Clinical Practice Guideline Forefoot Disorders et al. 2009a), flexor-to-extensor tendon transfer, where the FDL is transferred to the dorsum of the proximal phalanx (Clinical Practice Guideline Forefoot Disorders et al. 2009a; Good and Fiala 2010; Kwon and De Asla 2011), extensor tenotomy (Good and Fiala 2010) or tendon lengthening (Clinical

Practice Guideline Forefoot Disorders et al. 2009a), extensor tendon transfer, where the EDL is transferred to the tarsal region (American College of Foot and Ankle Surgeons Preferred Practice Guidelines Committee 1999), and plantar plate repair (Lui 2007; Nery et al. 2012; Yu et al. 2002). Bone procedures alone or in combination with soft-tissue procedures are typically performed for semi-rigid or rigid deformities. Commonly employed bone procedures include partial or complete IPJ or MTPJ arthroplasty (Clinical Practice Guideline Forefoot Disorders et al. 2009a; Good and Fiala 2010; O'Kane and Kilmartin 2005), distal metatarsal osteotomy (Weil osteotomy; Good and Fiala 2010; Singh and Briggs 2012), and IPJ arthrodesis (Konkel et al. 2007; Miller 2002; O'Kane and Kilmartin 2005). Other soft-tissue and bone procedures may be performed to correct associated pathology [e.g. hallux valgus (Chadwick and Saxby 2011; Clinical Practice Guideline Forefoot Disorders et al. 2009a)].

There are no high-quality data on the incidence of adverse effects of surgery for digit deformities. Potential adverse effects include pain (American College of Foot and Ankle Surgeons Preferred Practice Guidelines Committee 1999), persistent oedema (Angirasa et al. 2011; Lancaster et al. 2008), residual, recurrent, or new deformity (American College of Foot and Ankle Surgeons Preferred Practice Guidelines Committee 1999; Angirasa et al. 2011; Konkel et al. 2007; Kwon and De Asla 2011; Lancaster et al. 2008; Molloy and Shariff 2011), infection (American College of Foot and Ankle Surgeons Preferred Practice Guidelines Committee 1999; Konkel et al. 2007), hardware or implant failure (American College of Foot and Ankle Surgeons Preferred Practice Guidelines Committee 1999; Angirasa et al. 2011; Konkel et al. 2007; Kwon and De Asla 2011), and neurological or vascular compromise (American College of Foot and Ankle Surgeons Preferred Practice Guidelines Committee 1999; Kwon and De Asla 2011; Lancaster et al. 2008).

Evidence of the effectiveness of surgery for lesser digit deformities is limited to anecdotal and case series reports. Ratings of surgical success differ widely between studies and the usefulness of direct comparison is severely limited by large differences in patient populations, concurrent interventions, outcome measures, completeness of follow-up, and follow-up duration. Well-designed and reported randomized controlled trials are required to evaluate the effectiveness of surgical (and non-surgical) interventions for lesser digit deformities.

FUTURE DIRECTIONS

The forefoot is a small area of the body that endures large mechanical stress throughout activities of daily life. This chapter has detailed four common chronic musculoskeletal pathologies of the forefoot. Successful clinical management of these conditions is underpinned by sound anatomical and biomechanical knowledge, careful diagnostic testing, and diligent synthesis of research evidence with clinical experience and patient preference to deliver gold-standard evidence-based treatment.

INVITED COMMENTARY

Forefoot problems account for over 85% of my surgical case load, with 55% of my surgical activity accounted for by hallux valgus and hallux rigidus. Hallux valgus and hallux rigidus / limitus will present in mild, moderate, and severe forms but symptoms may not correlate with clinical findings and the greatest challenge remains the mild deformity with pain well out of proportion to the degree of deformity or joint degeneration. In mild hallux valgus there is a risk of overcorrection and joint stiffness whereas in early hallux limitus the surgical options are limited, with no procedure able to ensure the restoration of normal range of pain-free movement. The evidence basis for conservative and surgical treatment of first-MPJ pain and deformity continues to grow but, although it is clear that hallux valgus patients now have effective treatment options, the outcomes for hallux rigidus remain disappointing. Is it time that treatment moved on from salvage procedures that seek to immobilize the joint to interventions that will renew the joint surface and restore a normal range and quality of movement?

The pain associated with Morton's neuroma can be intense and disabling. Many clinicians will use injection therapy as the first line of treatment because it seems to be successful with few risks, but the evidence base is poor and sufferers of the condition will often lose patience with slow improvement in their symptoms, demanding surgical excision instead. However, surgical outcomes are variable. Failure will often leave patients with intractable pain that can be treated only with further injection therapy or exploratory-type surgery. More outcomes research is urgently required to improve the evidence basis for injection therapy, while a radical rethink of surgical treatment is long overdue because of the unpredictable nature of surgical excision. Is there really no other way than excising the digital nerve as it passes between and distal to the metatarsophalangeal joints, leaving the patient with profound numbness and the possibility of further problems with the cut end of the nerve?

Accurate diagnosis of neuroma is vital, and in my experience neuroma is vastly overdiagnosed, whereas capsulitis of the MTPJ is vastly underdiagnosed. Certainly when pain is focused around the second and third MTPJ area then capsulitis is much more likely. The place for diagnostic ultrasound remains contentious because it is so observer-dependent. For me, ultrasound contributes toward an accurate diagnosis but is less important than good history taking. Where ultrasound is most important, however, is in sizing the lesion. 'Neuroma' less than 6 mm in size should be considered normal nerve tissue and the diagnosis reviewed.

Lesser digit deformities are one of the inconveniences of life, making footwear-fitting difficult as well as causing cosmetic concerns. Often apparent in early childhood, the effectiveness of splinting and strapping the child's digital deformity is poorly researched. Traditionally the surgical approach involves fusing the interphalangeal joints but this will leave the toe very straight, compromising function as the normal human toe must have some flexion in order to purchase the ground. Loss of toe purchase will increase the risk of metatarsalgia as during propulsion the body weight is usually shared between the toes and the metatarsal heads.

The length of the toes is critical to the cosmetic appearance of the foot, while the length of the metatarsals is critical to the function of the foot. Shortening or elevating a metatarsal through surgery or trauma will leave the foot at grave risk of developing transfer metatarsalgia. It is frustrating for clinicians and patients alike that plantar corns remain very resistant to conservative treatment, but the surgical options are fraught with risk of creating a new problem under an adjacent metatarsal head.

Although it is disappointing that so many of the common forefoot problems remain difficult to resolve, our best hope for the future is to continue building our evidence base. Excluding treatments that do not work and basing our advice to patients on the known outcomes of those treatments that offer minimal risk and maximal pain relief is what this chapter aims to provide.

Tim Kilmartin PhD, FCPodS
Consultant Podiatric Surgeon, Hillsborough Private Clinic,
Belfast and Ilkeston Hospital, Ilkeston, Derbyshire;
Lecturer, School of Podiatry, Ulster University, Derry, UK

REFERENCES

Adams, W.R. 2nd, 2010. Morton's neuroma. Clinics in Podiatric Medicine and Surgery 27 (4), 535–545.

Addante, J., Peicott, P., Wong, K., et al., 1986. Interdigital neuromas. Results of surgical excision of 152 neuromas. Journal of the American Podiatric Medical Association 76 (9), 493–495.

Akin, O.F., 1925. The treatment of hallux valgus: a new operative procedure and its results. Medical Sentinel 33, 678–679.

Alvarez, R., Haddad, R.J., Gould, N., et al., 1984. The simple bunion: anatomy at the metatarsophalangeal joint of the great toe. Foot and Ankle International 4 (5), 229–240.

American College of Foot and Ankle Surgeons Preferred Practice Guidelines Committee, 1999. Hammer toe syndrome: preferred practice guidelines. Journal of Foot and Ankle Surgery 38 (2), 166–178.

Angirasa, A.K., Augoyard, M., Coughlin, M.J., et al., 2011. Hammer toe, mallet toe, and claw toe. Foot and Ankle Specialist 4 (3), 182–187.

Arai, K., Toh, S., Tsubo, K., et al., 2002. Complications of vascularized fibula graft for reconstruction of long bones. Plastic and Reconstructive Surgery 109, 2301–2306.

Atinga, M., Dodd, L., Foote, J., et al., 2011. Prospective review of medium term outcomes following interpositional arthroplasty for hammer toe deformity correction. Journal of Foot and Ankle Surgery 17 (4), 256–258.

Banks, A.S., Hsu, Y., Mariash, S., et al., 1994. Juvenile hallux abducto valgus association with metatarsus adductus. Journal of the American Podiatric Medical Association 84 (5), 219–224.

Barouk, L., 2000. Scarf osteotomy for hallux valgus correction: local anatomy, surgical technique, and combination with other forefoot procedures. Foot and Ankle Clinics 6, 105–112.

Barrett, S., Jarvis, J., 2005. Equinus deformity as a factor in forefoot nerve entrapment: treatment with endoscopic gastrocnemius recession. Journal of the American Podiatric Medical Association 95 (5), 464–468.

Barret, S., Pignetti, T., 1994. Endoscopic decompression for intermetatarsal nerve entrapment – the EDIN technique: preliminary study with cadaveric specimens; early clinical results. Journal of Foot and Ankle Surgery 33 (5), 503–508.

Barrett, S., Walsh, A., 2006. Endoscopic decompression of intermetatarsal nerve entrapment: a retrospective study. Journal of the American Podiatric Medical Association 96, 19–23.

Bartolomei, F., Wertheimer, S., 1983. Intermetatarsal neuromas: distribution and etiologic factors. Journal of Foot Surgery 22 (4), 279–282.

Basadonna, P., Rucco, V., Gasparini, D., et al., 1999. Plantar fat pad atrophy after corticosteroid injection for an interdigital neuroma: a case report. American Journal of Physical Medicine and Rehabilitation 78, 283–285.

Beeson, P., 2004. The surgical treatment of hallux limitus/rigidus: a critical review of the literature. The Foot 14 (1), 6–22.

Beeson, P., Phillips, C., Corr, S., et al., 2008. Classification systems for hallux rigidus: a review of the literature. Foot and Ankle International 29 (4), 407–414.

Beeson, P., Phillips, C., Corr, S., et al., 2009. Cross-sectional study to evaluate radiological parameters in hallux rigidus. Foot (Edinb) 19 (1), 7–21.

Beggs, I., 1999. Sonographic appearances of nerve tumors. Journal of Clinical Ultrasound 27, 363–368.

Bennett, G., Graham, C., Mauldin, D., et al., 1995. Morton's interdigital neuroma: a comprehensive treatment protocol. Foot and Ankle International 16 (12), 760–763.

Bennett, P.J., Patterson, C., Wearing, S., et al., 1998. Development and validation of a questionnaire designed to measure foot-health status. Journal of the American Podiatric Medical Association 88 (9), 419–428.

Benvenuti, F., Ferrucci, L., Guralnik, J.M., et al., 1995. Foot pain and disability in older persons: an epidemiologic survey. Journal of the American Geriatrics Society 43 (5), 479.

Bergin, S.M., Munteanu, S.E., Zammit, G.V., et al., 2012. Impact of first metatarsophalangeal joint osteoarthritis on health related quality of life. Arthritis Care and Research 64 (11), 1691–1698.

Bonney, G., Macnab, I., 1952. Hallux valgus and hallux rigidus. Journal of Bone and Joint Surgery 34, 366–385.

Botek, G., Anderson, M.A., 2011. Etiology, pathophysiology, and staging of hallux rigidus. Clinics in Podiatric Medicine and Surgery 28 (2), 229–243, vii.

Boulton, A., 1996. The pathogenesis of diabetic foot problems: an overview. Diabetic Medicine 13 (Suppl. 1), 12–16.

Bourke, G., Owen, J., Machet, D., 1994. Histological comparison of the third interdigital nerve in patients with Morton's metatarsalgia and control patients. Australian and New Zealand Journal of Surgery 64 (6), 421–424.

Brantingham, J.W., Chang, M.N., Gendreau, D.F., et al., 2007. The effect of chiropractic adjusting, exercises and modalities on a 32-year-old professional male golfer with hallux rigidus. Clinical Chiropractic 10 (2), 91–96.

Bratkowski, B., 1978. Differential diagnosis of plantar neuromas: a preliminary report. Journal of Foot and Ankle Surgery 17, 99–102.

Brewster, M., 2010. Does total joint replacement or arthrodesis of the first metatarsophalangeal joint yield better functional results? A systematic review of the literature. Journal of Foot and Ankle Surgery 49 (6), 546–552.

Bryant, A., Tinley, P., Singer, K., 1999. Plantar pressure distribution in normal, hallux valgus and hallux limitus feet. The Foot 9 (3), 115–119.

Bryant, A., Tinley, P., Singer, K., 2000. A comparison of radiographic measurements in normal, hallux valgus, and hallux limitus feet. Journal of Foot and Ankle Surgery 39 (1), 39–43.

Bryant, A., Mahoney, B., Tinley, P., 2001. Lateral intermetatarsal angle: a useful measurement of metatarsus primus elevatus? Journal of the American Podiatric Medical Association 91 (5), 251–254.

Budiman-Mak, E., Conrad, K.J., Roach, K.E., et al., 1995. Can foot orthoses prevent hallux valgus deformity in rheumatoid arthritis? A randomized clinical trial. Journal of Clinical Rheumatology 1 (6), 313.

Bus, S.A., Maas, M., de Lange, A., et al., 2005. Elevated plantar pressures in neuropathic diabetic patients with claw/hammer toe deformity. Journal of Biomechanics 38 (9), 1918–1925.

Bus, S.A., Maas, M., Michels, R.P.J., et al., 2009. Role of intrinsic muscle atrophy in the etiology of claw toe deformity in diabetic neuropathy may not be as straightforward as widely believed. Diabetes Care 32 (6), 1063–1067.

Camasta, C.A., 1996. Hallux limitus and hallux rigidus. Clinical examination, radiographic findings, and natural history. Clinics in Podiatric Medicine and Surgery 13 (3), 423–448.

Canseco, K., Long, J., Marks, R., et al., 2008. Quantitative characterization of gait kinematics in patients with hallux rigidus using the Milwaukee foot model. Journal of Orthopaedic Research 26 (4), 419–427.

Canseco, K., Rankine, L., Long, J., et al., 2010. Motion of the multisegmental foot in hallux valgus. Foot and Ankle International 31 (2), 146–152.

Caporusso, E., Fallat, L., Savoy-Moore, R., 2002. Cryogenic neuro-ablation for the treatment of lower extremity neuromas. Journal of Foot and Ankle Surgery 41, 286–290.

Cashley, D., 2000. Manipulative therapy in the treatment of plantar digital neuritis (Morton's neuroma). British Journal of Podiatry 3 (3), 67–69.

Chadwick, C., Saxby, T., 2011. Hammertoes/clawtoes: metatarsophalangeal joint correction. Foot and Ankle Clinics 16 (4), 559–571.

Chiodo, C.P., Schon, L.C., Myerson, M.S., 2004. Clinical results with the Ludloff osteotomy for correction of adult hallux valgus. Foot and Ankle International 25 (8), 532–536.

Cho, N.H., Kim, S., Kwon, D.J., et al., 2009. The prevalence of hallux valgus and its association with foot pain and function in a rural Korean community. Journal of Bone and Joint Surgery, British Volume 91 (4), 494–498.

Claisse, P.J., Binning, J., Potter, J., 2004. Effect of orthotic therapy on claw toe loading: results of significance testing at pressure sensor units. Journal of the American Podiatric Medical Association 94 (3), 246–254.

Clinical Practice Guideline Forefoot Disorders, Thomas, P.J.L., Blitch, E.L. 4th, et al., 2009a. Diagnosis and treatment of forefoot disorders. Section 3. Morton's intermetatarsal neuroma. Journal of Foot and Ankle Surgery 48 (2), 251–256.

Clinical Practice Guideline Forefoot Disorders, Thomas, P.J.L., Blitch, E.L. 4th, et al., 2009b. Diagnosis and treatment of forefoot disorders. Section 1. Digit deformities. Journal of Foot and Ankle Surgery 48 (2), 257–263.

Coetzee, J.C., 2003. Scarf osteotomy for hallux valgus repair: the dark side. Foot and Ankle International 24 (1), 29–33.

Cohn, I., Kanat, I., 1984. Functional limitation of motion of the first metatarsophalangeal joint. Journal of Foot Surgery 23 (6), 477.

Colgrove, R., Huang, E., Barth, A., et al., 2000. Interdigital neuroma: intermuscular neuroma transposition compared with resection. Foot and Ankle International 21, 206–211.

Connor, J.C., Berk, D.M., 1994. Continuous passive motion as an alternative treatment for iatrogenic hallux limitus. Journal of Foot and Ankle Surgery 33 (2), 177–179.

Cook, E., Cook, J., Rosenblum, B., et al., 2009. Meta-analysis of first metatarsophalangeal joint implant arthroplasty. Journal of Foot and Ankle Surgery 48 (2), 180–190.

Coombs, R., Schaden, W., Zhou, S., 2000. Introduction. In: Coombs, R. (Ed.), Musculoskeletal shockwave therapy, Greenwich Medical Media, London, p. 37.

Corless, J.R., 1976. A modification of the Mitchell procedure. Journal of Bone and Joint Surgery, British Volume 58B (1), 138.

Corrigan, J.P., Moore, D.P., Stephens, M.M., 1993. Effect of heel height on forefoot loading. Foot and Ankle International 14 (3), 148–152.

Coughlin, H., 1984. Mallet toes, hammer toes, claw toes, and corns. Postgraduate Medicine 75 (5), 191–198.

Coughlin, M., 1995. Operative treatment of the mallet toe deformity. Foot and Ankle International 16 (3), 109–116.

Coughlin, M.J., 1987. Crossover second toe deformity. Foot and Ankle International 8 (1), 29–39.

Coughlin, M.J., 1995. Juvenile hallux valgus: etiology and treatment. Foot and Ankle International 16 (11), 682–697.

Coughlin, M.J., 1997. Hallux valgus in men: effect of the distal metatarsal articular angle on hallux valgus correcting. Foot and Ankle International 18 (8), 463–470.

Coughlin, M.J., Shurnas, P.S., 2003a. Hallux rigidus. Grading and long-term results of operative treatment. Journal of Bone and Joint Surgery, American Volume 85-A (11), 2072–2088.

Coughlin, M.J., Shurnas, P.S., 2003b. Hallux rigidus: demographics, etiology, and radiographic assessment. Foot and Ankle International 24 (10), 731–743.

Coughlin, M.J., Jones, C.P., 2007. Hallux valgus: demographics, etiology, and radiographic assessment. Foot and Ankle International 28 (7), 759–777.

Coughlin, M.J., Grebing, B.R., Jones, C.P., 2005. Arthrodesis of the first metatarsophalangeal joint for idiopathic hallux valgus: intermediate results. Foot and Ankle International 26 (10), 783–792.

Dananberg, H.J., 1986. Functional hallux limitus and its relationship to gait efficiency. Journal of the American Podiatric Medical Association 76 (11), 648–652.

Dananberg, H.J., 1993. Gait style as an etiology to chronic postural pain. Part I. Functional hallux limitus. Journal of the American Podiatric Medical Association 83 (8), 433–441.

Dananberg, H.J., 1999. Sagittal plane biomechanics. In: Subotnik, S.I. (Ed.), Sports medicine and the lower extremity. Churchill Livingstone, New York, p. 137.

David, R., Delagoutte, J., Renard, M., 1989. Anatomical study of the sesamoid bones of the first metatarsal. Journal of the American Podiatric Medical Association 79 (11), 536–544.

Davies-Colley, N., 1887. On contraction of the metatarsophalangeal joint of the great toe (hallux flexus). Transactions of the Clinical Society of London 20, 165–171.

DeCarbo, W.T., Lupica, J., Hyer, C.F., 2011. Modern techniques in hallux rigidus surgery. Clinics in Podiatric Medicine and Surgery 28 (2), 361–383, ix.

DeFrino, P.F., Brodsky, J.W., Pollo, F.E., et al., 2002. First metatarsophalangeal arthrodesis: a clinical, pedobarographic and gait analysis study. Foot and Ankle International 23 (6), 496–502.

Deland, J.T., Williams, B.R., 2012. Surgical management of hallux rigidus. Journal of the American Academy of Orthopaedic Surgeons 20 (6), 347–358.

Delbridge, L., Ctercteko, G., Fowler, C., et al., 1985. The aetiology of diabetic neuropathic ulceration of the foot. British Journal of Surgery 72, 1–6.

Delius, M., 1994. Medical applications and bioeffects of extracorporeal shock waves. Shock Waves 4, 55.

Dellon, A., 1992. Treatment of Morton's neuroma as a nerve compression. The role for neurolysis. Journal of the American Podiatric Medical Association 82, 399–402.

Deschamps, K., Birch, I., Desloovere, K., et al., 2010. The impact of hallux valgus on foot kinematics: a cross-sectional, comparative study. Gait and Posture 32 (1), 102–106.

Dockery, G., 1999. The treatment of intermetatarsal neuromas with 4% alcohol sclerosing injections. Journal of Foot and Ankle Surgery 38, 403–408.

Donatelli, R., 1985. Normal biomechanics of the foot and ankle. Journal of Orthopaedic and Sports Physical Therapy 7 (3), 91.

Drago, J.J., Oloff, L., Jacobs, A.M., 1984. A comprehensive review of hallux limitus. Journal of Foot Surgery 23 (3), 213–220.

Drury, A.L., 2011. Use of homeopathic injection therapy in treatment of Morton's neuroma. Alternative Therapies in Health and Medicine 17 (2), 48.

du Plessis, M., Zipfel, B., Brantingham, J.W., et al., 2011. Manual and manipulative therapy compared to night splint for symptomatic hallux abducto valgus: an exploratory randomised clinical trial. Foot (Edinb) 21 (2), 71–78.

Durrant, B., Chockalingam, N., 2009. Functional hallux limitus: a review. Journal of the American Podiatric Medical Association 99 (3), 236–243.

Durrant, M., Siepert, K., 1993. Role of soft tissue structures as an etiology of hallux limitus. Journal of the American Podiatric Medical Association 83 (4), 173–180.

Easley, M.E., Davis, W.H., Anderson, R.B., 1999. Intermediate to long-term follow-up of medial-approach dorsal cheilectomy for hallux rigidus. Foot and Ankle International 20 (3), 147–152.

Ellington, J., 2011. Hammertoes and clawtoes: proximal interphalangeal joint correction. Foot and Ankle Clinics 16 (4), 547–558.

Enklaar, J., 1956. Hübscher's maneuver in the nosis of flatfoot. Maandschrift Voor Kindergeneeskunde 24 (9), 189.

Espinosa, N., Brodsky, J.W., Maceira, E., 2010. Metatarsalgia. Journal of the American Academy of Orthopaedic Surgeons 18 (8), 474–485.

Espinosa, N., Seybold, J.D., Jankauskas, L., et al., 2011. Alcohol sclerosing therapy is not an effective treatment for interdigital neuroma. Foot and Ankle International 32 (6), 576–580.

Eustace, S., O'Byrne, J., Stack, J., et al., 1993. Radiographic features that enable assessment of first metatarsal rotation: the role of pronation in hallux valgus. Skeletal Radiology 22 (3), 153–156.

Fazal, M.A., Khan, I., Thomas, C., 2012. Ultrasonography and magnetic resonance imaging in the diagnosis of Morton's neuroma. Journal of the American Podiatric Medical Association 102 (3), 184–186.

Ferrari, J., Malone-Lee, J., 2002. The shape of the metatarsal head as a cause of hallux abductovalgus. Foot and Ankle International 23 (3), 236–242.

Ferrari, J., Hopkinson, D.A., Linney, A.D., 2004. Size and shape differences between male and female foot bones: is the female foot predisposed to hallux abducto valgus deformity? Journal of the American Podiatric Medical Association 94 (5), 434–452.

Ferrari, J., Higgins, J.P., Prior, T.D., 2009. Interventions for treating hallux valgus (abductovalgus) and bunions. Cochrane Database of Systematic Reviews (2), CD000964.

Finney, W., Wiener, S., Catanzariti, F., 1989. Treatment of Morton's neuroma using percutaneous electrocoagulation. Journal of the American Podiatric Medicine Association 79 (2), 615–618.

Flavin, R., Stephens, M.M., 2004. Arthrodesis of the first metatarsophalangeal joint using a dorsal titanium contoured plate. Foot and Ankle International 25 (11), 783–787.

Freed, J., 1993. The increasing recognition of medullary lysis, cortical osteophytic proliferation, and fragmentation of implanted silicone polymer implants. Journal of Foot and Ankle Surgery 32 (2), 171–179.

Fridman, R., Cain, J.D., Weil, L. Jr., 2009. Extracorporeal shockwave therapy for interdigital neuroma: a randomized, placebo-controlled, double-blind trial. Journal of the American Podiatric Medical Association 99 (3), 191–193.

Friscia, D., Strom, D., Parr, J., et al., 1991. Surgical treatment for primary interdigital neuroma. Orthopedics 14 (6), 669–672.

Fuhrmann, R.A., Roth, A., Venbrocks, R.A., 2005. [Metatarsalgia. Differential diagnosis and therapeutic algorithm]. Der Orthopade 34 (8), 767–768, 769–772, 774–775.

Fuller, E.A., 2000. The windlass mechanism of the foot. A mechanical model to explain pathology. Journal of the American Podiatric Medical Association 90 (1), 35–46.

Garrow, A.P., Papageorgiou, A., Silman, A.J., et al., 2001. The grading of hallux valgus: The Manchester Scale. Journal of the American Podiatric Medical Association 91 (2), 74–78.

Garth, W.P. Jr., Miller, S.T., 1989. Evaluation of claw toe deformity, weakness of the foot intrinsics, and posteromedial shin pain. American Journal of Sports Medicine 17 (6), 821–827.

Geldwert, J.J., Rock, G., McGrath, M., et al., 1992. Cheilectomy: still a useful technique for grade I and grade II hallux limitus/rigidus. Journal of Foot Surgery 31 (2), 154–159.

Genon, M.P., Chin, T.Y., Bedi, H.S., et al., 2010. Radio-frequency ablation for the treatment of Morton's neuroma. Australia and New Zealand Journal of Surgery 80 (9), 583–585.

Gibbs, R.C., Boxer, M.C., 1982. Abnormal biomechanics of feet and their cause of hyperkeratoses. Journal of the American Academy of Dermatology 6 (6), 1061–1069.

Gibson, J.N.A., Thomson, C.E., 2005. Arthrodesis or total replacement arthroplasty for hallux rigidus: a randomized controlled trial. Foot and Ankle International 26 (9), 680–690.

Gilheany, M.F., Landorf, K.B., Robinson, P., 2008. Hallux valgus and hallux rigidus: a comparison of impact on health-related quality of life in patients presenting to foot surgeons in Australia. Journal of Foot and Ankle Research 1, 14.

Golightly, Y.M., Hannan, M.T., Dufour, A.B., et al., 2012. Racial differences in foot disorders and foot type. Arthritis Care and Research 64 (11), 1756–1759.

Good, J., Fiala, K., 2010. Digital surgery: current trends and techniques. Clinics in Podiatric Medicine and Surgery 27 (4), 583–599.

Goodfellow, J., 1966. Aetiology of hallux rigidus. Proceedings of the Royal Society of Medicine 59 (9), 821.

Goucher, N.R., Coughlin, M.J., 2006. Hallux metatarsophalangeal joint arthrodesis using dome-shaped reamers and dorsal plate fixation: a prospective study. Foot and Ankle International 27 (11), 869–876.

Govsa, F., Bilge, O., Ozer, M.A., 2005. Anatomical study of the communicating branches between the medial and lateral plantar nerves. Surgical and Radiologic Anatomy 27 (5), 377–381.

Grace, T., Sunshein, K., Jones, R., et al., 1993. Metatarsus proximus and digital divergence. Association with intermetatarsal neuromas. Journal of the American Podiatric Medical Association 83, 406–411.

Grady, J.F., Axe, T.M., Zager, E.J., et al., 2002. A retrospective analysis of 772 patients with hallux limitus. Journal of the American Podiatric Medical Association 92 (2), 102–108.

Granberry, W., Noble, P., Bishop, J., et al., 1991. Use of a hinged silicone prosthesis for replacement arthroplasty of the first metatarsophalangeal joint. Journal of Bone and Joint Surgery, American Volume 73 (10), 1453–1459.

Greenberg, G., 1979. Relationship of hallux abductus angle and first metatarsal angle to severity of pronation. Journal of the American Podiatry Association 69 (1), 29–34.

Greenfield, J., Rea, J., Ilfield, F., 1984. Morton's interdigital neuroma: indications for treatment by local injections versus surgery. Clinical Orthopaedics and Related Research 185, 142–144.

Gregg, J.M., Schneider, T., Mark, P., 2008. MR imaging and ultrasound of metatarsalgia – the lesser metatarsals. Radiologic Clinics of North America 46 (6), 1061–1078, vi–vii.

Hall, C., Nester, C.J., 2004. Sagittal plane compensations for artificially induced limitation of the first metatarsophalangeal joint a preliminary study. Journal of the American Podiatric Medical Association 94 (3), 269–274.

Halstead, J., Redmond, A.C., 2006. Weight-bearing passive dorsiflexion of the hallux in standing is not related to hallux dorsiflexion during walking. Journal of Orthopaedic and Sports Physical Therapy 36 (8), 550–556.

Halstead, J., Turner, D.E., Redmond, A.C., 2005. The relationship between hallux dorsiflexion and ankle joint complex frontal plane kinematics: a preliminary study. Clinical Biomechanics 20 (5), 526–531.

Hanft, J.R., Mason, E.T., Landsman, A., et al., 1993. A new radiographic classification for hallux limitus. Journal of Foot and Ankle Surgery 32 (4), 397–404.

Hansen, S. Jr., 2000. Functional reconstruction of the foot and ankle. Lippincott Williams and Wilkins, Philadelphia, PA.

Hardy, R., Clapham, J., 1951. Observations on hallux valgus. Journal of Bone and Joint Surgery, British Volume 33 (3), 376–391.

Hart, E.S., deAsla, R.J., Grottkau, B.E., 2008. Current concepts in the treatment of hallux valgus. Orthopaedic Nursing 27 (5), 274–280.

Heden, R., Sorto, L. Jr., 1981. The Buckle point and the metatarsal protrusion's relationship to hallux valgus. Journal of the American Podiatry Association 71 (4), 200.

Helal, B., Gupta, S., Gojaseni, P., 1974. Surgery for adolescent hallux valgus. Acta Orthopedica Scandinavica 45 (2), 271–295.

Hicks, J., 1954. The mechanics of the foot: II. The plantar aponeurosis and the arch. Journal of Anatomy 88 (Pt 1), 25.

Hodor, L., Barkal, K., Hatch-Fox, L., 1997. Cryogenic denervation of the intermetatarsal space neuroma. Journal of Foot and Ankle Surgery 36, 311–314.

Holewski, J., Moss, K., Stess, R., et al., 1989. Prevalence of foot pathology and lower extremity complications in a diabetic outpatient clinic. Journal of Rehabilitation Research and Development 26, 35–44.

Hopson, M., McPoil, T., Cornwall, M., 1995. Motion of the first metatarsophalangeal joint. Reliability and validity of four measurement techniques. Journal of the American Podiatric Medical Association 85 (4), 198–204.

Horton, G., Park, Y.-W., Myerson, M., 1999. Role of metatarsus primus elevatus in the pathogenesis of hallux rigidus. Foot and Ankle International 20 (12), 777.

Hsi, W.-L., Kang, J.-H., Lee, X.-X., 2005. Optimum position of metatarsal pad in metatarsalgia for pressure relief. American Journal of Physical Medicine and Rehabilitation 84 (7), 514–520.

Hughes, R.J., Ali, K., Jones, H., et al., 2007. Treatment of Morton's neuroma with alcohol injection under sonographic guidance: follow-up of 101 cases. American Journal of Roentgenology 188 (6), 1535–1539.

Humbert, J., Bourbonniere, C., Laurin, C., 1979. Metatarsophalangeal fusion for hallux valgus: indications and effect on the first metatarsal ray. Canadian Medical Association Journal 120 (8), 937.

Iagnocco, A., Coari, G., Palombi, G., et al., 2001. Sonography in the study of metatarsalgia. Journal of Rheumatology 28 (6), 1338–1340.

Iida, M., Basmajian, J.V., 1974. Electromyography of hallux valgus. Clinical Orthopaedics and Related Research 101, 220–224.

Jack, E., 1940. The aetiology of hallux rigidus. British Journal of Surgery 27 (107), 492–497.

Jack, E.A., 1953. Naviculo-cuneiform fusion in the treatment of flat foot. Journal of Bone and Joint Surgery, British Volume 35, 75.

John, M.M., Kalish, S., Perns, S.V., et al., 2011. Dynamic splinting for postoperative hallux limitus: a randomized, controlled trial. Journal of the American Podiatric Medical Association 101 (4), 285–288.

Judge, M., LaPointe, S., Yu, G., et al., 1999. The effect of hallux abducto valgus surgery on the sesamoid apparatus position. Journal of the American Podiatric Medical Association 89 (11), 551–559.

Juriansz, A.M., 1996. Conservative treatment of hallux valgus: a randomised controlled clinical trial of hallux valgus night splints. King's College, University of London, London.

Kankanala, G., Jain, A., 2007. The operational characteristics of ultrasonography for the diagnosis of plantar intermetatarsal neuroma. Journal of Foot and Ankle Surgery 46, 213–217.

Kappel-Bargas, A., Woolf, R.D., Cornwall, M.W., et al., 1998. The windlass mechanism during normal walking and passive first metatarsalphalangeal joint extension. Clinical Biomechanics 13 (3), 190–194.

Keller, W.L., 1904. The surgical treatment of bunions and hallux valgus. New York Medical Journal 80 (741), 16.

Kernbach, K.J., 2012. Hammertoe surgery: arthroplasty, arthrodesis or plantar plate repair? Clinics in Podiatric Medicine and Surgery 29 (3), 355–366.

Kilmartin, T., Wallace, W., 1994. Effect of pronation and supination orthosis on Morton's neuroma and lower extremity function. Foot and Ankle International 15 (5), 256–262.

Kilmartin, T., Barrington, R., Wallace, W., 1992. The x-ray measurement of hallux valgus: an inter-and intra-observer error study. The Foot 2 (1), 7–11.

Kilmartin, T., Barrington, R., Wallace, W., 1994. A controlled prospective trial of a foot orthosis for juvenile hallux valgus. Journal of Bone and Joint Surgery, British Volume 76 (2), 210–214.

Komeda, T., Tanaka, Y., Takakura, Y., et al., 2001. Evaluation of the longitudinal arch of the foot with hallux valgus using a newly developed two-dimensional coordinate system. Journal of Orthopaedic Science 6 (2), 110–118.

Konkel, K., Menger, A., Retzlaff, S., 2007. Hammer toe correction using an absorbable intramedullary pin. Foot and Ankle International 28, 916–920.

Kunze, B., Wulker, N., 2011. Problem cases of metatarsalgia]. Der Orthopade 40 (5), 399–402, 404–406.

Kwon, J.Y., De Asla, R.J., 2011. The use of flexor to extensor transfers for the correction of the flexible hammer toe deformity. Foot and Ankle Clinics 16 (4), 573–582.

Kwon, O.Y., Tuttle, L.J., Johnson, J.E., et al., 2009. Muscle imbalance and reduced ankle joint motion in people with hammer toe deformity. Clinical Biomechanics 24 (8), 670–675.

Laird, P., 1972. Functional hallux limitus. The Illinois Podiatrist 9, 4.

Lallemand, B., Care, G., Franck, T., et al., 2003. [How I explore … a Morton's neuroma]. Revue Medicale de Liege 58 (10), 638–640.

Lancaster, S.C., Sizensky, J.A., Young, C.C., 2008. Acute mallet toe. Clinical Journal of Sport Medicine 18 (3), 298–299.

Landorf, K.B., 2009. Extracorporeal shockwave therapy for interdigital neuroma: a randomized, placebo-controlled, double-blind trial. Journal of the American Podiatric Medical Association 99 (5), 472–473.

Lapidus, P., 1934. Operative correction of the metatarsus varus primus in hallux valgus. Surgery in Gynecology and Obstetrics 58, 183–191.

Lazarides, S., Hildreth, A., Prassanna, V., et al., 2005. Association amongst angular deformities in hallux valgus and impact of the deformity in health-related quality of life. Foot and Ankle Surgery 11 (4), 193–196.

Lee, J.-H., Han, S.-H., Ye, J.-F., et al., 2012. Effective zone of botulinum toxin a injections in hallux claw toe syndrome: an anatomical study. Muscle and Nerve 45 (2), 217–221.

Lee, K.S., 2009. Musculoskeletal ultrasound: how to evaluate for Morton's neuroma. AJR. American Journal of Roentgenology 193 (3), W172.

Lee, K.T., Lee, Y.K., Young, K.W., et al., 2009. Results of operative treatment of double Morton's neuroma in the same foot. Journal of Orthopaedic Science 14 (5), 574–578.

Leveille, S.G., Guralnik, J.M., Ferrucci, L., et al., 1998. Foot pain and disability in older women. American Journal of Epidemiology 148 (7), 657–665.

Lichniak, J.E., 1997. Hallux limitus in the athlete. Clinics in Podiatric Medicine and Surgery 14 (3), 407–426.

Ludloff, K., 1918. Die Beseitigung des Hallux Valgus durch die schrage planta-dorsale Osteotomie des Metatarsus. I. Archiv für Klinische Chirurgie 110, 364–387.

Lui, T., 2007. Arthroscopic-assisted correction of claw toe or overriding toe deformity: plantar plate tenodesis. Archives of Orthopaedic and Trauma Surgery 127 (9), 823–826.

Magnan, B., Marangon, A., Frigo, A., et al., 2005. Local phenol injection in the treatment of interdigital neuritis of the foot (Morton's neuroma). La Chirurgia Degli Organi Di Movimento 90, 371–377.

Maher, A., Metcalfe, S., 2008. First MTP joint arthrodesis for the treatment of hallux rigidus: results of 29 consecutive cases using the foot health status questionnaire validated measurement tool. The Foot 18 (3), 123–130.

Makki, D., Haddad, B.Z., Mahmood, Z., et al., 2012. Efficacy of corticosteroid injection versus size of plantar interdigital neuroma. Foot and Ankle International 33 (9), 722–726.

Mancuso, J.E., Abramow, S.P., Landsman, M.J., et al., 2003. The zero-plus first metatarsal and its relationship to bunion deformity. Journal of Foot and Ankle Surgery 42 (6), 319–326.

Mann, R.A., Coughlin, M.J., 1981. Hallux valgus – etiology, anatomy, treatment and surgical considerations. Clinical Orthopaedics and Related Research 157, 31–41.

Mann, R.A., Pfeffinger, L., 1991. Hallux valgus repair: DuVries modified McBride procedure. Clinical Orthopaedics and Related Research 272, 213–218.

Mann, R., Rudicel, S., Graves, S., 1992. Repair of hallux valgus with a distal soft-tissue procedure and proximal metatarsal osteotomy. A long-term follow-up. Journal of Bone and Joint Surgery, American Volume 74 (1), 124–129.

Markovic, M., Crichton, K., Read, J.W., et al., 2008. Effectiveness of ultrasound-guided corticosteroid injection in the treatment of Morton's neuroma. Foot and Ankle International 29 (5), 483–487.

Martinez-Nova, A., Sanchez-Rodriguez, R., Perez-Soriano, P., et al., 2010. Plantar pressures determinants in mild hallux valgus. Gait and Posture 32 (3), 425–427.

McBride, E., 1928. A conservative operative for bunions. Journal of Bone and Joint Surgery 10, 735–739.

McMaster, M., 1978. The pathogenesis of hallux rigidus. Journal of Bone and Joint Surgery, British Volume 60 (1), 82–87.

Mendicino, S., Rockett, M., 1997. Morton's neuroma. Update on diagnosis and imaging. Clinics in Podiatric Medicine and Surgery 14, 303–311.

Menz, H.B., Lord, S.R., 2001. The contribution of foot problems to mobility impairment and falls in community dwelling older people. Journal of the American Geriatrics Society 49 (12), 1651–1656.

Menz, H.B., Lord, S.R., 2005. Gait instability in older people with hallux valgus. Foot and Ankle International 26 (6), 483–489.

Menz, H.B., Munteanu, S.E., 2005. Radiographic validation of the Manchester scale for the classification of hallux valgus deformity. Rheumatology 44 (8), 1061–1066.

Menz, H.B., Tiedemann, A., Kwan, M.M.-S., et al., 2003. Reliability of clinical tests of foot and ankle characteristics in older people. Journal of the American Podiatric Medical Association 93 (5), 380–387.

Menz, H.B., Roddy, E., Thomas, E., et al., 2011. Impact of hallux valgus severity on general and foot-specific health-related quality of life. Arthritis Care and Research 63 (3), 396–404.

Meyer, M., 1926. Eine neue Modifikation der Hallux valgus Operation. Zeitbildung Chirurgie 53, 3265–3268.

Mickle, K.J., Munro, B.J., Lord, S.R., et al., 2011. Gait, balance and plantar pressures in older people with toe deformities. Gait and Posture 34 (3), 347–351.

Miller, S.J., 2002. Hammer toe correction by arthrodesis of the proximal interphalangeal joint using a cortical bone allograft pin. Journal of the American Podiatric Medical Association 92 (10), 563–569.

Minami, A., Kasashima, T., Iwasaki, N., et al., 2000. Vascularised fibular grafts: an experience of 102 patients. Journal of Bone and Joint Surgery, British Volume 82, 1022–1025.

Mitchell, C.L., Fleming, J.L., Allen, R., et al., 1958. Osteotomy-bunionectomy for hallux valgus. The Journal of Bone and Joint Surgery 40 (1), 41–60.

Molloy, A., Shariff, R., 2011. Mallet toe deformity. Foot and Ankle Clinics 16 (4), 537–546.

Moore, J.L., Rosen, R., Cohen, J., et al., 2012. Radiofrequency thermoneurolysis for the treatment of Morton's neuroma. Journal of Foot and Ankle Surgery 51 (1), 20–22.

Mulder, J., 1951. The causative mechanism in Morton's metatarsalgia. Journal of Bone and Joint Surgery, British Volume 33B, 94–95.

Mulier, T., Steenwerckx, A., Thienpont, E., et al., 1999. Results after cheilectomy in athletes with hallux rigidus. Foot and Ankle International 20 (4), 232–237.

Munuera, P.V., Dominguez, G., Castillo, J.M., 2007. Radiographic study of the size of the first metatarso-digital segment in feet with incipient hallux limitus. Journal of the American Podiatric Medical Association 97 (6), 460–468.

Munuera, P.V., Domínguez, G., Lafuente, G., 2008. Length of the sesamoids and their distance from the metatarsophalangeal joint space in feet with incipient hallux limitus. Journal of the American Podiatric Medical Association 98 (2), 123–129.

Musson, R.E., Sawhney, J.S., Lamb, L., et al., 2012. Ultrasound guided alcohol ablation of Morton's neuroma. Foot and Ankle International 33 (3), 196–201.

Nashi, M., Venkatachalam, A., Muddu, B., 1997. Surgery of Morton's neuroma: dorsal or plantar approach? Journal of the Royal College of Surgeons (Edinburgh) 42 (1), 36–37.

Nawoczenski, D.A., Ludewig, P.M., 2004. The effect of forefoot and arch posting orthotic designs on first metatarsophalangeal joint kinematics during gait. Journal of Orthopaedic and Sports Physical Therapy 34 (6), 317.

Nawoczenski, D.A., Baumhauer, J.F., Umberger, B.R., 1999. Relationship between clinical measurements and motion of the first metatarsophalangeal joint during gait. Journal of Bone and Joint Surgery, American Volume 81 (3), 370–376.

Nery, C., Coughlin, M.J., Baumfeld, D., et al., 2012. Lesser metatarsophalangeal joint instability: prospective evaluation and repair of plantar plate and capsular insufficiency. Foot and Ankle International 33 (4), 301–311.

Nguyen, U.-S., Hillstrom, H.J., Li, W., et al., 2010. Factors associated with hallux valgus in a population-based study of older women and men: the MOBILIZE Boston Study. Osteoarthritis and Cartilage 18 (1), 41–46.

Nilsonne, H., 1930. Hallux rigidus and its treatment. Acta Orthopaedica 1 (1–4), 295–303.

Nix, S., Smith, M., Vicenzino, B., 2010. Prevalence of hallux valgus in the general population: a systematic review and meta-analysis. Journal of Foot and Ankle Research 3 (1), 21.

Nix, S.E., Vicenzino, B.T., Collins, N.J., et al., 2013. Gait parameters associated with hallux valgus: a systematic review. Journal of Foot and Ankle Research 6 (1), 9.

Nunan, P., Giesy, B., 1997. Management of Morton's neuroma in athletes. Clinics in Podiatric Medicine and Surgery 14 (3), 489–501.

O'Kane, C., Kilmartin, T., 2005. Review of proximal interphalangeal joint excisional arthroplasty for the correction of second hammer toe deformity in 100 cases. Foot and Ankle International 26 (4), 320–325.

Okuda, R., Kinoshita, M., Yasuda, T., et al., 2007. The shape of the lateral edge of the first metatarsal head as a risk factor for recurrence of hallux valgus. Journal of Bone and Joint Surgery 89 (10), 2163–2172.

Oliver, T.P., Armstrong, D.G., Harkless, L.B., et al., 1996. The combined hammer toe-mallet toe deformity with associated double corns: a retrospective review. Clinics in Podiatric Medicine and Surgery 13 (2), 263–268.

Oloff, L.M., Jhala-Patel, G., 2008. A retrospective analysis of joint salvage procedures for grades III and IV hallux rigidus. Journal of Foot and Ankle Surgery 47 (3), 230–236.

Owens, R., Gougoulias, N., Guthrie, H., et al., 2011. Morton's neuroma: clinical testing and imaging in 76 feet, compared to a control group. Journal of Foot and Ankle Surgery 17 (3), 197–200.

Park, H.-J., Kim, S.S., Rho, M.-H., et al., 2011. Sonographic appearances of Morton's neuroma: differences from other interdigital soft tissue masses. Ultrasound in Medicine and Biology 37 (8), 1204–1209.

Pastides, P., El-Sallakh, S., Charalambides, C., 2012. Morton's neuroma: A clinical versus radiological diagnosis. Journal of Foot and Ankle Surgery 18 (1), 22–24.

Pavol, M.J., Owings, T.M., Foley, K.T., et al., 1999. Gait characteristics as risk factors for falling from trips induced in older adults. Journals of Gerontology Series A: Biological Sciences and Medical Sciences 54 (11), M583–M590.

Payne, C., Dananberg, H., 1997. Sagittal plane facilitation of the foot. Australasian Journal of Podiatric Medicine 31 (1), 7–11.

Payne, C., Chuter, V., Miller, K., 2002. Sensitivity and specificity of the functional hallux limitus test to predict foot function. Journal of the American Podiatric Medical Association 92 (5), 269–271.

Perera, A.M., Mason, L., Stephens, M.M., 2011. The pathogenesis of hallux valgus. Journal of Bone and Joint Surgery, American Volume 93 (17), 1650–1661.

Perini, L., Del Borrello, M., Cipriano, R., et al., 2006. Dynamic sonography of the forefoot in Morton's syndrome: correlation with magnetic resonance and surgery. Radiologia Medica 111 (7), 897–905.

Phillips, R., Law, E., Ward, E., et al., 1996. Functional motion of the medial column joints of the foot during propulsion. Journal of the American Podiatric Medical Association 86 (10), 474–486.

Piggott, H., 1960. The natural history of hallux valgus in adolescence and early adult life. Journal of Bone and Joint Surgery, British Volume 42 (4), 749–760.

Pique-Vidal, C., Sole, M.T., Antich, J., 2007. Hallux valgus inheritance: pedigree research in 350 patients with bunion deformity. Journal of Foot and Ankle Surgery 46 (3), 149–154.

Pons, M., Alvarez, F., Solana, J., et al., 2007. Sodium hyaluronate in the treatment of hallux rigidus. A single-blind, randomized study. Foot and Ankle International 28 (1), 38–42.

Pulavarti, R.S., McVie, J.L., Tulloch, C., 2005. First metatarsophalangeal joint replacement using the bio-action great toe implant: intermediate results. Foot and Ankle International 26 (12), 1033–1037.

Raymakers, R., Waugh, W., 1971. The treatment of metatarsalgia with hallux valgus. Journal of Bone and Joint Surgery, British Volume 53 (4), 684–687.

Reddy, P., Zelicof, S., Ruotolo, C., et al., 1995. Interdigital neuroma: local cutaneous changes after corticosteroid injection. Clinical Orthopaedics and Related Research 317, 185–187.

Resch, S., Stenstrom, A., Egund, N., 1989. Proximal closing wedge osteotomy and adductor tenotomy for treatment of hallux valgus. Foot and Ankle International 9 (6), 272–280.

Richardson, E., Brotzman, S., Graves, S., 1993. The plantar incision for procedures involving the forefoot. An evaluation of one hundred and fifty incisions in 115 patients. Journal of Bone and Joint Surgery 75 (5), 726–731.

Robinson, A.H.N., Limbers, J.P., 2005. Modern concepts in the treatment of hallux valgus. Journal of Bone and Joint Surgery, British Volume 87 (8), 1038–1045.

Roddy, E., Zhang, W., Doherty, M., 2007. Validation of a self-report instrument for assessment of hallux valgus. Osteoarthritis and Cartilage 15 (9), 1008–1012.

Roddy, E., Zhang, W., Doherty, M., 2008. Prevalence and associations of hallux valgus in a primary care population. Arthritis Care and Research 59 (6), 857–862.

Root, M.L., Orien, W.P., Weed, J.H., 1977. Motion at specific joints of the foot. In: Root, S.A. (Ed.), Normal and abnormal function of the foot, Clinical Biomechanics Corporation, Los Angeles CA, pp. 46–60.

Rosenberg, G., Sferra, J., 1998. Morton's neuroma: primary and recurrent and their treatment. Foot and Ankle Clinics 3, 473–484.

Roukis, T.S., Scherer, P., Anderson, C., 1996. Position of the first ray and motion of the first metatarsophalangeal joint. Journal of the American Podiatric Medical Association 86 (11), 538–546.

Roukis, T.S., Jacobs, P.M., Dawson, D.M., et al., 2002. A prospective comparison of clinical, radiographic, and intraoperative features of hallux rigidus: short-term follow-up and analysis. Journal of Foot and Ankle Surgery 41 (3), 158–165.

Rout, R., Tedd, H., Lloyd, R., et al., 2009. Morton's neuroma: diagnostic accuracy, effect on treatment time and costs of direct referral to ultrasound by primary care physicians. Quality in Primary Care 17 (4), 277–282.

Sahrmann, S., 2002. Diagnosis and movement of movement impairment syndrome, Mosby, St Louis.

Sammarco, G.J., Idusuyi, O.B., 2001. Complications after surgery of the hallux. Clinical Orthopaedics and Related Research 391, 59–71.

Sammarco, G., Brainard, B., Sammarco, V., 1993. Bunion correction using proximal chevron osteotomy: a single incision technique. Foot and Ankle 14 (1), 8–14.

Saygi, B., Yildirim, Y., Saygi, E., et al., 2005. Morton neuroma: comparative results of two conservative methods. Foot and Ankle International 26 (7), 556–559.

Scherer, P.R., Sanders, J., Eldredge, D.E., et al., 2006. Effect of functional foot orthoses on first metatarsophalangeal joint dorsiflexion in stance and gait. Journal of the American Podiatric Medical Association 96 (6), 474–481.

Schreiber, K., Khodaee, M., Poddar, S., et al., 2011. Clinical inquiry. What is the best way to treat Morton's neuroma? Journal of Family Practice 60 (3), 157–158, 168.

Schrier, J.C.M., Verheyen, C.C.P.M., Louwerens, J.W., 2009. Definitions of hammer toe and claw toe: an evaluation of the literature. Journal of the American Podiatric Medical Association 99 (3), 194–197.

Schurman, D.J., Smith, R.L., 2004. Osteoarthritis: current treatment and future prospects for surgical, medical, and biologic intervention. Clinical Orthopaedics and Related Research 427, S183–S189.

Seibert, N.R., Kadakia, A.R., 2009. Surgical management of hallux rigidus: cheilectomy and osteotomy (phalanx and metatarsal). Foot and Ankle Clinics 14 (1), 9–22.

Shamus, J., Shamus, E., Gugel, R.N., et al., 2004. The effect of sesamoid mobilization, flexor hallucis strengthening, and gait training on reducing pain and restoring function in individuals with hallux limitus: a clinical trial. Journal of Orthopaedic and Sports Physical Therapy 34 (7), 368–376.

Sharp, R., Wade, C., Hennessy, M., et al., 2003. The role of MRI and ultrasound imaging in Morton's neuroma and the effect of size of lesion on symptoms. Journal of Bone and Joint Surgery 85 (7), 999–1005.

Shaw, A., 1974. The biomechanics of hallux valgus in pronated feet. Journal of the American Podiatry Association 64 (4), 193–201.

Shereff, M.J., Baumhauer, J.F., 1998. Hallux rigidus and osteoarthrosis of the first metatarsophalangeal joint. Journal of Bone and Joint Surgery 80 (6), 898–908.

Shereff, M.J., Bejjani, F., Kummer, F., 1986. Kinematics of the first metatarsophalangeal joint. Journal of Bone and Joint Surgery, American Volume 68 (3), 392–398.

Shine, L., 1965. Incidence of hallux valgus in a partially shoe-wearing community. British Medical Journal 1 (5451), 1648.

Silver, D., 1923. The Operative Treatment of Hallux Valgus. Journal of Bone and Joint Surgery 5, 225.

Singh, A.K., Briggs, P.J., 2012. Metatarsal extension osteotomy without plantar aponeurosis release in cavus feet. The effect on claw toe deformity a radiographic assessment. Journal of Foot and Ankle Surgery 18 (3), 210–212.

Smith, D., Barnes, B., Sands, A., et al., 1997. Prevalence of radiographic foot abnormalities in patients with diabetes. Foot and Ankle International 18, 342–346.

Smith, R.W., Reynolds, J.C., Stewart, M.J., 1984. Hallux valgus assessment: report of research committee of American Orthopaedic Foot and Ankle Society. Foot and Ankle International 5 (2), 92–103.

Smith, S.M., Coleman, S.C., Bacon, S.A., et al., 2012. Improved ankle push-off power following cheilectomy for hallux rigidus: a prospective gait analysis study. Foot and Ankle International 33 (6), 457–461.

Solan, M.C., Calder, J.D., Bendall, S.P., 2001. Manipulation and injection for hallux rigidus. Is it worthwhile? Journal of Bone and Joint Surgery, British Volume 83 (5), 706–708.

Steinberg, M., 1955. The use of vitamin B-12 in Morton's neuralgia. Journal of the American Podiatric Medical Association 45, 566–567.

Stuck, R., Moore, J., Patwardhan, A., et al., 1988. Forces under the hallux rigidus foot with surgical and orthotic intervention. Journal of the American Podiatric Medical Association 78 (9), 465–468.

Sullivan, J., 1967. Neuroma diagnosis by means x-ray evaluation. Journal of Foot and Ankle Surgery 6, 45–46.

Summers, A., 2010. Diagnosis and treatment of Morton's neuroma. Emergency Nurse 18 (5), 16–17.

Sung, W., Weil, L. Jr., Weil, L.S. Sr., et al., 2012. Diagnosis of plantar plate injury by magnetic resonance imaging with reference to intraoperative findings. Journal of Foot and Ankle Surgery 51 (5), 570–574.

Suzuki, J., Tanaka, Y., Takaoka, T., et al., 2004. Axial radiographic evaluation in hallux valgus: evaluation of the transverse arch in the forefoot. Journal of Orthopaedic Science 9 (5), 446–451.

Symeonidis, P.D., Iselin, L.D., Simmons, N., et al., 2012. Prevalence of interdigital nerve enlargements in an asymptomatic population. Foot and Ankle International 33 (7), 543–547.

Tai, C., Ridgeway, S., Ramachandran, M., et al., 2008. Patient expectations for hallux valgus surgery. Journal of Orthopaedic Surgery of Hong Kong 16 (1), 91.

Takakura, Y., Yajima, H., Tanaka, Y., et al., 2000. Treatment of extrinsic flexion deformity of the toes associated with previous removal of a vascularized fibular graft. Journal of Bone and Joint Surgery, American Volume 82, 58–61.

Tamir, E., McLaren, A.-M., Gadgil, A., et al., 2008. Outpatient percutaneous flexor tenotomies for management of diabetic claw toe deformities with ulcers: a preliminary report. Canadian Journal of Surgery 51 (1), 41–44.

Taranto, J., Taranto, M.J., Bryant, A.R., et al., 2007. Analysis of dynamic angle of gait and radiographic features in subjects with hallux abducto valgus and hallux limitus. Journal of the American Podiatric Medical Association 97 (3), 175–188.

Tehraninasr, A., Saeedi, H., Forogh, B., et al., 2008. Effects of insole with toe-separator and night splint on patients with painful hallux valgus: a comparative study. Prosthetics and Orthotics International 32 (1), 79–83.

Thomas, P.J., Smith, R.W., 1999. Proximal phalanx osteotomy for the surgical treatment of hallux rigidus. Foot and Ankle International 20 (1), 3–12.

Thomas, S., Barrington, R., 2003. Hallux valgus. Current Orthopaedics 17 (4), 299–307.

Thomson, C., Gibson, J., Martin, D., 2004. Interventions for the treatment of Morton's neuroma. Cochrane Database of Systematic Reviews (3), CD003118.

Threthowan, J., 1923. Hallux valgus. In: Choyce, C.C. (Ed.), A system of surgery. PG Hoeber, New York, pp. 1046–1049.

Timins, M., 2000. MR imaging of the foot and ankle. Foot and Ankle Clinics 5, 83–101.

Tokita, F., Obara, N., Miyano, S., et al., 1991. A study on the distribution of foot sole pressure of hallux valgus. Hokkaido Journal of Orthopaedic Trauma Surgery 35, 33–37.

Torkki, M., Malmivaara, A., Seitsalo, S., et al., 2001. Surgery vs orthosis vs watchful waiting for hallux valgus. Journal of the American Medical Association 285 (19), 2474–2480.

Torkki, M., Malmivaara, A., Seitsalo, S., et al., 2003. Hallux valgus: immediate operation versus 1 year of waiting with or without orthoses: a randomized controlled trial of 209 patients. Acta Orthopaedica 74 (2), 209–215.

Trivedi, B., Marshall, M., Belcher, J., et al., 2010. A systematic review of radiographic definitions of foot osteoarthritis in population-based studies. Osteoarthritis and Cartilage 18 (8), 1027–1035.

Trnka, H., Muhlbauer, M., Zembsch, A., et al., 1999. Basal closing wedge osteotomy for correction of hallux valgus and metatarsus primus varus: 10- to 22-year follow-up. Foot and Ankle International 20 (3), 171–177.

Uchiyama, E., Kitaoka, H.B., Luo, Z.-P., et al., 2005. Pathomechanics of hallux valgus: biomechanical and immunohistochemical study. Foot and Ankle International 26 (9), 732–738.

Uludag, B., Tataroglu, C., Bademkiran, F., et al., 2010. Sensory nerve conduction in branches of common interdigital nerves: a new technique for normal controls and patients with morton's neuroma. Journal of Clinical Neurophysiology 27 (3), 219–223.

Valente, M., Crucil, M., Alecci, V., 2008. Operative treatment of interdigital Morton's neuroma. Chirurgia Degli Organi di Movimento 92 (1), 39–43.

Van Gheluwe, B., Dananberg, H.J., Hagman, F., et al., 2006. Effects of hallux limitus on plantar foot pressure and foot kinematics during walking. Journal of the American Podiatric Medical Association 96 (5), 428–436.

Van Saase, J., Van Romunde, L., Cats, A., et al., 1989. Epidemiology of osteoarthritis: Zoetermeer survey. Comparison of radiological osteoarthritis in a Dutch population with that in 10 other populations. Annals of the Rheumatic Diseases 48 (4), 271–280.

Vanore, J., O'Keefe, R., Pikscher, I., 1984. Silastic implant arthroplasty. Complications and their classification. Journal of the American Podiatry Association 74 (9), 423–433.

Vanore, J.V., Christensen, J.C., Kravitz, S.R., et al., 2003a. Diagnosis and treatment of first metatarsophalangeal joint disorders. Section 2: Hallux rigidus. Journal of Foot and Ankle Surgery 42 (3), 124–136.

Vanore, J.V., Christensen, J.C., Kravitz, S.R., et al., 2003b. Diagnosis and treatment of first metatarsophalangeal joint disorders. Section 1: Hallux valgus. Journal of Foot and Ankle Surgery 42 (3), 112.

Villas, C., Florez, B., Alfonso, M., 2008. Neurectomy versus neurolysis for Morton's neuroma. Foot and Ankle International 29 (6), 578–580.

Vito, G., Talarico, L., 2003. A modified technique for Morton's neuroma. Decompression with relocation. Journal of the American Podiatric Medical Association 93, 190–194.

Ware, J.E. Jr., Sherbourne, C.D., 1992. The MOS 36-item short-form health survey (SF-36): I. Conceptual framework and item selection. Medical Care 473–483.

Weil, L., Borelli, A., 1991. Modified Scarf bunionectomy: our experience in more than 1000 cases. Journal of Foot Surgery 30, 609–622.

Welsh, B.J., Redmond, A.C., Chockalingam, N., et al., 2010. A case-series study to explore the efficacy of foot orthoses in treating first metatarsophalangeal joint pain. Journal of Foot and Ankle Research 3, 17.

Wheeler, R., McDougall, A., 1954. The anatomy of hallux valgus. Journal of Bone and Joint Surgery, British Volume 36-B, 272–293.

Wilson, J.N., 1963. Oblique displacement osteotomy for hallux valgus. Journal of Bone and Joint Surgery, British Volume 45-B (3), 552–556.

Wu, K., 1996. Morton's interdigital neuroma: a clinical review of its etiology, treatment and results. Journal of Foot and Ankle Surgery 35 (2), 112–119.

Yap, L.P., McNally, E., 2012. Patient's assessment of discomfort during ultrasound-guided injection of Morton's neuroma: selecting the optimal approach. Journal of Clinical Ultrasound 40 (6), 330–334.

Yu, G., Johng, B., Freireich, R., 1987. Surgical management of metatarsus adductus deformity. Clinics in Podiatric Medicine and Surgery 4 (1), 207.

Yu, G., Judge, M., Hudson, J., et al., 2002. Predislocation syndrome. Progressive subluxation/dislocation of the lesser metatarsophalangeal joint. Journal of the American Podiatric Medical Association 92, 182–199.

Zammit, G.V., Menz, H.B., Munteanu, S.E., et al., 2008. Plantar pressure distribution in older people with osteoarthritis of the first metatarsophalangeal joint (hallux limitus/rigidus). Journal of Orthopaedic Research 26 (12), 1665–1669.

Zammit, G.V., Menz, H.B., Munteanu, S.E., 2009. Structural factors associated with hallux limitus/rigidus: a systematic review of case control studies. Journal of Orthopaedic and Sports Physical Therapy 39 (10), 733–742.

Zammit, G.V., Munteanu, S.E., Menz, H.B., et al., 2011. Development of a diagnostic rule for identifying radiographic osteoarthritis in people with first metatarsophalangeal joint pain. Osteoarthritis and Cartilage 19 (8), 939–945.

Zelent, M., Kane, R., Neese, D., et al., 2007. Minimally invasive Morton's intermetatarsal neuroma decompression. Foot and Ankle International 28, 263–265.

Zgonis, T., Jolly, G.P., Garbalosa, J.C., et al., 2005. The value of radiographic parameters in the surgical treatment of hallux rigidus. Journal of Foot and Ankle Surgery 44 (3), 184–189.

Chapter 5

Rearfoot Entities

Bill Vicenzino

Chapter Outline

This chapter deals with pain in the heel that might have several local differential diagnoses, these being plantar fasciitis or plantar heel pain, tibialis posterior tendon dysfunction or adult-acquired flatfoot, tarsal tunnel syndrome and calcaneal fractures. Several authors have suggested that plantar fasciitis, tibialis posterior tendon dysfunction and tarsal tunnel syndrome should be viewed as a triad, hence the focus of this chapter. Calcaneal stress fractures, much like the foregoing conditions, are of insidious onset. Non-specific heel pain such as

fat-pad contusion/bruising has not been covered in this chapter because, although it might be a differential diagnosis, its presentation is quite non-specific with little research coverage.

PLANTAR FASCIITIS/PLANTAR HEEL PAIN

INTRODUCTION

Plantar fasciitis is a common cause of foot pain that is estimated to affect 1 in 10 people over a lifetime (Crawford and Thomson 2003) and cost over a quarter of a billion dollars a year (Riddle and Schappert 2004; Tong and Furia 2010). A recent systematic review of running-related musculoskeletal injuries reported prevalence and incidence rates as high as 17.5% and 10%, respectively (Lopes et al. 2012), whereas the incidence in a military population was found to be 10.5 in 1000 person-years incidence (Scher et al. 2009). Two-thirds of those experiencing plantar fasciitis present to their family physician (Riddle and Schappert 2004) and 16% of a sample of athletes from local athletic and university sports clubs visited a healthcare practitioner for this condition (Rome et al. 2001). Plantar fasciitis is managed by a wide spectrum of healthcare professions, including podiatrists, orthotists, medical practitioners, rheumatologists, orthopaedic surgeons, physiotherapists and osteopaths (Crawford and Thomson 2003). Clinically, the condition is quite easily recognized by site of pain and first-step pain, which contrasts with the uncertainty surrounding risk factors, underlying pathology or cause, and the best course of treatment.

PREDISPOSING FACTORS

Physical Predisposing Factors

It would seem that this condition occurs mainly in the fifth to seventh decades of life (Butterworth et al. 2012; Irving et al. 2006; Riddle et al. 2003), not unlike some of the tendinopathies (e.g. Achilles, tennis elbow) that can also occur in substantial numbers in non-athletic populations.

The load taken through lower limb musculoskeletal structures has been increasingly considered as an associated or risk factor to a number of musculoskeletal conditions. In this respect, weight, height, and body mass index (BMI) have been evaluated in a number of studies (Butterworth et al. 2012; Irving et al. 2006). Butterworth et al. (2012) reviewed 25 papers on the association between BMI and foot disorders and found no prospective cohort studies that could conclusively identify risk factors predisposing to the onset of chronic plantar heel pain. They identified nine matched case–control and three cross-sectional studies that showed at least a large effect size of association between cases of chronic plantar heel pain and controls (Cohen $d \geq 0.75$) in six of the eight studies of non-athletic populations [e.g. odds ratio (OR) of 5.6 [95% confidence interval (CI): 1.9 to 16.6] for those

with a BMI > 30 kg/m^2 in a non-athletic population (Riddle et al. 2003). Significant heterogeneity prevented meta-analysis (Butterworth et al. 2012). A recent prospective risk factor study for the development of lower extremity tendinopathy and plantar fasciitis in United States military personnel also identified a higher risk of plantar fasciitis in those who were overweight and obese, as well as some other factors (e.g. recent deployment, older age, serving in the army, history of tendinopathy or fracture) (Owens et al. 2013). The association between chronic plantar heel pain and BMI, height and weight appears not to be present in an athletic population (Irving et al. 2006).

A wide range of physical factors and functional characteristics of the ankle, foot and lower limb (e.g. talocrural and first metatarsophalangeal joint motion, plantar fascia thickness, calf muscle strength and flexibility, leg length discrepancy, stance phase duration and more) have been evaluated in terms of their relationship to chronic plantar heel pain (Irving et al. 2006). In their systematic review, Irving et al. (2006) found some evidence that limited ankle dorsiflexion and first metatarsophalangeal joint extension was associated with chronic plantar heel pain, but that the association with static or dynamic foot form was inconclusive. A recent study of non-obese (BMI < 25 kg/m^2) individuals with plantar fasciitis found reduced ankle dorsiflexion and a tendency towards valgus in relaxed stance position to be independent predictors of the patient group compared with healthy controls (Lee et al. 2011). When non-weightbearing passive ankle dorsiflexion (with knee extended) is less than $0°$, and between $1°$ and $5°$, the odds ratios are 23.3 and 8.2 respectively, which are substantial effects (Riddle et al. 2003). However, none of these studies employed prospective longitudinal designs and so it is difficult to state conclusively that ankle dorsiflexion, great toe extension and a valgus heel preceded the signs and symptoms.

Psychosocial Predisposing Factors

Not much seems to have been studied on potential psychosocial risk factors associated with chronic plantar heel pain. In a retrospective chart review study of 155 patients attending a physiotherapy clinic for foot- and ankle-related problems of whom 13% had heel pain, the Tampa Scale of Kinesiophobia (TSK-11) was one of the factors contributing to the self-reported disability (Lentz et al. 2010). Other factors were age, duration of symptoms, and deficiency in range of motion. Pain-related fear of movement might plausibly be associated with higher BMI, which together might need addressing in some clients presenting with plantar heel pain.

DIAGNOSIS

A diagnosis of plantar fasciitis is frequently made on clinical signs and symptoms. Classically, the patient reports pain on the first steps on arising in the morning or after sustained low/non-weightbearing postures (usually getting out of a chair after sitting for a while) and physical examination elicits reproduction of pain to palpation of the medial calcaneal tuberosity and in some patients along the plantar fascia (Tu and Bytomski 2011). Additionally, ankle and great toe extension might elicit discomfort or the patient's symptoms. Given that there are a number of structures underlying the clinician's palpating digit (e.g. flexor digitorum brevis, abductor halluces, medial head of quadratus plantae, plantar vessels and nerves) that could be stressed with great toe extension, the condition is increasingly labelled chronic plantar heel pain so as not to presume a structure that has not been conclusively identified to be the source of the symptoms. The lack of inflammatory markers adds further to the argument that the term 'chronic plantar heel pain' should be used instead of 'plantar fasciitis', because the suffix 'itis' denotes an underlying inflammatory process (Lemont et al. 2003).

Ultrasonography and MRI are not commonly required to make the diagnosis, though in recalcitrant cases it would be prudent to undertake such examinations in order to rule out other likely causes of the symptoms (Goff and Crawford 2011). Should imaging be undertaken, there is some good evidence of its utility. A meta-analysis of three papers ($n=161$ cases and 116 controls) revealed that chronic plantar heel pain was associated with a proximal plantar fascia thickness of >4.0 mm on ultrasonography [OR: 105.11 (95% CI: 3.09 to 3577.28)] (McMillan et al. 2009). Meta-analysis identified 3.35 mm (1.80 to 4.89) thicker proximal plantar fascia in the chronic plantar heel pain cases on MRI ($n=78$ cases and 163

controls) and 2.16 mm (1.60 to 2.17) on ultrasonography ($n=379$ cases and 434 controls) (McMillan et al. 2009). A patient presenting with the above clinical exam features and proximal plantar fascia thickness >4.0 mm on ultrasound examination is highly likely to have what is commonly referred to as plantar fasciitis.

The presence of calcaneal spurs on X-ray is sometimes the focus of attention by patients and clinicians, though their relationship to plantar fasciitis or stress of the fascia has recently been questioned. A radiographic, gross morphological and histological study of 64 heels in 32 human cadavers reported that the bony trabeculae of the spurs are aligned in the direction of weightbearing stress on the calcaneus during gait and standing, rather than in line with the plantar fascia or muscles (Li and Muehleman 2007). The authors proposed the spur to be more of a skeletal response to protect bone against stresses that might lead to microfracture, rather than a longitudinal traction of the fascia at its enthesis. This proposition is consistent with findings from another study of weightbearing lateral foot radiographs in 216 people that showed spurs are related to obesity [OR 7.9 (3.6 to 17)] in older men and women, but not with radiographic measures of foot posture (Menz et al. 2008). This study reported an OR of 4.6 (2.3 to 9.4) of having a history of heel pain.

IMPAIRMENTS

Impairments commonly considered in clinical practice relate to pain either with or without stress testing and other contributing factors such as abnormal biomechanics of joints (e.g. overpronation) and soft tissues (e.g. triceps surae).

Pain

Pain is the primary presenting feature of chronic plantar heel pain, especially on first step. Pain is a complex entity and is measured clinically with visual analogue scales (VAS, 0 to 100 mm) or numerical rating scales (NRS, categories from 0 to 10) with the 0 anchor representing no pain and 10 the worst pain imaginable. Landorf et al. (2010) evaluated the minimally important difference of the VAS for average pain and on first-step pain by using an anchor-based approach in a study of 184 patients with plantar heel pain undergoing two clinical trials involving taping and stretching. They reported that the minimally important difference for the average pain VAS was −8 mm (95% CI: −12 to −4) and for first-step pain VAS −19 mm (−25 to −13) (Landorf et al. 2010). These data could be useful in evaluating effects of treatment and possibly the severity of the condition relative to others. Though these two measures both capture key features of plantar heel pain and are easy to use in clinic, it is somewhat surprising to note that reporting of such pain scales is not a regular feature of clinical or laboratory trials of this condition. In the trials that do report these pain ratings it would seem that the baseline pain (average or on first step) approximates 50% of the scale (VAS or NRS) (Ribeiro et al. 2011; Stratton et al. 2009; Wearing et al. 2004). The clinician should also consider foot health quality of life questionnaires [Foot Health Status Questionnaire (FHSQ)] and indices [Foot Function Index (FFI)], which include pain sub-scales that canvas the patient's perception of pain under more activities/conditions. These scales are dealt with in the section on quality of life below.

The Jack Test or Windlass Mechanism. A commonly performed physical test in clinic is to extend the first metatarsophalangeal (MTP) joint in either weightbearing or non-weightbearing to determine whether it elicits the patient's plantar heel pain (McPoil et al. 2008). It appears to be a derivation of what was first described by Jack (1953), though his description has the test done in weightbearing, to see whether the arch could be restored in through what has been termed the 'windlass effect/mechanism' on the plantar fascia (Hicks 1954). Increased strain has been demonstrated at the plantar fascia with this test in cadaveric specimens (Alshami et al. 2007) and might be the mechanism by which plantar heel pain is elicited from sensitized plantar structures. Both the non-weightbearing and weightbearing tests have high specificity (100%) but low sensitivity (<32%) (De Garceau et al. 2003), and as such are probably not useful if used in isolation from other signs and symptoms. Limitation in active and passive range of motion on the non-weightbearing test was shown in a small group of runners with plantar fasciitis (n=6, controls n=12) (Creighton and Olson 1987). However, this

was not the case in an age- and sex-matched control study of 20 patients with plantar heel pain of an average 19.9 (33.2) months' duration (Allen and Gross 2003), which again cautions against weighing too highly impairments of first metatarsophalangeal joint extension in the examination of plantar heel pain.

Plantar Fascia Tightness

Clinicians frequently stretch and massage the plantar structures on the rationale that they have limited extensibility. There is some evidence that the plantar fascia is shorter in plantar heel pain. Lateral radiographs of 64 feet with plantar heel pain compared with 80 feet without heel pain taken in weightbearing and non-weightbearing showed that the plantar fascia was shorter in the plantar heel pain group in both weightbearing [approximately 7 mm (control length was 151 mm)] and non-weightbearing [approximately 5 mm (control length was 136 mm)]. The difference between weightbearing and non-weightbearing was 12.8 mm for plantar heel pain, compared with 15.4 mm for control (Sahin et al. 2010), indicating lower extensibility under loading. The implication being that there is a limitation of plantar fascia length and extensibility, which might need to be considered in the treatment plan.

Rearfoot Posture

Ankle and foot posture, notably (over)pronation, is often clinically regarded as a related impairment, though it is difficult to find definitive evidence for foot posture impairments in plantar heel pain. For example, Irving et al. (2007) reported that a more pronated foot posture (FPI 4 to 10) and high BMI (30 to 46.3 kg/m²) were independently associated with chronic plantar heel pain (median duration 12 months) on multivariate analyses of data from 80 patients compared with age- and sex-matched controls. This contrasts to reports of no differences in foot posture in a number of other studies. Allen et al. (2003) found no differences in longitudinal arch angle and rearfoot–tibia angle between patients (n=20, average duration 19.9 months) and age- and sex-matched controls. Ribeiro et al. (2011) likewise did not find differences in rearfoot alignment in 45 runners (30 current and 15 with greater than 2 months' remission, compared with 60 controls) with plantar heel pain [pain VAS 5 (SD 2) cm]. Wearing et al. (2004) examined 25 runners with a recent past history of plantar heel pain [duration since diagnosis of 2.8 years (SD 2.4) but no pain on running for 2 months] and reported no differences in rearfoot angle compared with age- and sex-matched controls, but they did show a lower arch height.

In terms of ankle and foot relationships (posture) during dynamic tasks, such as walking or running, there appears to be no evidence of impairments in those with plantar heel pain. In their case–control study of 25 runners, Pohl et al. (2009) did not find any differences in motion at the rearfoot or ankle, but they did report greater rate of vertical loading and impact peak in plantar heel pain. Wearing et al. (2004) used digital fluoroscopy to capture dynamic lateral images from 10 patients with plantar heel pain [mean duration 9 (SD 6) months, mean pain VAS 4 (SD 2) cm] and 10 controls of similar age, sex and BMI. They found no differences in arch angle or change in arch angle during the gait cycle, but did show a greater peak extension at the first metatarsophalangeal joint [4.6° (1.44 to 7.76)].

Ankle Dorsiflexion and Triceps Surae Involvement

Ankle range of motion is routinely examined in clinical evaluation of a patient with plantar heel pain. It would seem that a prevailing clinical dogma is that ankle dorsiflexion will be limited in plantar fasciitis, often assumed as reflecting tightness (contracture) of the triceps surae muscles (Bolivar et al. 2013). Somewhat surprisingly, ankle joint structures are seldom considered as a possible limitation of dorsiflexion. A 2006 systematic review (Irving et al. 2006) of factors associated with chronic plantar heel pain reported that there was some evidence of limited ankle dorsiflexion. For example, in a study of 50 cases compared with 100 controls, Riddle et al. (2003) reported odds ratios of 23.3, 8.2 and 2.9 for dorsiflexion less than 0°, 1–5° and 6–10° respectively. Recently, Bolivar et al. (2013) reported a substantial limitation in non-weightbearing dorsiflexion [knee extended: 15.6° (14.04 to 17.16) and flexed: 15.1° (13.33 to 16.87), $n=50$/group] compared with a control group (equivalent in age and BMI, sex matching was unreported and there was no description of duration or severity of plantar heel pain). By using ROC curve analyses, Bolivar et al. (2013) determined that 10° dorsiflexion was the lower

limit of normal range of dorsiflexion (when the knee was extended). An intriguing feature of the data that Bolivar et al. reported was that the difference in dorsiflexion between the knee-flexed and knee-extended tests was similar in both groups [plantar heel pain 5.1° (3.63 to 6.57) and control 4.6° (2.75 to 6.45)]. Measuring dorsiflexion with knee flexed reduces the gastrocnemius muscle's influence as a limiting factor on the measured range of motion. That both groups exhibited similar differences between knee-extended and knee-flexed states implies that the gastrocnemius is no greater a factor in plantar heel pain than it is in healthy controls. This leaves the question of what might be the reason for the substantial ankle dorsiflexion limitation found by these authors (i.e. soleus muscle, other extrinsic muscles of the foot and ankle, or ankle joint structures). From a clinical perspective, the limiting factor to dorsiflexion could influence the impairment-based treatment techniques that are selected (e.g. ankle joint manipulation or soleus versus gastrocnemius muscle stretches).

In contrast to findings of limited dorsiflexion are studies that indeed find greater dorsiflexion as a feature of plantar heel pain. For example, Pohl et al. (2009) reported greater non-weightbearing dorsiflexion in runners [mean difference with knee extended: 3.8° (0.85 to 6.75), knee flexed 4.6° (1.41 to 7.7), $n=25$/group] and Irving et al. (2007) reported greater weightbearing dorsiflexion [4.6 (2.46 to 6.74), $n=80$/group]. Then there are several reports of either no significant differences between patients and controls (Messier and Pittala 1988; Rome 1997), or only a minority of subjects categorized as having a tight gastrocnemius soleus complex, in a retrospective case audit (Taunton et al. 2002).

The evidence on dorsiflexion with plantar heel pain indicates that there might be a high level of heterogeneity in clinical presentation. For example, this can be seen from a comparison of the quantity of motion measured in the control group of two different studies. Bolivar et al. (2013), who reported substantial limitation in dorsiflexion, recorded dorsiflexion of 24.8° (4.7) and 20.2° (4.6) for knee-flexed and knee-extended tests respectively, whereas Pohl et al. (2009), who reported greater dorsiflexion, recorded dorsiflexion of 9.2° (5.4) and −0.4° (3.9) respectively for knee-flexed and knee-extended tests.

Muscle Performance

It is common to measure the force development capacity of muscles local to an injury (e.g. toe flexors and calf plantarflexors). Allen et al. (2003) showed that there was a lower capacity to generate isometric toe flexor force in a plantar heel pain group compared with an age-, sex- and BMI-equivalent control group [mean deficit of 39 N (3.86 to 74.14), $n=20$/group], but not between the affected and unaffected side [8 N (−20.28 to 36.28)]. Consistent with this poorer force generation performance is evidence of atrophy in the intrinsic plantar foot muscles (Chang et al. 2012). Irving et al. (2007) measured the number of heel raises to fatigue and showed an impairment in chronic heel pain patients of 2.9 raises (0.02 to 5.78), though this was not a sufficiently large enough effect to be retained in the multivariate model, which showed BMI and FPI as being associated with chronic plantar heel pain.

Tightness of the hamstring muscles has also been associated with plantar heel pain. Bolivar et al. (2013) reported straight leg raise to be 29.1° (24.86 to 33.34) less in a group of 50 patients with plantar heel pain compared with a control group. They calculated 70° to be the normal value for this measure. This is reasonably consistent with findings from another study of Labovitz et al. (2011) in which they measured popliteal angle at end-range knee extension with the hip at 90° flexion and scored ≤160° as being tight ([OR 8.7 (4.4 to 17.2), $n=103$ feet with plantar heel pain and 107 without heel pain].

In summary, patient presentation features that should be measured are pain, Jack's test, foot posture, and the extensibility of soft tissues (e.g. plantar ankle and foot structures). It must be remembered that there appears to be heterogeneity in presentation of these features from reports in the literature, which behoves the clinician to be wary of potential for expectation bias in clinical reasoning. This is especially cogent because in the literature on this condition there is a notable absence of an explicit statement on blinding of the rater to the pain/injury status of the participant, which introduces a potential source of bias.

FUNCTION

There are several measurement tools that capture the function levels of patients with plantar heel pain, such as the Foot and Ankle Ability Measure (FAAM), Foot Health Status Questionnaire (FHSQ) and Foot Function Index (FFI), which have been shown to satisfy adequate content and construct validity, reliability, and responsiveness (Martin and Irrgang 2007) and have been recommended for use by clinicians in measuring outcomes from physical treatments and status of plantar heel pain (McPoil et al. 2008). However, only the FAAM deals solely with function, whereas the FHSQ and FFI have other subscales (e.g. pain, activity) and as a total score are often referred to as health-related quality-of-life tools. The FHSQ and FFI are covered within the following section on quality of life.

The FAAM has been reported as an outcome measure in several studies of physical interventions for plantar heel pain (Cleland et al. 2009; Drake et al. 2011) and of its sensitivity to change (Martin and Irrgang 2007; Martin et al. 2005) has been recommended for use in a physical therapy setting in guidelines (McPoil et al. 2008). It is solely a function-based survey (i.e. no questions on pain intensity) as it covers a comprehensive list of physical activities/tasks and consists of a 21-item activities of daily living subscale and an 8-item sports subscale. Each item is rated on a five-point Likert scale ['unable to do (0)' through to 'no difficulty (4)'] and then expressed as a percentage of a total possible score, allowing for some items to be rated 'not applicable' (N/A) (Martin et al. 2005). The FAAM is a reliable instrument (minimal detectable change based on 95% confidence interval was ±6 and ±12 points for Activity of Daily Living (ADL) and Sports subscale respectively) with a minimally clinically important difference of 8 and 9 points on the ADL and sport subscales respectively as determined by the difference in those improved versus not improved in a study of a 4-week physical therapy programme (Martin et al. 2005).

QUALITY OF LIFE

There are two questionnaires designed to measure foot-health-related quality of life: the FFI and FHSQ questionnaires. The FFI is the oldest and most reported of the two and was specifically designed in relation to treatment of the rheumatoid foot with orthoses (Budiman-Mak et al. 1991). The FHSQ was developed and tested within a context of foot surgery in a podiatry practice (Bennett and Patterson 1998; Bennett et al. 1998). There is a need to further develop surgery-context-specific foot-health-related quality of life tools (Parker et al. 2003).

The FFI is a multifaceted index of foot health that has been extensively used [78 studies (mostly in the USA (41%)] across many conditions of the foot, with 11 (14%) studies of plantar heel pain (Budiman-Mak et al. 2013). The FFI has undergone some revision over time and the most recent version comprises five subscales: pain, stiffness, difficulty, activity limitation, and social issues, all which are rated against four response categories (either: no, mild, moderate, severe for pain, stiffness and difficulty; or none, a little, some or most for activity limitation and social issues). It can be used in a long or short form, in which the numbers of items for each subscale are respectively: pain 11 or 7, stiffness 8 or 7, difficulty 20 or 11, activity limitation 9 or 3, and social issues 19 or 6 (Budiman-Mak et al. 2013). The FFI is scored as a percentage of total possible points, either for each subscale or in total. A recent comprehensive review of English language papers from the last 20 years of studies using the FFI (Budiman-Mak et al. 2013) showed that it is a simple self-administered survey with minimal administrative burden and an easy scoring, being written to a grade 8 school reading level.

A study of 175 patients with heel pain enrolled in two clinical trials was used to calculate a patient-rated anchor-based minimally important difference for the FFI and its subscales (Landorf and Radford 2008). The minimally important difference was 7 (−0.1 to 13.1) for the total FFI, 12 points (3.8 to 20.7) for the pain subscale, and 7 (−1.5 to 15) for the disability subscale.

The FHSQ consists of 13 items grouped into four domains: four items each for pain and function, three items for footwear, and the remaining two covering general foot health (Martin and Irrgang 2007). Each item is rated on a Likert scale and a proprietary computer program is used to generate scores ranging from 0 to 100 points, with lower scores representing poorer status (Bennett and Patterson 1998; Bennett et al. 1998). This questionnaire is not freely available and along with the need for proprietary software is less attractive than the FFI to use clinically.

In a study of conservative treatments (taping and stretching, $n=184$), which determined a patient-orientated anchor-based minimally important difference

for the FHSQ subscales, the minimally important difference for pain was 13 points (6 to 19), function 7 points (1 to 13), footwear −2 points (−8 to 4), and general foot health 0 points (−7 to 6) (Landorf et al. 2010). The findings for pain and function are consistent with previous work (Landorf and Radford 2008). The findings for footwear and general foot health subscales are probably indicative of a poor sensitivity to detect change (Landorf and Keenan 2002) and the authors recommend further work in this domain (Landorf et al. 2010).

Foot-heath-related quality of life as measured with the FHSQ is substantially poorer in chronic plantar heel pain [median duration of 12 months (range, 6–96 months), $n=80$] when compared with age-matched controls ($n=80$) who had similar co-morbidities but significantly lower BMI [by 2.3 kg/m^2 (0.69 to 3.91)] and lower obesity rate (approximately half as many with BMI > 30 kg/m^2) (Irving et al. 2008). The chronic plantar heel pain group was worse by 51.7 (46.52 to 56.88) points on pain, 38.3 (32.26 to 44.34) points on function, 20.7 (12.24 to 29.16) points on footwear and 39.9 (31.84 to 47.96) on general foot health (Irving et al. 2008). The poorer quality of life in the chronic plantar heel pain group was not influenced by BMI, age or sex.

MANAGEMENT STRATEGIES
Overview of Approach to Management

General medical management of this condition tends to have three levels (Goff and Crawford 2011). First self-treatments such as activity modification (including complete rest if required), ice, oral analgesics, and stretching are trialled. If there is no change over several weeks then the second level of interventions would include physical therapy, foot orthoses, night splinting and steroid injections. There is an expectation that 90% of patients would respond to these, but should the pain be recalcitrant after 6 or more months then the third level would involve extracorporeal shock wave therapy (ESWT) or plantar fasciotomy (Goff and Crawford 2011).

It would seem that orthoses (custom-made or prefabricated) had most evidence in support of a likely beneficial effect (McPoil et al. 2008; Landorf and Menz 2008). This evidence was reported in a systematic review of publications (January 2007 census date) of the clinical efficacy of custom-made (casted) orthoses, corticosteroid injections (±nonsteroidal anti-inflammatory medication), ESWT, heel cups, heel pads, laser, local anaesthetic injections (±corticosteroid injection), night splints plus non-steroidal anti-inflammatory drugs, stretching exercises, surgery, taping, and ultrasound (Landorf and Menz 2008). This conclusion has independent confirmation in contemporaneous reviews (Hawke et al. 2008; Lee et al. 2009) and guidelines of the Orthopedic Section of the American Physical Therapy Association (McPoil et al. 2008), with Lee et al. (2009) showing a 15–35% advantage of orthoses over night splints (census date December 2007).

However, the evidence in favour of orthoses was not supported in a hypothetical case survey of 116 orthopaedic surgeons [responses from 84 (72%)]. This survey determined the surgeons' preferences for conservative and surgical management of a hypothetical 42-year-old female information technology analyst with a 4-month duration of recalcitrant right plantar heel pain (DiGiovanni et al. 2012). The patient's physician had prescribed ice, NSAIDs, Achilles stretching and activity modification (including cessation of her 6 miles per week run), but to no avail. The patient wore an over-the-counter medial arch support for the previous year. The surgeons were questioned about their treatment prescription at this stage and most favoured plantar fascia specific stretching (37, 44%), followed by supervised physical therapy (20, 24%), night splinting (17, 20%), steroid injection (5, 6%), custom orthotics 3, 4%), and cast/boot immobilization (2, 2%) (DiGiovanni et al. 2012). Interestingly, custom orthoses were not favoured, which contrasts with evidence from systematic reviews (Landorf and Menz 2008; Lee et al. 2009). What remained unanswered is the impact on surgeon's decisions of the patient-selected use of arch supports over the preceding 12 months. Perhaps the surgeons discounted orthoses on the basis that the arch supports had not prevented the plantar heel pain. If 6 months later there was no improvement from their prescribed treatments, the surgeons indicated that their next choice was surgery or ESWT (62 (74%)). Even though there is insufficient research on surgery (League 2008), the most popular surgery was gastrocnemius recession

(±other procedures) and open partial plantar fascia release with nerve decompression.

Pharmacological Strategies

Corticosteroid Injections. Corticosteroid injections are commonly prescribed in general practice. Landorf and Menz's (2008) systematic review of treatment studies, which compared injections with orthoses, no active treatment, heel pads, and analgesic, concluded that the evidence did not support the use of corticosteroid injections. However, all reviewed studies (January 2007 census date) received a low GRADE score, which essentially meant that further research is very likely to change the conclusion that corticosteroid injections ought not be used (Guyatt et al. 2008). A recent study of a higher quality than previously reviewed by Landorf and Menz (2008) compared an ultrasound guided injection of 1 mL saline (placebo) with 1 mL of 4 mg/mL dexamethasone sodium phosphate, both preceded by an ultrasound-guided tibial nerve block with 2% lidocaine hydrochloride (McMillan et al. 2010). McMillan et al. (2012) found a superior effect for the steroid injection at 4 weeks, but not at 8 and 12 weeks. At 4 weeks, the mean difference in pain relief as measured on the pain domain of the FHSQ was 11 points, which although statistically significant was slightly less than the 13-point minimally important difference. The outcome of the clinical trial was more impressive when categorizing those with a change of greater than 19.5 points as having a real improvement, in which case the numbers needed to treat (NNT) was 2.93 (2.76 to 3.12). A statistically significant reduction in plantar fascia thickness also occurred with the mean difference of 0.35 mm (0.03 to 0.67), but this was not greater than the 0.7 mm measurement error. However, when categorizing a real improvement as greater than 0.7 mm the NNT was 3.15 (2 to 7.35), which represents a strong effect. Unlike pain, the plantar fascia thickness was significantly reduced at all follow-up time points [e.g. 0.43 mm (0.01 to 0.85) at 12 weeks], which reflects the relatively weak relationship between pain and fascia thickness (e.g. $r=0.3$, $p=0.007$ at 4 weeks). A significant reduction in plantar fascia thickness and perifascial oedema, but not echogenicity or fat pad thickness, following steroid injection has been reported previously in a case series of 31 consecutive cases (Kayhan et al. 2011).

The use of ultrasound-guided injections has been increasingly advocated. A recent steroid injection study of 35 heels found no difference between ultrasound, palpation, and scintigraphy guidance in terms of outcomes in plantar fascia thickness and pain severity (Yucel et al. 2009). The authors recommended ultrasound- or palpation-guided injections as they were more clinically accessible.

The rate of adverse events following steroid injection appears to be low, ranging from 2.4% ($n=120$) (Kim et al. 2010) to 6% ($n=765$) (Acevedo and Beskin 1998) in retrospective case audits and none in the clinical trial of McMillan et al. (2012). Kim et al. (2010) reported that patients with an injection-related rupture had an average of 2.67 injections and an average BMI of 38.6 kg/m^2, which might guide clinicians in their clinical decision making.

Other Injection Types. Despite scant tangible clinical evidence of an appropriate quality, blood or platelet-rich plasma (PRP) has increasingly been injected in tendinopathies and plantar fasciitis (Kaux and Crielaard 2013). Emblematic of the low standard of trial methodology reported for these injections is the study of Aksahin et al. (2012) who treated 30 consecutive patients with a local injection of 2 mL of 40 mg methylprednisolone and then a second lot of 30 consecutive patients with 3 mL of PRP, all being injected concurrently with 2 mL of 2% prilocaine. Both injections improved the plantar fasciitis at 3 and 26 weeks (Aksahin et al. 2012), with no significant differences between injection type. This was not borne out in a similar study of autologous blood in which four groups of 25 consecutive cases were injected with: (a) 2 mL of autologous blood alone; (b) 2 mL of lidocaine combined with peppering; (c) 2 mL of triamcinolone alone, or (d) 2 mL of triamcinolone combined with peppering. Injections of autologous blood and lidocaine were inferior to the corticosteroid injection at 3 and 26 weeks, with peppering being the superior of the corticosteroid injections (Kalaci et al. 2009).

Botulinum toxin type A has also been increasingly injected for musculoskeletal conditions, for which there seems to be a dearth of evidence or in some cases biologically plausible mechanisms. Diaz-Llopis et al. (2012) conducted a 1-month follow-up clinical trial in which they randomized 28 patients to either 100 U of botulinum toxin type A were diluted in 1 mL of normal saline and 70 U were injected: 40 U in the tender region of the heel medial to the insertion of the plantar fascia and 30 U in the area between one inch (2.5 cm) distal to the talar insertion of the plantar fascia and the midpoint of the plantar arc in the midpoint of the plantar arch or 2 mL of betamethasone 6 mg/mL as acetate and disodium phosphate plus 0.5 mL of 1% mepivacaine in the area of the calcaneal tuberosity. Although they reported favourable results for the botulinum toxin A injection at 4 months, their data did not exhibit statistically significant differences (i.e. $p=0.069$), though with small patient numbers their study might have been underpowered to detect the approximate 12 points of difference in improvement between treatments ($34.24 \pm SD\ 21.10$ versus 22.12 ± 27.42 for botulinum toxin A versus corticosteroid injections, respectively). They allowed those who had no change or deterioration in FHSQ to cross over after 1 month (i.e. it was no longer a randomized trial) and reported superiority of the botulinum toxin A group for the 1- to 6-month time period.

Injection of an irritant solution such as hyperosmolar dextrose under the prolotherapy premise of stimulating an inflammatory response followed by tissue healing has also been advocated. Ryan et al. (2009) performed a case series of ultrasound-guided injections in which 20 patients presented for a median of 3 sessions (range: 1 to 12) over a mean 22 weeks (SD 15). Although 75% of patients required only 1 session, some required up to an average of 5.6 (SD 2) sessions until it had been determined they were satisfactorily treated or that they were not responding. All but four had responded favourably to treatment on follow-up some 12 months later.

Physical Strategies

Since the systematic reviews (Hawke et al. 2008; Landorf and Menz 2008; Lee et al. 2009) and guideline (McPoil et al. 2008) there has been some further work that might contribute to the clinical decision making in implementing physical strategies.

Foot Orthoses. Whether to prescribe custom or prefabricated foot orthoses appears to be a prevailing concern that, in the main, has not been comprehensively addressed by clinical trials (see above). A recent randomized clinical trial that compared a casted custom foot orthoses ($n=35$) with a prefabricated orthosis ($n=34$) showed that both interventions similarly reduced foot pain and disability significantly, as measured on the Manchester Foot Pain and Disability Questionnaire (Ring and Otter 2013). The authors recommended the prefabricated orthosis because it was 38% cheaper.

A study by Stolwijk et al. (2011) qualitatively evaluated plantar pressure distribution and insole shape in participants with heel pain (38 feet) and forefoot pain (metatarsalgia, 170 feet) who wore orthoses obtained from a podiatrist, pedorthist, or orthotist. They reported that insoles generally redistributed plantar pressure by significantly reducing it at the heel and metatarsal heads while increasing it under the medial and lateral midfoot region. This occurred regardless of the area of pain, which was not the case with the shape of the device. Compared with the forefoot pain group, the devices in the heel pain group had a significantly higher heel cup and lower midfoot support in both sagittal and transverse directions. The authors concluded that the clinicians (who were recognized experts in foot management) fabricated an insole that was similar between foot condition type and that the minor yet statistically significant variation in shape (customization) did not alter pressure distribution. This is consistent with findings of increased midfoot contact area and a fivefold reduction in heel peak plantar pressure with a prefabricated foot orthoses compared with three heel devices (silicon heel cup, soft-foam heel cup and heel lift) in 36 elderly patients with planar heel pain (Bonanno et al. 2011). It would seem that if plantar pressure redistribution is a goal of therapy it is not critical to fabricate custom orthoses. This is not to say that other features and effects of custom orthoses are not critical to their clinical efficacy.

A recent study comparing corticosteroid injection with a full-length silicone insole in patients with approximately 6.7 cm pain on VAS of 7 months' duration [(groups equally balanced on age, sex, BMI (approximately 30 kg/m^2)] showed that there was very little difference in outcomes at 1-month follow-up (Yucel et al. 2013). The authors recommend a trial of insoles as first-line treatment.

Taping. Van de Water and Speksnijder (2010) conducted a systematic review of controlled trials of taping for plantar fasciosis and identified five trials, three of

which were of high methodological quality but sufficiently heterogeneous to prevent meta-analysis. There is strong evidence of a short-term (1-week) effect of pain relief but inconclusive results on disability, which supports the use of taping such as the low Dye technique (Dye 2007) in the early management of plantar heel pain.

Stretching and Manual Therapy. In a systematic review of stretching of the calf muscles or plantar fascia, Sweeting et al. (2011) found six studies with significant heterogeneity to prevent meta-analysis. There were insufficient studies to assess whether stretching was superior to control or other interventions for pain and disability (Sweeting et al. 2011), but specific stretching of the plantar fascia might be better than calf (Achilles tendon) stretching alone in the short term on the FFI (DiGiovanni et al. 2003).

Combining orthoses, electrotherapy, or manual therapy with stretching is reasonably common in clinical practice, but research in support of such practice is nascent. For example, Drake et al. (2011) showed that combining 2 weeks of a temporary custom foot orthosis with stretching exercises (calf, plantar fascia, ankle) produced substantial improvements in pain and FAAM (far greater than minimally clinical important difference) in a case series of 15 patients with plantar heel pain of 20 months' duration (87% female, average age 37.6 years). Cleland et al. (2009) have shown that adding manual therapy to stretches of the plantar fascia, soleus, and gastrocnemius muscles proved to be superior to adding electrotherapy (ultrasound, iontophoresis with dexamethasone) in pain (NRS) and function (FAAM) at 4 weeks and the latter at 26 weeks.

Extracorporeal Shock Wave Therapy (ESWT). There is very-low-quality evidence that, when compared with placebo, ESWT marginally reduces plantar heel pain (Landorf and Menz 2008). A sensitivity analysis of the impact of the quality of the trial indicated that higher-quality trials do not detect significant effects of ESWT, whereas the lower-quality trials do (Thomson et al. 2005). A subsequent randomized clinical trial comparing ESWT with placebo ESWT ($n=20$/group) reported an advantage with ESWT in change from baseline of 1.5 point (−0.05 to 3.05) on pain Numeric Rating Scale (NRS), which does not reach the minimally clinically important difference (Vahdatpour et al. 2012). The study highlights some of the issues with research of this treatment (e.g. only measure pain on NRS, small sample size). Recently a randomized clinical trial showed that the improvement in pain VAS 3 months following ESWT (53/100 mm) was equivalent to that following a corticosteroid injection (40 mm) with similarly low rates of adverse effects (Yucel et al. 2010), which prompted the authors to recommend the injection as it was less expensive and likely more accessible.

One of the issues with ESWT has been that it is likely that there will be different levels of clinical efficacy with different dosing regimens. Chang et al. (2012) undertook a systematic review and meta-analysis of randomized clinical trials that compared shock wave therapy (focused and radial) with placebo. They recommended using radial shock wave therapy because it is least expensive and probably more effective. If using focused shock wave therapy, the analysis revealed superiority when using the highest tolerable energy output within medium intensity ranges (Morton et al. 2013).

Surgical Strategies

Surgical options are usually reserved for those with persistent pain of over 6 months' duration that have failed conservative management. Surgery may include release (partial or total) of the plantar fascia in isolation or combined with a range of other procedures, such as excision of abnormal tissue including any spur or nerve decompression (League 2008). Some have recommended endoscopic release to reduce postoperative morbidity and facilitate quicker recovery (Morton et al. 2013). Cryosurgery, in which a probe is inserted into the plantar surface of the most tender point of the plantar fascia at the calcaneus for application of two 3-minute freeze cycles with a 30-second thawing period interspersed, has been reported in a case series with promising results (Cavazos et al. 2009). As is characteristic of musculoskeletal surgery generally, there is no high-level randomized controlled trial that might be used as a guide to direct decisions of the patient and consultant (League 2008). In consulting with patients who are considering a plantar fasciotomy, it would be salient to consider that cadaveric

and in vivo studies have shown a loss of integrity of the medial longitudinal arch and an excessive medial shift of centre of pressure, being greater in cases of total fasciotomy (Tweed et al. 2009).

Lifestyle and Education Strategies

The relationship between high BMI and chronic plantar heel pain in non-athletes would plausibly lead to an emphasis on strategies that reduce BMI, though there is limited evidence in support of weight loss reducing foot pain (Butterworth et al. 2012).

FUTURE DIRECTIONS

A patient presenting to a clinic with pain in the plantar heel that is tender on palpation and symptomatic on first step will in all probability be diagnosed as plantar fasciitis. The increasing availability of diagnostic imaging modalities such as ultrasound has helped in better understanding the structures likely responsible for the symptoms. Although structural identification has improved, there is a need to better evaluate predisposing risk factors and head-to-head testing of treatments with high-quality longitudinal prospective studies. This should advance management of plantar heel pain through either preventative programmes or improved treatment protocols.

In applying evidence-based practice in implementing physical treatments, a clinician will usually address the patient's presenting physical impairments that have been identified from a clinical examination. For example, in-shoe foot orthoses would be considered if the patient exhibited excessive pronation and manual therapy would be considered to mobilize or stretch restricted joints and soft tissues. Further high-quality research on impairments using reliable measures and appropriate blinding is required in order to better understand the apparent heterogeneity in the current literature.

TIBIALIS POSTERION TENDON DYSFUNCTION (ADULT-ACQUIRED FLATFOOT)

INTRODUCTION

Posterior tibial tendon dysfunction (disorder or rupture) is a term that covers a constellation of signs and symptoms that was first reported in 1953 by Key

(1953). It is increasingly referred to as adult-acquired flatfoot deformity (Egol et al. 2010). Although the exact aetiology and risk factors are unknown, a system of staging based on clinical signs, imaging findings, and symptoms has emerged (Durrant et al. 2011). The staging system helps to direct treatments, with surgery being advocated for later progressed stages. Conservative treatment is advocated early and it has been suggested, with limited high-quality evidence, that non-operative treatment can improve pain, function, and disability as well as prevent need for surgery (Durrant et al. 2011).

There is scant evidence of its prevalence generally. A small validation study of a questionnaire (see diagnosis below) identified the condition in 6 of 65 (9%) elderly patients attending a clinic for an unrelated matter. A larger follow-up study of a random sample of 1000 over-40-year-old females registered to a general medical practice in Hertfordshire, England identified a prevalence of 3.3% (Kohls-Gatzoulis et al. 2009). An important feature of this study was that all the patients identified had had prolonged symptoms and were undiagnosed (Kohls-Gatzoulis et al. 2009). The condition is likely to affect females in substantially greater proportions than males (Barske et al. 2013; Durrant et al. 2011; Holmes and Mann 1992; Neville and Lemley 2012; O'Connor et al. 2010).

PREDISPOSING FACTORS

There has been inadequate research into the predisposing factors to posterior tibial tendon disorder. The condition is frequently reported to occur in middle-aged women (Rabbito et al. 2011). A case review of 67 patients aged on average 57 years reported a prevalence of co-morbidities (60%), such as obesity, diabetes, and hypertension, as well as previous exposure to steroids (oral or intramuscular) or previous trauma or surgery to the medial side of the foot and ankle (Holmes and Mann 1992). This is substantiated in part by a systematic review of 28 studies ($n = 19\,949$) that found adiposity, of which obesity is an extreme, has been linked as a risk factor to tendinopathy (Gaida et al. 2009). The mechanism underpinning this link is undetermined, but two hypotheses exist: either direct mechanical overload due to higher weight of the individual, or systemically through the effect of bioactive peptides or metabolic alterations on tendon

structure. Gaida et al. (2009) reasoned that it was not likely to be a mechanical loading mechanism because there were no differences between those with upper or lower limb tendinopathies. Notwithstanding those findings, the direct mechanical overloading of the foot structure is likely a significant predisposing factor given that the condition's phenotype includes flatfoot deformity in obese individuals (see diagnosis). Aurichio et al. (2011) reported that the arch index (area of mid-third of foot visualized on a podograph expressed as proportion of whole foot area) was significantly larger (flatfoot) in women [$n = 227$, age 69.9 (6.8) years, BMI 28.45 (5.12) kg/m^2] categorized as obese [$n = 75$ (33%), BMI > 30 kg/m^2], whereas FPI was larger (pronated) in men [$n = 172$, age 69.4 (6.7) years, BMI 27.0 (4.24) kg/m^2] who were categorized as obese [$n = 42$ (24.4%)].

DIAGNOSIS

Posterior tibial tendon disorder represents a continuum of dysfunction from early stages of tendinopathy to increasingly fixed flatfoot deformity with eventual breakdown and destruction of the subtalar and talocrural joints (Myerson 1996). Adult-acquired flatfoot deformity has recently been used as the diagnostic term (Egol et al. 2010), possibly because the condition is more complex and involved than simply a dysfunction of the tibialis posterior muscle and tendon.

Kohls-Gatzoulis et al. (2004a, 2009) developed and implemented a screening survey that will probably assist in identifying this condition. The survey consists of line drawings of feet (medial/lateral and right/left) on which the patient shades out areas of pain and swelling, and six closed-ended questions (yes/no) asking whether: (i) arch becoming flatter, (ii) heel turning out (walking more on inside of foot), (iii) pain on inside of foot, (iv) swelling on inside border of foot, (v) walking less because of foot, and (vi) difficulty walking on uneven surfaces due to foot. The authors determined that posterior tibial tendon dysfunction was present if there was: (a) medial pain or swelling on feet maps plus a positive response to anyone of the six questions on the survey, or (b) a positive response to two or more questions on the survey. This rating criteria was found to be highly specific and sensitive compared with a clinician's diagnosis (Kohls-Gatzoulis et al. 2004a).

The condition is usually categorized into four stages [recently with subclassifications (Bluman et al. 2007)], mainly constructed in order to assist in directing its management (Bluman et al. 2007; Chhabra et al. 2011; Weinraub et al. 2000). Stage 1 is pain±swelling at the medial malleolus posteriorly over the posterior tibial tendon, which is manifesting itself during or after walking, or prolonged weightbearing activities. Many clinically based classification systems include difficulty with performing five single-heel raises along with diminished muscle power and pain on testing the tibialis posterior muscle, but they do not refer to an everted/pronated rearfoot type (Kohls-Gatzoulis et al. 2004b). However, Rabbito et al. (2011), who conducted an age-, sex- and BMI-matched kinematic study of stage 1 symptomatic runners (n=12, approximate mean age 29 years, BMI 23.5 kg/m^2), reported no ankle invertor weakness, but a greater peak rearfoot eversion over longer periods during gait as well as lower arch height in 10% (not 50%) weightbearing.

It is postulated that there is a tendinopathy occurring at this stage, which might be evident on MRI (Chhabra et al. 2011) and ultrasound (Jain et al. 2011) scans. In a retrospective review of US scans from 217 consecutive cases, Jain et al. (2011) highlight that it is important to also visualize supra- and retromalleolar parts of the posterior tibial tendon, because the more severe tears and presence of tenosynovitis were identified in this area in 16.6% of cases, the majority of which were in females (Jain et al. 2011).

Stage 2 is pain over the posterior tibial tendon, possibly more distally and involving the insertion (Rabbito et al. 2011), swelling of the posterior tibial tendon sheath, and pain and difficulty with single-limb heel raise (Chhabra et al. 2011; Houck et al. 2009a). There might be some sinus tarsi pain in advanced stage 2 (Bluman et al. 2007). Classically it is in this stage that a key feature is reported to be acquired flatfoot deformity (Kohls-Gatzoulis et al. 2004b) with lowered medial longitudinal arch (Houck et al. 2009b). The deformity is still flexible in this stage with non-fixed rearfoot valgus and excessive forefoot abduction (too many toes sign) (Chhabra et al. 2011; Houck et al. 2009; Kohls-Gatzoulis et al. 2004b). The tibialis posterior muscle tests weak (Houck et al. 2008). Greater rearfoot eversion, ankle plantarflexion, and forefoot dorsiflexion have been reported in a kinematic case–control study of gait in 30 patients (FFI: activity 15, disability 34, pain 36%) and 15 controls (approximate age 58 years, BMI 30 kg/m^2) (Houck et al. 2009b). Characteristic radiographic changes in this stage are largely reflective of the kinematic changes, with loss of calcaneal pitch, rearfoot valgus, talonavicular uncovering and forefoot abduction (Bluman et al. 2007).

Stages 3 and 4 are characterized by more fixed acquired deformity and increasing joint degenerative changes at the subtalar joint in stage 3 and then involving the talocrural joint in the latter stage (Bluman et al. 2007; Kohls-Gatzoulis et al. 2004b; Smith and Bluman 2012). It is not surprising then that pain will now include these joints with pain over the sinus tarsi both medially and laterally. MRI findings in stage 3 include severe tendon tears and tenosynovitis, superficial deltoid and spring ligament abnormality, talar uncovering, early signs of talocalcaneal and calcaneofibular impingement and subtalar osteoarthritis (Chhabra et al. 2011). In stage 4 there are additional widespread changes on MRI in soft tissue (e.g. deltoid ligament) and joint structures (e.g. impingement and osteoarthritis of the talocrural, subtalar joints) (Chhabra et al. 2011).

IMPAIRMENTS

The impairments associated with this condition are the key features in establishing the diagnosis, such as a poor performance on heel raising, weak tibialis posterior muscle, and pronated/flatfoot type. A matter relevant to the validity of this condition being identified in the clinical setting, especially in the earlier stages, is that many of the impairments of the phenotype rely on measurements of foot posture and motion that require the clinician to perform a physical skill with some level of precision. It is therefore of concern that a recent study reported low levels of reliability in the clinical application of many of the tests commonly used to quantify or categorize foot posture and motion (Jarvis et al. 2012). The salient message from that study is that visual estimation through observation is not satisfactory.

Heel-rise Test

A classic sign of an incompetent posterior tibialis muscle is poor performance of heel rise (Egol et al.

2010; Myerson 1996), exhibited by a range of possible indicators such as lack of calcaneal inversion at peak of rise, inability to complete full plantarflexion range or a reduced endurance capacity (lower repetitions than unaffected side). Houck et al. (2009a) studied the kinematics of bilateral heel-rise tests in 30 patients with stage 2 posterior tibial tendon disorder (age 59.8 years, BMI 29.9 kg/m^2) compared with 15 healthy controls with normal medial longitudinal arch height (age 56.5 years, BMI 30.6 kg/m^2). They showed that the general pattern of the motion of the hind- and midfoot and the first metatarsophalangeal joints is similar between the groups, but that the pre-rise position was offset in the posterior tibial tendon disorder group (i.e. ankle and hallux plantarflexed, first metatarsal dorsiflexed and rearfoot everted relative to control). During heel rise there was less hallux dorsiflexion [6.7° (1.7 to 11.8)], greater first metatarsal dorsiflexion [9.0° (3.7 to 14.4)], and more rearfoot plantarflexion [7.3° (5.1 to 9.5)] (Houck et al. 2009a). At peak heel rise there was no difference in frontal plane position of the rearfoot, which is usually reported by clinicians as a key distinguishing feature. The authors indicated that an implication of their data was that the medial longitudinal arch is probably a more sensitive key point of observation than the rearfoot (i.e. lack of calcaneal inversion).

Recording the number of repetitions of heel raising is a physical exam test that is probably less prone to issues of reliability and validity than is visualizing poor movement patterning. Kulig et al. (2011) compared the number of repetitions of heel raising between a group of female patients with posterior tibial tendon disorder (n = 17, age 52.1 years, BMI 29.5 kg/m^2) and a matched control group (n = 17, age 50.7 years, BMI 26.9 kg/m^2). The control group completed on average 20.1 (SD 10.3) heel rises, which was 12.7 (7.26 to 18.14) times more than the patient group (Kulig et al. 2011). Although the groups were matched on age and BMI, there was a significant difference in arch height ratio [arch height/truncated foot length, mean difference 0.063 (0.04 to 0.09)] with the patient group having 29% lower arch height. Given this difference in medial longitudinal arch profile and the implications of the kinematic data of Houck et al. (2009a), clinicians might prioritize measures of the medial longitudinal arch in their clinical reasoning process.

Kulig et al. (2011) also evaluated hip abductor and extensor muscle strength and endurance capacity. There was a significant bilateral reduction in hip abductor and extensor strength (28.4% and 33.8%, respectively) and endurance (27.1% and 38.5%, respectively) in the patient group. These data indicate that clinicians ought to also test hip abductor and extensor muscle strength and endurance in the management of posterior tibial tendon disorder.

Posterior Tibialis Muscle Performance

Validly measuring the performance of the posterior tibialis muscle in isolation is not easy, given that there are other posterior (deep and superficial) compartment muscles that can substitute its function (Houck et al. 2008). Houck et al. (2008) built a device that positioned the foot in some plantarflexion (30–45°) and measured foot adduction force while the patient maintained a plantarflexion moment, rearfoot inversion, and their medial longitudinal arch. They used this device to compare 24 patients with posterior tibial tendon disorder (age 61 years, BMI 30 kg/m^2) with 15 control participants (age 55 years, BMI 28 kg/m^2) and identified approximately 29% deficit in strength [0.29 N/kg (0.13 to 0.45)]. The affected/unaffected side ratio was 0.77 (0.25) (Houck et al. 2008). Interestingly, although age, sex, and BMI were matched between groups, the patients with posterior tibial tendon disorder exhibited a 0.04 (0.02 to 0.06) deficit in arch height index (Houck et al. 2008), which is larger than the standard error of the measurement of 0.003 (Williams and McClay 2000). That is, these patients have a substantially lower medial longitudinal arch height, which might reasonably be associated with poor muscle function. It appears that medial longitudinal arch height is important to measure clinically.

Medial Longitudinal (Midfoot) Arch Height

Measuring arch height can be used to aid diagnosis, treatment planning, and for tracking progression of the condition over time (to validate treatment or to show the need to change management approach). Measurement of the arch height, taken from the dorsum of the midfoot (=half length of foot) is clinically possible without the need for sophisticated equipment or resource. To accommodate variation in arch height in feet of different lengths (i.e. in normal feet, the longer feet would have higher arches) the arch height can be expressed as a proportion of the truncated length of the foot (posterior heel to first metatarsophalangeal joint line). This is termed the 'arch height index' (Williams and McClay 2000). The arch height index has high levels of intra- and inter-rater reliability (>0.93 and 0.8, respectively) and has been validated against X-ray images (Williams and McClay 2000). It ought to be routinely measured at the initial examination as it has been shown to be different in posterior tibial tendon disorder compared with controls (e.g. Houck et al. 2008; Kulig et al. 2011; Neville et al. 2007; Rabbito et al. 2011) and is one of the characteristic features of the condition. As indicated above, studies that report arch height index usually find it is significantly lower in the posterior tibial tendon disorder group than in comparator groups. However, there is variation beyond 0.003 [i.e. the standard error of measurement (Williams and McClay 2000)] in the actual arch height reported by different studies, which make their data difficult to use in diagnosing the condition. For example, Houck et al. (2008) reported the arch height index to be 0.35 (SD 0.03, $n=15$) compared with the arch height index of 0.311 (SD 0.036, $n=17$) reported by Neville et al. (2007) in cohorts of similar BMI ($\sim$30 kg/m^2) and stage (stage 2). There is a need for larger normative data on arch height index stratifying for such things as age, sex, BMI and symptoms before this primary phenotype feature is able to be quantified validly and used in diagnosis. In the meantime it is recommended that medial longitudinal arch height be measured as an impairment, to be used as a target for treatment and in monitoring progress.

FUNCTION

Gait Performance

Gait performance can be measured in clinic by simply measuring the distance walked and pain exacerbated. In their study of hip and calf muscle performance, Kulig et al. (2011) reported that, on a 6-minute walk test, patients with posterior tibial tendon disorder walked 74.4 m (17.52 to 131.28) less and reported more pain [21.7 mm (9.84 to 33.56)]. Though minimal detectable change has not been calculated for this population, the deficit in distance walked is beyond the minimally clinically important difference of 61.34 mm in hip and knee osteoarthritis (Kennedy et al. 2005). These data are consistent with a kinematic study that showed reduced walking speed (0.33 m/s), cadence (7.97 steps/min) and stride length (0.31 m), but longer stance duration (3.53%) in a group of 34 patients (age 52.8 years, BMI 32.0 kg/m^2) compared with 25 controls (age 41.3 years, BMI 26.3 kg/m^2) (Ness et al. 2008).

Compared with measuring distance walked and pain response to walking, the phenotypical flatfoot posture (rearfoot eversion, forefoot abduction, lowered medial longitudinal arch) observed clinically during non-static weightbearing activities (e.g. gait) is difficult to quantify clinically without sophisticated equipment. A number of studies using such equipment have quantified differences in gait between participants with posterior tibial tendon disorder and healthy asymptomatic controls. Kinematic data have shown reduced dorsiflexion and increased eversion of the rearfoot, decreased plantarflexion and increased abduction of the forefoot, and reduced hallux extension (Houck et al. 2009; Ness et al. 2008). A further subclassification of posterior tibial tendon dysfunction occurs with those who test weak [affected/unaffected ratio: 0.64 (0.2)] exhibiting significantly greater rearfoot eversion, forefoot abduction, and lower medial longitudinal arch (Neville et al. 2010). Neville et al. (2007) demonstrated that the posterior tibial tendon length (modelled from kinematic data) was significantly greater throughout the range, especially in loading response and pre-swing phases. EMG activity of the posterior and anterior tibialis, gastrocnemius and fibularis longus muscles were also shown to be substantially higher (Ringleb et al. 2007), indicating that foot posture disadvantages muscle function (Murley et al. 2009).

QUALITY OF LIFE

It is not difficult to conceive that a person with an inability to raise onto the forefoot on a single limb with an adult-acquired and dysfunctional posterior tibial tendon in advanced stages will have a poorer than expected quality of life (Durrant et al. 2011). However, there is not much in the way of evidence to either quantify or validate such an impression. The association with the adiposity-related diseases would further contribute to the lower than expected quality of life.

There are few studies reporting quality of life or using validated instruments. FFI appears to be the most often used in studies of posterior tibial tendon disorder, interestingly mainly in studies of non-surgical approaches to management (Augustin et al. 2003; Bek et al. 2012; Kulig et al. 2009a, 2009b; Lin et al. 2008). The FFI was outlined in the section on plantar heel pain above. Currently there are no data in this condition on FFI in terms of validation or minimal clinical difference, though it has shown responsiveness to change in treatment studies (see following section on treatment).

MANAGEMENT STRATEGIES

The treatment of this condition focuses heavily on reversing the abnormal alignment in the rear- and midfoot with physical treatments involving orthoses and exercises. Failing satisfactory resolution of the condition through conservative approaches, surgery to address misalignment is then contemplated. Although there is a staging system to classify this condition, largely designed to direct treatment, there is very little research validating at what stage a treatment is most efficacious, or to the extent that any one treatment is more efficacious than others or the natural history.

Pharmacological Strategies

There is no research into specific pharmacological strategies for this condition, though anti-inflammatory, pain- and systemic-disease-specific pharmacotherapy is usually recommended as part of a management plan (Bluman et al. 2007; Egol et al. 2010; Myerson 1996). Corticosteroid injections around the tendon or administered systemically are probably not recommended, as they have been associated as a predisposing factor (Bluman et al. 2007; Holmes and Mann 1992; Myerson 1996).

Physical Strategies

Considering that the primary characteristics of this condition revolve around an incompetent tibialis posterior muscle and a flat-footed posture, it is not surprising that the most commonly proposed physical therapies are exercises and orthoses, often in combination. Unfortunately, there is a dearth of high-quality clinical research into the efficacy and effects of exercise programmes and orthoses, with a predominance of

case series and only two randomized clinical trials. In the main these studies are poorly reported and with significant methodological flaws (e.g. no intention to treat analysis, loss to follow-up of 20% or more, and variable reporting of outcomes and baseline patient characteristics such as BMI and the duration of symptoms) and are not that useful in directing decisions regarding treatments. The studies evaluate either orthoses or exercises combined with orthoses. The following is a description of the commonly prescribed orthoses and exercises combined with orthoses, along with some of the research findings.

Orthoses. There are two basic types of orthoses that could be used in the management of posterior tibial tendon disorder: an in-shoe foot orthosis worn under the foot in the shoe, and an ankle–foot orthosis that has stirrup-like bracing extending up the distal leg. There have been no studies that have directly compared these two types of orthoses, but there have been a number of clinical trials (mainly case series) that have studied the orthoses separately. Bek et al. (2003) reported a series of 25 cases (age 30.7 years, i.e. a reasonably young cohort) for which a pragmatic clinical approach to prescribing a custom-made orthosis was used (88% in-shoe devices). At 6-week follow-up there was approximately a 50% improvement in FFI pain and disability ratings (Bek et al. 2003). Interestingly, it has been shown that anti-pronation orthoses, either custom or prefabricated, alter electromyographic amplitude of the tibialis posterior and fibularis longus, with the latter approximating normal activation pattern (Murley et al. 2010).

The type of foot orthosis for posterior tibial tendon disorder will most likely involve upright stirrups extending up the leg. Lin et al. (2008) studied a double upright ankle foot orthosis in a case series study of 32 patients who had stage 2 posterior tibial tendon disorder, with a long-term follow-up averaging 8.6 years. The double upright ankle–foot orthosis improved the condition sufficiently enough for 70% of the patients to be device-free and avoiding surgery (Lin et al. 2008). This is consistent with another case series study of a similar brace, the Arizona brace, in 21 patients with stages 1 to 3 posterior tibial tendon disorder (Augustin et al. 2003); it showed significant improvements of 26.7 and 26.6 points on the FFI pain and activity subscales respectively over a 2-year follow-up period. The Arizona brace is a custom-moulded leather and polypropylene orthosis extending from the metatarsal heads to mid-tibia with either a lace-up or Velcro closure. It is fabricated from casting of the foot with the calcaneus positioned in its neutral anatomical alignment and uses a three-point fixation mechanism of maintaining rearfoot to tibia alignment (Augustin et al. 2003). Customizing this type of orthosis might provide for an improved outcome in terms of alignment and perceived correction of deformity by the patient (Neville and Houck 2009). A kinematic gait analysis study ($n=15$, 10 females, stage 2, age 61.8 years, BMI 31.8 kg/m^2) of a hinged Arizona brace, a no-hinge Arizona device, a fixed ankle–foot orthosis and a shoe-only condition showed that hindfoot inversion control was greater in the hinged device only, whereas all devices increased forefoot plantarflexion compared with the shoe-only condition during all phases of gait. Forefoot adduction was not corrected by any of the devices (Neville and Lemley 2012).

Surgical Strategies

There are a variety of surgical approaches to this condition and very little evidence-based guidelines to aid clinical decision making. Compounding matters is the lack of research-based evidence validating the underlying causes of the condition (Pinney and Van Bergeyk 2003). Some of the surgical options are tenosynovectomy, soft-tissue reconstruction (e.g. flexor digitorum longus (FDL) transfer, deltoid and spring ligaments, tightening of the plantar fascia), calcaneal osteotomy (to medialize the calcaneum), medial cuneiform (Cotton) wedge osteotomy, lateral column lengthening (preferably by calcaneal osteotomy/lengthening procedure), and arthrodesis (of rear- and midfoot joints) (Bluman et al. 2007; Feibel and Donley 2006; Hiller and Pinney 2003; Pinney and Van Bergeyk 2003; Zaw and Calder 2010). A stage-based approach is often advocated in applying these surgical options, with soft-tissue surgery in earlier stages [e.g. FDL transfer±medializing calcaneal osteotomy in stage 2 (Zaw and Calder 2010)] and more aggressive bony/articular surgery in latter more advanced stages with increasingly fixed deformities (Bluman et al. 2007; Weinraub and Heilala 2000). There is a contemporary trend to

preserve joint integrity to allow more normal articular mechanics and to focus on correcting bony deformities to minimize overload on soft tissues (Hiller and Pinney 2003; Pinney and Van Bergeyk 2003).

Surgery attempts to correct mechanical imbalances and deformities – for example, the FDL transfer to augment posterior tibial tendon and a medializing calcaneal osteotomy to overcome a valgus rearfoot deformity (usually advocated for stage 2), or correcting forefoot abduction deformity with medial and lateral column procedures (Zaw and Calder 2010). The ability of such surgical procedures to correct mechanical imbalances has been evaluated in a nascent body of research. A kinematic study of walking gait evaluated 20 patients (18 females, age 60.3 years, stage 2) a minimum 1 year after a FDL transfer, spring ligament reconstruction, and medial displacement calcaneal osteotomy (Brodsky et al. 2009). Comparisons were made with the unaffected side and with a control group (18 females, age 60.9 years) similar in sex, age, and height but not weight (operated group 82.9 kg versus control 72.5 kg, BMI not supplied), because the kinematic analysis system was not available before the surgery. There was no significant difference between affected side and control, or between affected and unaffected sides, in rearfoot sagittal and frontal plane motion or ankle power in terminal stance. There was a bilateral reduction in single-support time in the operated group compared with the control group (Brodsky et al. 2009). Brilhault and Noel (2012) reported a case series of 17 feet with stage 2 posterior tibial tendon disorder in which 13 were able to achieve an inverted calcaneum on single-limb heel raise on average 4 years after rearfoot reconstruction surgery (involved Evans calcaneal opening wedge osteotomy, triceps surae and peroneus brevis tendon lengthening). A more rigorous kinematic analysis of walking on average 24.6 months after a similar procedure revealed less favourable outcomes with significant differences between the operated ($n=13$, 92% female, age 57.8 years, BMI 32.2 kg/m^2) and control ($n=13$, 77% female, age 57.2 years, BMI 25.5 kg/m^2) groups for first metatarsal dorsiflexion and rearfoot eversion (Barske et al. 2013). Again there was no pre-operative kinematic data with which to compare post-operative status, which limits translation of these findings to advice a clinician might wish to provide to patients.

Some indication of those who might be likely to go to surgery can be seen from the findings of a retrospective case audit of a reasonably representative cohort (O'Connor et al. 2010). The audit compared the initial examination findings between those who had an operation ($n=41$, 71% female, median BMI 25–30 kg/m²) and those who did not ($n=125$, 78% female, median BMI > 30 kg/m²). The operated group had significantly greater BMI, longer duration of symptoms (operated median > 12 months, non-operated < 6 months), were more likely to have had a cortisone injection and have worn orthoses and were generally more severe (operated versus non-operated: stage 3: 22% versus 12%; stage 2: 75% versus 67%; stage 1: 3% versus 21%) (O'Connor et al. 2010).

Lifestyle and Education Strategies

Exercise Programmes. Consistent features of studies of exercise for this condition are that: (i) they invariably include an orthosis intervention, mostly the kind that incorporates a leg component, and (ii) there is substantial variability in the exercises performed and presence of other co-interventions. The exercises range from specific eccentric or concentric exercises for tibialis posterior (Kulig et al. 2009a, 2009b) to exercises for all muscles in the leg region (Alvarez et al. 2006). Some of the other co-interventions are joint manipulations, electrotherapy, and bandaging (Bek et al. 2012).

In one of the few randomized clinical trials, Kulig et al. (2009b) randomly allocated 40 patients into three groups: (i) concentric exercise (age 55.3 years, BMI 32 kg/m², $n=13$, 1 loss to follow-up), (ii) eccentric exercise [age 49.4 years, BMI 28.5 kg/m², $n=15$, 3 loss to follow-up (20%)] or (iii) no concentric/eccentric exercise (age 51.3 years, BMI 28.7 kg/m², $n=12$) for 12 weeks. In addition, all participants did calf stretching and wore a custom-made in-shoe foot orthosis. The exercise programme were performed in a custom-built rig and with elastic resistance bands, both of which involved inversion/adduction of the foot while maintaining slight pressure through the ball of the foot onto the supporting surface (Kulig et al. 2009a). The exercises accentuated foot adduction and were performed while wearing shoes and orthoses as this has been shown to best facilitate posterior tibial muscle activity (Kulig et al. 2004, 2005). All

participants had weekly visits to a physiotherapist to check, monitor and progress exercises. All groups exhibited significant and substantial improvements on the FFI total [mean difference (95% Confidence Interval (95%CI)) 18.5 (5.42 to 31.58)], pain [24.7 (10.46 to 38.94)] and disability [24.5 (5.98 to 43.02)] subscale and pain after the 5-minute walk test [20.9 mm (5.9 to 35.9)], but not on the FFI activity limitation subscale or the 5-minute walk test. The eccentric group performed better than the other groups for FFI total, pain, and disability. It should be noted that analyses did not proceed on an intention-to-treat basis and the loss to follow-up occurred solely in the exercise groups [reasons being: surgery (1), failed to return for testing (1), renovating house and excluded as violating inclusion criteria (1), continued sport with increase in symptoms and was immobilized by her physician (1)]. This, along with the loss to follow-up of 20% in the eccentric exercise, compromises the quality of the study and its outcomes. Interestingly, in a small case series study [$n=10$, age 52 (6.5) years, BMI 29.6 (7.1) kg/m²], Kulig et al. (2009a) showed a similar lack of improvement in 5-minute walk test and the FFI activity limitation subscale. Their programme consisted of prescribed custom orthoses and calf stretches, combined with a 2-week unloading phase followed by a 10-week tendon-specific eccentric exercise programme. There were substantial improvements in the number of heel rises performed, but the ultrasound scan findings for the tendon remained unchanged at follow-up from baseline (Kulig et al. 2009a).

Mechanistically, the strengthening of the tibialis posterior muscle might be effective through the normalization of abnormal plantar loading patterns in terminal stance phase of gait (Neville et al. 2013). This is based on evidence from a case–control study showing that patients who tested weak on isometric foot adduction–inversion (<80% affected/unaffected ratio) exhibited reduced plantar loading in terminal stance (patients: $n=16$, age 58.2 years, BMI 30.8 kg/m²; controls $n=15$, age 56.5 years, BMI 30.6 kg/m²) (Neville et al. 2013). So if exercises result in strength gains in tibialis posterior muscle then the plantar loading patterns might be normalized.

In addition to prescribing exercises that seek to strengthen tibialis posterior muscle specifically in relative isolation, to the extent that it is possible, a clinician might consider a more comprehensive strengthening of all leg muscles. In one of the larger case series undertaken, Alvarez et al. (2006) studied a four-phase comprehensive strengthening programme of the posterior tibial, peroneals, anterior tibial and gastrocnemius/soleus muscles that used isokinetics [KinCom 57500 (Chattanooga Group, Hixson, Tennessee)], exercise band, heel rises (double and single support) and toe walking. A pre-treatment phase was first instituted, comprising non-weightbearing exercises at home, sole to sole in slight plantarflexion (25 reps by 4 sets progressing to 12 sets at 2 weeks). Then phase 1 involved patient education and exercise band for dorsiflexion, inversion, and eversion ensuring slow controlled eccentric phases (target 200 repetitions). Phase 2 involved two to six clinic visits to perform isokinetic inversion and eversion exercises at 30° and 60° per second at a sufficiently low resistance to allow 200 repetitions in a session, plus addition to the home programme of single-stance heel raising (aiming for 50 repetitions), toe ambulation [aim for 100 feet (30 m)] and balance board training, followed by heel cord stretching and ice if required. Phase 3 started between the fifth and seventh sessions and basically involved progression of the previous phase and assessment to see whether the patient could do 200 repetitions of exercise band, 50 single-stance heel raises, toe walking over 100 feet (30 m) and isokinetic evaluation showing less than 10% difference between sides. The comprehensive exercise programme also included two different types of foot orthoses. Depending on the duration and severity of the symptoms, an articulated leg–foot orthosis was used if symptom duration exceeded 3 months or the patient was unable to perform a single-stance heel raise or ambulate more than one block ($n=33$). An in-shoe foot orthosis device was prescribed if the symptoms were present for less than 3 months and the patient could perform a single-stance heel raise and walk more than a block ($n=14$). When symptoms had subsided and strength was within 15% of the contralateral side, the articulated leg–foot device was replaced by the in-shoe device (Alvarez et al. 2006); the study followed 47 patients (stages 1 and 2, average age 50 years, female 37, duration of symptoms 19 weeks, BMI not reported) over a minimum 1-year period. Patients were in the treatment phase for a median of 120 days (range 28 to 392) and attended a median of 10 (3 to 17) physiotherapy sessions spread over a mean of 33 days (13 to 79). They reported 83% (39) as successfully treated – defined as the patients being satisfied plus having no persistent tenderness, pain on toe walking or requiring ongoing bracing. Five patients (11%) were dissatisfied with treatment and went to surgery and a further three, while satisfied, were recorded as non-successes because of persistent tenderness, toe-walking pain or needing ongoing bracing (Alvarez et al. 2006).

In one of the only other randomized clinical trials, Bek et al. (2012) studied the benefits of adding a comprehensive clinic-based treatment (15 treatments in 3 weeks) to a home exercise programme. The clinic-based treatment was cold application; posterior tibial muscle-strengthening exercises with elastic resistance bands and proprioceptive neuromuscular facilitation techniques; ankle, subtalar, and midtarsal joint mobilizations; Achilles and plantar fascia stretching; high-voltage pulsed galvanic current neuromuscular stimulation; bandaging; proprioceptive training and customized shoe inserts. The home programme involved 15 minutes' cold application, gastrocnemius–soleus stretching both manually and with a supinator wedge for the foot, heel rising on one and two feet, posterior tibial muscle strengthening with elastic resistance, intrinsic foot muscle exercises, and recommendations for appropriate shoes. Twenty-eight patients (age 33.56 years) were randomized to the combined clinic–home programme group and 21 (age 28.57 years) to the home-based group (stage 1 to 3, BMI not reported). A wide range of outcomes was measured (methods and units of measure incompletely reported), but only posterior tibial muscle strength gains were significantly greater in the centre-based programme [0.72 units (0.34 to 1.10) centre-based versus 0.34 units (−0.51 to 1.19)] (Bek et al. 2012). Both groups reported significant improvements in pain severity (>2 cm on 10 cm VAS), which supports either of them as a physical treatment approach. The quality of this study suffers due to the incomplete information about the outcome measures and the apparent post-hoc exclusion of a substantial proportion [7/28 (25%)] of the home-based programme.

Notwithstanding the shortcomings of these studies, their findings lend support to the prescription of orthoses in combination with exercises to strengthen the tibialis posterior muscle, either in isolation or in more comprehensive programmes involving other leg muscles and physical therapy modalities. Combining both orthoses and exercises in treatment is substantiated by a biomechanical study of gait (patients: $n=30$, stage 2, age 58.1 years, BMI 30.6 kg/m^2; matched controls $n=15$) that reported the postural flatfoot deformity could occur in the absence of strength deficits of the deep posterior compartment muscles, but that the severity of the deformity was greater with strength deficits (Neville et al. 2010). Clinical best practice for physical therapy would then favour a combination of support with orthoses and strengthening with exercises.

Dietary Strategies. A characteristic feature highlighted by many authors is that the condition is progressive and often presents at a late stage (Barske et al. 2013; Kohls-Gatzoulis et al. 2004b). At the advanced stages there are quite profound articular and bony changes, the amelioration of which would only seem appropriately managed by surgery (Durrant et al. 2011). Given that the condition appears to be related to adiposity-related diseases (e.g. obesity, diabetes, hypertension), it would seem advisable that programmes to counter these are promoted generally and aggressively in people with stage 1 or 2 of the disorder, while still being advocated in advanced stages. Addressing more general and systemic health issues would then appear good practice for all clinicians consulting a patient with this condition. Included in this ought to be consideration of statin medication usage as one of its side effects is tendinopathy (Marie et al. 2008).

FUTURE DIRECTIONS

A feature of most narrative reviews or clinical opinion pieces is that the authors recount that the diagnosis is usually missed in its earlier stages, leaving fewer opportunities for conservative management and requiring reconstructive surgeries, even possibly arthrodesis (Bodill and Concannon 2012; Durrant et al. 2011). This highlights the difficulties inherent in the posterior tibial tendon disorder/adult-acquired phenotype, and that is that the diagnosis in its earlier stages is yet to be validated (Durrant et al. 2011). That is, at what stage does a normal variant of foot

posture become a significant risk factor for this condition? To answer this, large-scale, population-wide foot-profiling studies [e.g. using arch height index (Williams and McClay 2000), FPI (Redmond et al. 2008), or midfoot width measures (McPoil et al. 2009)] are required, ensuring to capture essential data as age, sex and BMI, which appear important to this condition.

TARSAL TUNNEL SYNDROME

INTRODUCTION

Tarsal tunnel syndrome (TTS) appears to be less common than its apparent upper limb analogue, carpal tunnel syndrome (Preston et al. 2013), which is a likely explanation for there being comparatively less evidence regarding its management. Tarsal tunnel syndrome is essentially numbness or tingling in the plantar aspect of the foot accompanied by nerve-like pain attributable to branches of the tibial nerve (Jolly et al. 2005). The nerve is compromised at the tunnel between the flexor retinaculum and the underlying bones (calcaneus and talus). Its prevalence is not readily discernible from the literature and is likely distorted by observer bias (Preston et al. 2013).

PREDISPOSING FACTORS

There are a myriad of potential candidates for predisposing factors, none of which has been verified by research. The extrinsic factors could include direct insult to the nerve through trauma, overly tight shoes/laces, or from generalized lower limb swelling (Ahmad et al. 2012; Toth et al. 2005). Abnormal rearfoot posture or motion (e.g. excessive pronation) along with unaccustomed overuse [e.g. long-distance running (Jackson and Haglund 1992)] or overload (Kinoshita et al. 2006) might also be a contributing factor in the compromise of the tibial nerve within the tarsal tunnel (McCrory et al. 2002; Meyer et al. 2002).

DIAGNOSIS

The diagnosis of TTS remains largely based on clinical presentation (Ahmad et al. 2012). It is characteristically recognized clinically as plantar heel pain that extends from the tarsal tunnel down into the distribution of the lateral and medial plantar nerves accompanied by neural-like symptoms of burning, sharp, shooting, shock-like, electric sensations in the same distribution of the lateral and medial plantar nerves (Alshami et al. 2008a; Jackson and Haglund 1991). Pain and associated neural symptoms in the proximal half of the heel are probably not associated with TTS but rather the medial calcaneal nerve, which branches from the tibial nerve prior to the tarsal tunnel (flexor retinaculum) (Jolly et al. 2005). These symptoms are probably worse at night owing to venous stasis and congestion, as well as being aggravated during weight-bearing activities. Careful history taking and clinical examination are required to ensure that the symptoms are not due to the lumbar spine (e.g. nerve root compression or irritation) (Jolly et al. 2005). Not unlike plantar heel pain of plantar fascia origin, first-step pain is not uncommon (Jolly et al. 2005; Öztuna et al. 2002).

Physical examination relies predominantly on palpation of the neural structures in combination with physical manoeuvres that stress the tarsal tunnel and neural structures. Testing for sensory deficits should reveal diminished sensation in the region of the most involved branch of the tibial nerve, but most likely this will be in the distribution of the medial plantar nerve (Alshami et al. 2008a; Kinoshita et al. 2006). Tapping along the course of the nerve may reproduce symptoms (known as Tinel's sign), but it often is not good at identifying entrapment of the first branch of the lateral plantar nerve (Baxter's or inferior calcaneal nerve) (Jolly et al. 2005), which is the branch of the tibial nerve that most closely innervates the typical area of plantar fasciitis pain. In many patients, sustained passive dorsiflexion/eversion of the rear- and forefoot while holding the toes in full extension will elicit the symptoms (Kinoshita et al. 2001); however, if used in isolation this will not differentiate the source of the symptoms from that of plantar fasciitis (Alshami et al. 2008a). Adding other manoeuvres to increase strain in the neural tract but not the plantar fascia, such as hip flexion with knee extended, is one method recommended to aid in the differential diagnosis (Alshami et al. 2008a, 2008b). Plantarflexion–inversion positioning of the ankle and foot has also been used to implicate the tarsal tunnel, on the basis that it reduces the space within the tunnel and increases pressure on the nerve (Bracilovic et al. 2006; Trepman et al. 1999). The clinical utility of this plantar–inversion test, especially its sensitivity, is likely to be increased if manual compression over the tunnel is maintained by the clinician during the manoeuvre (Abouelela and Zohiery 2012).

Electrodiagnostic or electrophysiological tests in the form of nerve conduction or electromyography studies might be ordered as they could confirm the diagnosis (Ahmad et al. 2012; Dellon 2008). However, a recent systematic review concluded that they cannot be used as a definitive diagnosis of TTS owing to false-negative rates and unknown sensitivity and specificity for nerve conduction and needle electromyography tests (Patel et al. 2005). Diagnostic ultrasound in conjunction with electrodiagnostic testing might provide improved capability to inform the diagnosis (Padua et al. 2007), though verification is required through research (Ahmad et al. 2012; Alshami et al. 2008a; Ibrahim et al. 2013; Therimadasamy et al. 2011).

IMPAIRMENTS

A key discriminatory feature between tarsal tunnel syndrome and other plantar foot conditions (e.g. plantar fasciitis, adult-acquired, heel fat pad syndrome) is the sensory disturbance related to the involvement of the branches of the tibial nerve around the flexor retinaculum. Thus, clinical examination should reveal impaired sensory responses to such testing as light touch and two-point discrimination. In the clinic this could be gleaned from a quick comparison between sides and regions of nerve distribution (e.g. medial and lateral plantar nerves). The sensory impairment could be quantified by two-point discrimination testers (e.g. Disk-Criminator, sharp-tipped sliding calipers) or a pressure-specifying sensory device (PSD) (Dellon et al. 1992). The clinical use of measuring devices that do not quantify the pressure applied to the skin has been questioned on the basis of their reliability (Catley et al. 2013; Lundborg and Rosen 2004) and variability within normal (Nolan 1983), though the lateral plantar foot region was amongst the more reliable tested sites (Catley et al. 2013). The PSD was designed to overcome rater-related issues such as the amount of pressure applied (Dellon et al. 1992; Lundborg and Rosen 2004). Tassler and Dellon (1996) quantified normal values for one-point static touch and static two-point discrimination by using the PSD in a group of 34 participants [20 female: average age 46.4 years (range 21 to 84))] and then compared them with a group of 22 patients with TTS [13 female, mean age: 37.5 years (range: 21–60)]. The one-point static touch pressure was on average (SD) 0.58 (0.34) g/mm^2 in controls and 10.9 (17.5) g/mm^2 in the TTS group [those with positive electrodiagnostic tests were substantially higher at 15 (21.1) g/mm^2], and similarly for two-point discrimination with controls registering 3.8 (1.0) mm and tarsal tunnel syndrome 10.7 (3.3) mm [again those positive on electrodiagnostic testing were more impaired 12.1 (3.3) mm] (Tassler and Dellon 1996).

MANAGEMENT STRATEGIES

There is a dearth of information in the literature regarding the management of tarsal tunnel syndrome. This might reflect a low prevalence of the condition or that it is poorly identified. Its analogue in the upper limb, carpal tunnel syndrome, would seem best managed by surgical release (Verdugo et al. 2008), but for TTS there is little by way of verification for this through randomized clinical trials. Given the lack of good evidence on surgical outcomes, a pragmatic approach would probably first involve a trial of a period of activity modification, anti-inflammatory medication, orthotic devices to correct any contributory poor foot and ankle alignment, followed by progressive mobilization, including a programme of neural mobilization/exercises (Ahmad et al. 2012; Alshami et al. 2008a; Jackson and Haglund 1991; Meyer et al. 2002).

Pharmacological Strategies

Anti-inflammatory medication, including corticosteroid injections into the tarsal tunnel and about the tibial nerve and its branches, has been suggested in order to reduce swelling and inflammation in and about the nerve (Ahmad et al. 2012). As has been recommended elsewhere, using ultrasound to guide the injection might well lead to better targeting of corticosteroid injection, improving outcome.

Physical Strategies

There appears to be little differentiation in the physical treatment approaches taken for TTS compared with plantar heel pain, probably reflecting some of the commonalities in diagnosis (e.g. pain with weight-bearing tasks, first-step pain) (Alshami et al. 2008a). A variety of techniques might be considered such as: external supports in the form of taping, splinting, orthoses and bracing, massage to remove any oedema within the tunnel, stretches of the Achilles tendon, and modalities geared at reducing inflammation (e.g. ice, ultrasound, extracorporeal shock wave therapy) (Ahmad et al. 2012; Alshami et al. 2008a). There is little in the way of any high-quality clinical trials that supports one or more of these modalities beyond each other or no treatment (Ahmad et al. 2012). It would be reasonable to prescribe anti-pronation orthoses in cases where there is excessive pronation linked to the symptoms (Jackson and Haglund 1992; McCrory et al. 2002).

There is a specific physical therapy in the form of neural mobilization that might be clinically useful in managing TTS (Alshami et al. 2008a), as it has been recommended in the treatment of other common peripheral neuropathies (e.g. carpal tunnel syndrome) (Page et al. 2012). The neural mobilization uses knee extension movements plus or minus hip flexion or slump of the trunk (Alshami et al. 2008a) in an attempt to improve nerve health by removing oedema and encouraging nutrition of the compromised nerve at the tarsal tunnel and/or beyond. There are a number of case studies reporting positive outcomes without adverse effects (Alshami et al. 2008a; Meyer et al. 2002) and one randomized clinical trial (Kavlak and Uygur 2011); Kavlak and Uygur randomized 28 patients into two treatment groups, both of which underwent stretching and strengthening exercises, orthoses, ice, and bandaging for those who had oedema. One of the groups additionally had tibial nerve mobilization exercises in the form of knee flexion–extension while the ankle and foot were dorsiflexed/everted and the trunk slumped (Meyer et al. 2002). The treatment period was 6 weeks, at which time the outcomes were measured. The group treated with additional tibial nerve mobilization had significant improvements in two-point discrimination, Tinel sign and tibial nerve stretch test, indicating that neural mobilization might specifically address features that are different to other forms of plantar heel pain. Interestingly, both groups demonstrated significant improvements in range of motion, muscle strength, and pain severity. Given the greater changes in the neurological-related signs (e.g. two-point discrimination, Tinel sign, and tibial nerve stretch test) it could be speculated that ongoing treatment over a longer period might translate into superior pain outcomes in the neural mobilization group.

Surgical Strategies

Surgical decompression is an option available should there be no response to conservative management (Ahmad et al. 2012). The surgery not only decompresses the tunnel at the level of the flexor retinaculum, but should follow the branches of the tibial nerve distally and remove the septum between medial and lateral plantar nerves as well as the fibrous roof (Dellon 2008). There are no systematic reviews that explore the safety and efficacy of various surgical approaches for TTS (Perera et al. 2013) and reported success rates vary widely (Hendrix et al. 1998; Jerosch et al. 2006). A recent literature review recommended that surgery proceed only in the event that a trial of conservative treatment had not improved the condition and that there was a definite point of nerve entrapment (Ahmad et al. 2012). It would appear that a diagnostic ultrasound scan, especially high definition, could be used to identify the nerve entrapment and its cause and location, as well as confirm diagnosis of the condition (Ahmad et al. 2012; Therimadasamy et al. 2011), thereby improving outcomes.

Lifestyle and Education Strategies

A recent literature review indicated that failed surgery might be due to intraneural fibrosis when decompression was performed too late (Ahmad et al. 2012), the implication being that conservative management should be initiated early and in a focused manner to enable decisions leading to better outcomes. Although this is a plausible approach, there is no research in its support.

FUTURE DIRECTIONS

Research needs to focus on the diagnostic utility of clinical examination and laboratory tests (e.g. electrodiagnostic, ultrasound, other imaging modalities) so as to facilitate early diagnosis and better-guided management. In order to advance understanding of this condition there is also a need for epidemiological studies to quantify the prevalence rates, as well as clinical trials to determine which are the best forms of conservative management and surgical approaches.

HIGH-ENERGY INJURY CALCANEAL FRACTURE

INTRODUCTION

Traumatic calcaneal fractures occur from high-energy axial loading that result in both shear and compression failure of bone (Daftary et al. 2005). They are frequently reported as the most commonly fractured tarsal bone and for being somewhat controversial with a poor reputation, yet comprise only up to 2% of all fractures (Daftary et al. 2005; Eastwood and Phipp 1997; Rammelt and Zwipp 2004; Sayed-Noor et al. 2011). The majority of traumatic calcaneal fractures are intra-articular, which contributes to the uncertainty of whether surgical or conservative approaches are better (Bruce and Sutherland 2013). Further fuelling the controversy is recent evidence of the poor reliability of X-rays, CT scans, and classification systems to identify the fracture (Roll et al. 2011; Sayed-Noor et al. 2011).

DIAGNOSIS

The key diagnostic feature of a calcaneal fracture is sudden onset of pain and disability following a high-energy traumatic incident. The typical patient is characterized as being male in the 30–60-year-old age bracket. Clinical presentation is one of a deformed, swollen, and painful heel, with an inability to ambulate normally. There are two main types of fracture: extra- and intra-articular. The majority are intra-articular, occur through the posterior facet, and are frequently displaced (Bruce and Sutherland 2013; Ibrahim et al. 2007). A review of radiological records in a Netherlands trauma centre (approximately 24 thousand patients annually) between 2003 and 2005 showed that overall extra-articular fractures represented 35% of calcaneal fractures (Schepers et al. 2008a). The extra-articular fractures occurred in younger people (32.7 versus 40.3 years, $p=0.04$) with a lower male predominance than the intra-articular fractures (63% versus 79%, $p=0.04$), which was inferred to be largely a function of the trauma mechanism (work-related high-energy trauma in relatively older males) (Schepers et al. 2008a).

CT scans and X-ray are the clinical mainstay of determining the type and extent of the fracture, which is arguably necessary for informed decisions on management (Guerado et al. 2012). As the fractures are usually complex geometrically, the three-dimensional representation gained from CT scans is often cited as being advantageous for planning surgery (Guerado et al. 2012; Sayed-Noor et al. 2011). A number of systems of calcaneal fracture classification based on X-rays and CT scans have been developed in order to assist decision making (e.g. Essex-Lopresti, Zwipp, Crosby, Sanders) (Schepers et al. 2009). Interestingly, Schepers et al. (2009) found that these systems showed positive correlations with outcome but not with treatment performed, and in the main had poor to moderate reliability. The latter is consistent with recent studies that generally report the reliability (inter-rater and inter-rater) of several classification schemes as being unsatisfactory (Guerado et al. 2012; Roll et al. 2011; Sayed-Noor et al. 2011), though not surprisingly less so in the hands of more experienced orthopaedic surgeons (Roll et al. 2011).

IMPAIRMENTS AND FUNCTION

A 2008 Netherlands-wide survey of traumatology and orthopaedic staff regarding intra-articular calcaneal fractures found very low utilization (7%) of outcome scores (Schepers et al. 2008b).

Schepers et al. (2008c) performed a systematic search of the literature and found that the most-cited clinical outcome scores for intra-articular calcaneal fractures were, in descending order, the American Orthopedic Foot and Ankle Society (AOFAS) hindfoot score, Maryland Foot Score (MFS) and the Creighton-Nebraska score (CN). They then evaluated the reliability and validity of these three scores on a series of cases with displaced intra-articular calcaneal fractures ($n = 48$, median age = 48 years, 72% male). All three measures showed high correlation with a VAS for overall patient satisfaction ($r = 0.72$ to 0.76), indicating sound criterion validity (Schepers et al. 2008c). In addition, the measures showed acceptable levels of content validity in scores on pain, return to work, subtalar range of motion, walking distance, ankle range of motion, and limping. The reliability as indicated by Chronbach's alpha was best for MFS (0.82), then AOFAS (0.78) and CN (0.61). Schepers et al. (2008c) recommended on balance choosing either the AOFAS or the MFS. In addition to reporting the total of the subcategories within the AOFAS and MFS, Tornetta et al. (2013) recommended reporting the individual components of the scores, largely due to the dominating presence of pain in explaining the total score.

The AOFAS is a 100-point scale, which consists of both patient and clinician ratings across a range of measures of pain, function, and alignment (American Orthopedic Foot and Ankle Society 2013). The pain subscale has four categories, with 40 points indicating no pain and 0 points indicating severe, almost always present pain. Function is out of 50, a combination of three patient-rated activities and four clinician-observed impairments. The three patient-rated activities are: (a) activity limitations with support required (four categories, with 10 points no limitation using no support and 0 indicating severe limitation daily, using ambulation aids other than a cane), (b) maximum walking distance in blocks (four categories, with 5 points if > 6 and 0 points if < 1), and (c) difficulty on walking surfaces (three categories, with 5 points for no difficulty on any surface and 0 points for severe difficulty on uneven terrain, stairs, inclines, and ladders). The four clinician-rated observations are: (a) gait abnormality, with three categories from 8 points for none or slight to 0 points for marked, (b) sagittal motion of flexion plus extension (three categories, with 8 points for ≥ 30° and 0 points for restriction < 15°), (c) hindfoot motion of inversion plus eversion (three categories, with 6 points for ≥ 75% of normal and 0 points for < 25%), and (d) ankle–hindfoot stability into anteroposterior and varus–valgus directions (either 8 points if stable or 0 points if definitely unstable). Finally there is a 10-point score for alignment, with three categories from good, plantigrade foot with well-aligned midfoot to 0 points for a poor, nonplantigrade foot with severe malalignment and symptoms. The Maryland Foot Score is also a score out of 100 with a pain subscale (45 points, ranging from no pain including with sports to 0 points for disabled, unable to work or shop) and a function subscale (55 points) (Sanders et al. 1993). The function subscale has a series of questions related to gait covering distance walked (10 points), shoes (10 points), and stability, support, limp, stairs, and terrain all having a maximum of 4 points each. Cosmesis is rated from 10 points for normal to 0 points for multiple deformities, and the clinician assesses motion at the ankle, subtalar, midfoot, and metatarsophalangeal from 5 points for normal to 0 points for ankylosed (Sanders et al. 1993).

QUALITY OF LIFE

There are reports of protracted periods of incapacitation following these injuries with partial impairment for several (3 to 5) years post-fracture (Bruce and Sutherland 2013). Calcaneal fractures tend to occur in younger people and generally require a considerable period of non-weightbearing and convalescence, which contributes to absence from work, activities of daily living, as well as sport and recreation. This along with residual pain and time required mobilizing impact considerably on quality of life of the patient. The impost on the community is not inconsiderable with an economic impact from extended hospital stays, costs of treatment and time lost from work (Schepers et al. 2008b). These negative impacts on the person and impost on society are exaggerated/compounded in cases prone to poor results (e.g. male, heavy manual work, comminuted fracture) (Bruce and Sutherland 2013; Sanders 2000).

MANAGEMENT STRATEGIES

In part, the controversy surrounding this condition arises from an uncertainty over whether a surgical approach is the best approach (Bruce and Sutherland 2013; Gougoulias et al. 2009; Guerado et al. 2012) and, if surgery is undertaken, which approach is most appropriate (Schepers 2011; Yang et al. 2012).

In the most recent Cochrane review on the matter of surgery versus conservative intervention, Bruce and Sutherland (2013) identified four trials (602 participants) that were suitable for inclusion. Three of these were small single-centre trials and the other was a multicentre study of 424 participants with displaced intra-articular fractures. Follow-up ranged from 1 to 15 years. All trials were at a high risk of bias as they failed to conceal allocation adequately and had incomplete follow-up. Pooling was not possible. Strongest evidence was formed from the larger trial, which

showed no clinically significant differences between surgery and conservative treatment at 3-year follow-up for a custom disease-specific score, chronic pain or health-related quality of life as measured on the SF-36. The reporting of complications in the large trial seemed haphazard, being reported over a number of different publications, but it would seem that the surgical group reported greater complications and issues (e.g. late arthrodesis, thromboemboli, superficial and deep wound infections, malposition of fixation and compartment syndrome). A current ongoing trial of 150 participants (recruitment finalized May 2012) should provide better information on the relative clinical efficacy of open reduction and internal fixation by the extensile lateral approach compared with elevation, ice, splinting, and early mobilization (Griffin 2013). The findings of the Cochrane review are largely similar to those of the previous systematic review on this topic (Gougoulias et al. 2009).

A recent systematic review that evaluated the efficacy of bone grafts in the treatment of displaced intra-articular calcaneal fractures included 1281 fractures from 32 primary studies (not limited to randomized clinical trials), of which only four were direct comparative studies (Yang et al. 2012). As indicated above the reporting of outcomes was highly variable, which along with substantial heterogeneity in surgical approaches and post-operative management impeded a meaningful synthesis of data. Notwithstanding these issues, the bone graft treatment allowed significantly quick return to full weightbearing (5.4 months compared with 10.5 months) and produced a significantly higher Bohler's angle. In terms of efficacy, there was a small benefit in the grafted group on the AOFAS (71.4 versus 80.5) compared with the non-grafted group, which was not closely reflected in the results on a categorical scale (grafted versus non-grafted: excellent 35% versus 34%, good 40% versus 42%, fair 21% versus 14%, poor 4% versus 10%) (Yang et al. 2012).

The percutaneous distraction and subsequent fixation of bony fragments through ligamentotaxis for intra-articular calcaneal fractures has evolved from 1855, but is less popular than open reduction and internal fixation methods (e.g. as above per systematic) (Schepers and Patka 2009). Schepers and Patka (2009) attempted a systematic review of the literature on this technique and identified eight studies that used this method, but were limited from meta-analysis due to substantial heterogeneity in classification systems, techniques, and outcome-scoring systems. These studies showed that reasonably good outcomes with only 10–29% of patients rating the outcome as fair or poor, complications due to infections and secondary arthrodesis each being in the order of 2–15%. Inability to return to work was between 10 and 26% (Schepers and Patka 2009). These findings were largely echoed by a systematic review of Pelliccioni et al. (2012), which showed favourable outcomes for percutaneous fixation using Kirschner wires compared with open reduction and internal fixation, but there was substantial heterogeneity and insufficient evidence to assert superiority of any one technique over another.

The issue of complications following intra-articular calcaneal fractures managed either surgically or conservatively should be considered by both clinician and patient when making management decisions. For example, there are higher rates of infection following surgery but possibly less need for subtalar arthrodesis due to arthritic changes (Bruce and Sutherland 2013). There is also the risk of arthrofibrosis of the subtalar joint and calcaneal non-union, which is infrequently reported but might be higher than expected (Schepers and Patka 2008).

FUTURE DIRECTIONS

There is a need for an improved method of systematically characterizing the type of fracture so that surgical and conservative management approaches can be better matched to specific fracture type. Further work is required on outcome measures, because a case has been made for the field to adopt and consistently use a small set of outcome measures uniformly in research and practice. Finally, the controversy of whether to operate and which operation to perform would probably be settled by high-quality clinical trials that adopt reliable and valid fracture qualification systems and outcome measures (Gougoulias et al. 2009).

CALCANEAL STRESS FRACTURE

INTRODUCTION

Heel pain can present as an overuse calcaneal stress fracture. Calcaneal stress fractures are reasonably common in specific populations and tend to be overlooked early in presentation (Berger et al. 2007), so a high index of suspicion should be exercised in long-distance runners, military recruits, jumpers, and osteoporotic people presenting with heel pain (Boden et al. 2001). A MRI study of a high-risk group – military recruits –with a total exposure of 117 149 person-years found an incidence of 2.6 (95% CI: 1.6 to 3.4) per 10 000 person-years (Sormaala et al. 2006). These data possibly represent relatively higher rates of occurrence of calcaneal stress fractures, owing to the use of the more sensitive MRI or bone scans instead of X-rays in earlier studies (Berger et al. 2007; Matheson et al. 1987; Sormaala et al. 2006; Spitz and Newberg 2002). In a prospective study of the evolution of bone-scan- or X-ray-determined stress fractures in 250 patients presenting with exercise-related leg pain, Greaney et al. (1983) reported the posterior calcaneus to be the single most common site (21%). In an analysis of 320 athletes with bone-scan-diagnosed stress fractures over a 3.5-year period, Matheson et al. (1987) reported that tarsal bones (25%) were the most common foot and ankle stress fractures, second only to tibial stress fractures (49%). This is consistent with more recent findings of talar and calcaneal stress fractures being the most common of the tarsal bones (Sormaala 2006).

PREDISPOSING FACTORS

It is difficult to find specific predisposing factors for stress fractures to the calcaneus. The most commonly cited risk factor for all stress fractures is participation in at-risk physical activities and undertaking a load or an increase in load that is beyond the person's capabilities and capacity. In terms of specific risk factors for calcaneal stress fractures, the frequently associated physical activities are marching (military), running (athletics, particularly long distance), and jumping (jump-related sports, gymnastics, ballet). A detailed evaluation of the biomechanics of gait, marching, and jumping should be undertaken so as to identify any excessive or pronounced heelstrike or unco-ordinated landing/foot contact, as these have been listed as possible factors contributing to the problem.

In terms of military recruits, there are a number of studies of possible risk factors. A prospective study of 179 Finnish male military recruits (aged 18–25 years) found that those who were taller, had poorer physical conditioning, low hip bone mineral content and density, as well as high serum parathyroid hormone levels were more likely to experience a stress fracture in their 6–12 months' military service (Välimäki et al. 2005). Consequently, and with the knowledge that Finnish recruits are low in vitamin D intake, the authors recommended supplementation with vitamin D so as to lower serum parathyroid hormone levels. In terms of stress fractures of the calcaneus, only 1 of the 15 injured recruits had a fracture of the calcaneus (10 metatarsal bone, 4 tibia), so it is difficult to determine whether the risk factors are site-specific. The finding of poor physical conditioning in the Finnish study was similar to a study of 693 female and 626 male US Marine Corps recruits, which reported that for both sexes there were deficits in fitness, muscle and bone parameters [measured on dual-energy X-ray absorptiometry (DXA) scans] in those with stress fractures (Beck et al. 2000). These authors pooled all fractures into the analyses and there was no indication whether any calcaneal fractures were in the study.

A case–control study of 31 US Naval Academy recruits showed that those who had a stress fracture underwent greater weight loss with the regular daily physical training (Armstrong et al. 2004). This study did not specify that there were any calcaneal fractures in the sample. Notwithstanding this, a recurring feature in most stress fractures is low body weight, specifically in females where it is important to be aware to the female triad of low body weight, dysmenorrhea, and low energy intake (Beck et al. 1996; Dugan and Weber 2007).

DIAGNOSIS

Diagnosis of a calcaneal stress fracture is made on the basis of a thorough history and physical examination with diagnostic imaging used to confirm the presence and location of the stress reaction/fracture (Boden et al. 2001). Clinical features that will increase the suspicion of a calcaneal stress fracture are insidious onset pain in the heel that has been without a specific traumatic incident in a patient who has performed substantial amounts of weightbearing activities, such as can be expected in the military (long marches), long-distance running, jumping and ballet dancing. Careful history taking will probably reveal recent

increases in loading, or resumption of previous level loads after a period of de-loading (e.g. break for short temporary illness or off-season). Patients will report that the pain is reproduced by the loading activities (e.g. marching, running, jumping) and relieved by rest in the earlier stages, but will progress to being present during rest and lesser loaded activities if not managed appropriately (Berger et al. 2007). A key physical examination finding is localized calcaneal bone pain on palpation. Squeezing the calcaneus simultaneously from the lateral and medial side is one way of eliciting this palpation sign. Pain on landing from a jump is also likely to be provocative. Pain during running and marching might not be reproducible in clinic in the early stages.

Radiography can be used to confirm the stress fracture, but is particularly unreliable for tarsal bones and not sensitive in the early stages (frequently cited as being the first 2–12 weeks) (Berger et al. 2007; Matheson et al. 1987; Sormaala et al. 2006). Until recently with the advent and advances in MRI, triple-phase technetium-99m biphosphate bone scintigraphy was the reference standard for stress fractures (Berger et al. 2007; Matheson et al. 1987; Spitz and Newberg 2002; Zwas et al. 1987). MRI has become the preferred imaging modality because it enables early identification of bone stress, its precise location and extent (Spitz and Newberg 2002).

The MRI study of a high-risk group of military recruits with a total exposure of 117 149 person-years reported the majority of calcaneal fractures to be located in the posterior (56%) and superior (79%) parts of the calcaneus (Sormaala et al. 2006). This postero-superior calcaneus site runs transverse to the calcaneal trabeculae just anterior to the apophyseal plate and is a differential diagnosis for retrocalcaneal bursitis and Achilles tendinopathy (Boden et al. 2001). The next most common site was the anterior calcaneus (26%) (Sormaala et al. 2006) adjacent to the medial tuberosity, a differential diagnosis for plantar fasciitis (Boden et al. 2001).

IMPAIRMENTS AND FUNCTION

It is difficult to find specific impairments and functional deficits for calcaneal stress fractures. As part of a comprehensive physical examination there are likely to be impairments and functional deficits as listed above for plantar fasciitis and possibly some of tibialis posterior tendon dysfunction impairments. For example, it is likely that there will be impaired ankle dorsiflexion and plantar fascia extensibility, as well as abnormal findings on gait and with tests of rear- and midfoot posture and motion

MANAGEMENT STRATEGIES

There is a void of literature and research regarding the rehabilitation of stress fractures in general and specifically calcaneal stress fractures (Dugan and Weber 2007). Calcaneal stress fractures are characterized as being low-risk stress fractures, which means that they have a good prognostic outcome if managed with activity limitation for 3 to 6 weeks (Boden et al. 2001). This is reflected in an 8-year retrospective study of 133 conscripts (385 stress injuries in 142 feet) undertaking military service, which found that the calcaneal stress injuries seemed to heal well, but that in some cases the patients had to be removed from physical training for up to some months (Sormaala 2006). Given that this injury probably occurs in individuals who are habituated to frequent long bouts of exercise, it is imperative that early education is undertaken to ensure the patient understands the pathology of stress fractures in relation to loading and the need to have a period of relative unloading of the rearfoot (Dugan and Weber 2007). As part of this education programme, the issue of possible risk factors related to the patient should be discussed and a plan to address these implemented. This education would be broadened in females to incorporate an understanding of the association between physical activity, nutrition, and menstrual history. It is critical in athletes to incorporate cross-training with exercise and activities that maintain fitness of the cardiovascular system and of other non-injured body parts, making sure not to load

the heel (e.g. swimming, upper limb ergometer, seated and lying weighted exercises). This will also help in the psychological adjustment to injury and convalescence that the person will undergo.

In patients who do not have pain with activities of daily living – that is, they are pain-free on walking about – then shoe inserts that help attenuate shock and impact through the rearfoot could be worn in order to assist in recovery. In the event that the patient has reached a stage where activities of daily living are symptomatic, it is then critical to offload the heel further by using walking aids (e.g. walking stick, crutches) for a short period (1–3 weeks). Shoe inserts could also be trialled to relieve symptoms and offload soft tissues that might also be sensitized. In addition to this, any identified physical impairments (e.g. reduced range of motion at the talocrural, subtalar or midtarsal joints, muscle weakness or tightness) should be addressed. In most cases, stretches to the calf and possibly the plantar fascia will be indicated.

When activities of daily living are pain-free and there is no longer localized pain over the calcaneus, the patient can be re-introduced into a graduated and progressive programme for their sport or activity, ensuring that there is no heel pain during or within 24 hours of exercising.

FUTURE DIRECTIONS

There is a lack of specific data relating to calcaneal stress fractures that should be addressed through studies of predisposing risk factors, impairments, and function. Clinical trials that evaluate different regimens of activity limitation then re-introduction along with physical modalities, along with studies of specific outcome measures, would be useful in assisting clinicians and patients in making clinical decisions regarding management.

INVITED COMMENTARY

This chapter deals with common rearfoot conditions including plantar fasciitis/plantar heel pain, tibialis posterior tendon dysfunction, tarsal tunnel syndrome and calcaneal fractures. Each condition is introduced with brief sections on epidemiology, predisposing factors and, importantly for the clinician, diagnosis. Following this, health status issues for each pathology are covered with sections on impairment and functional issues, and broader health-related quality of life issues, which provide a concise summary of how it affects people. Importantly, this information will assist clinicians in

Continued on following page

INVITED COMMENTARY (Continued)

their assessments of people with the above conditions. Finally, a review of the literature relating to treatment of these conditions is provided, with a plethora of information for clinicians actively treating patients with them.

The reader should be aware that the breadth of information presented is commendably vast. It is a substantial topic and one in which there is an extensive amount of research relating to it. Furthermore, much of the research is not homogeneous with different interventions or combinations of interventions being evaluated. Often, it can be a highly complex process for the author of a chapter like this to sort through various studies to provide 'sound bites' of information for the reader; that is, this is the condition, this is how you diagnose it, and this is how you treat it ... if only life were so simple!

With this in mind readers need to be aware of whether the research articles presented provide good evidence; that is, whether they provide results that are believable or not. It is a fundamental responsibility of clinicians to be able to relatively quickly determine whether a study is of high quality, because the researchers have used sound methods, or low quality, because it is plagued by bias (for example, due to a lack of blinding) and confounding (for example, due to issues like the Hawthorn effect, natural progression, regression to the mean, etc.) that may have over-inflated an intervention's effectiveness. This is the very essence of being a well-informed, evidence-based practitioner.

A further issue that requires reflection is that of the 'effect(s)' of an intervention and the 'effectiveness' of an intervention. Interventions have effects (for example, a foot orthosis causes significant redistribution of plantar pressures) but these effects do not always lead to effectiveness, where a patient's health status improves due to the intervention. Effects are of interest to explain how an intervention works, but effectiveness is crucial to ascertain whether an intervention is truly beneficial. Ideally, interventions will be supported by multiple high-quality randomised trials, or even systematic reviews, highlighting the health benefits of the intervention for a person with a condition. However, often this is not the case, and we are left with only laboratory-based studies (for example, plantar pressure or cadaver studies) where an effect has been found, but we do not know if that effect actually leads to real life benefits to a person; that is, the intervention is effective. Unfortunately, much of the research on foot-related musculoskeletal interventions is laboratory-based. Consequently, we know of some of the effects of the intervention, but we know very little about whether the intervention is truly effective. These principles mentioned above, quality of the evidence and effects versus effectiveness, are overriding principles of evidence for all interventions, but are of particular relevance to interventions for many lower limb conditions because of the relative infancy of the research.

Finally, other than the impressive coverage of information contained in this chapter, key points for readers to consider relate in particular to the future directions section at the end of each condition. Medical imaging is increasingly being used to diagnose and aide well-directed invasive interventions, such as injection therapy. In addition, the author considers future research to understand the aetiology and risk factors of these conditions, ensuring readers are abreast of where research is headed. Better understanding the conditions is vital because this may lead to cures, rather than just treating what has already developed.

Karl B. Landorf PhD
La Trobe University, Australia

REFERENCES

Abouelela, A.A.K.H., Zohiery, A.K., 2012. The triple compression stress test for diagnosis of tarsal tunnel syndrome. Foot (Edinb) 22 (3), 146–149.

Acevedo, J.I., Beskin, J.L., 1998. Complications of plantar fascia rupture associated with corticosteroid injection. Foot and Ankle International 19 (2), 91–97.

Ahmad, M., Tsang, K., Mackenney, P.J., et al., 2012. Tarsal tunnel syndrome: a literature review. Foot and Ankle Surgery 18 (3), 149–152.

Akşahin, E., Doğruyol, D., Yüksel, H.Y., et al., 2012. The comparison of the effect of corticosteroids and platelet-rich plasma (PRP) for the treatment of plantar fasciitis. Archives of Orthopaedic and Traumatic Surgery 132 (6), 781–785.

Allen, R.H., Gross, M.T., 2003. Toe flexors strength and passive extension range of motion of the first metatarsophalangeal joint in individuals with plantar fasciitis. Journal of Orthopaedic and Sports Physical Therapy 33 (8), 468–478.

Alshami, A.M., Babri, A.S., Souvlis, T., et al., 2007. Biomechanical evaluation of two clinical tests for plantar heel pain: the dorsiflexion-eversion test for tarsal tunnel syndrome and the windlass test for plantar fasciitis. Foot and Ankle International 28 (4), 499–505.

Alshami, A.M., Souvlis, T., Coppieters, M.W., 2008a. A review of plantar heel pain of neural origin: differential diagnosis and management. Manual Therapy 13 (2), 103–111.

Alshami, A.M., Babri, A.S., Souvlis, T., et al., 2008b. Strain in the tibial and plantar nerves with foot and ankle movements and the influence of adjacent joint positions. Journal of Applied Biomechanics 24 (4), 368.

Alvarez, R.G., Marini, A., Schmitt, C., et al., 2006. Stage I and II posterior tibial tendon dysfunction treated by a structured non-operative management protocol: an orthosis and exercise program. Foot and Ankle International 27 (1), 2–8.

American Orthopedic Foot and Ankle Society, 2013. Ankle–hindfoot scale. Online. Available: <http://www.eorif.com/ankle-foot-outcome-measures> (accessed 2 Sep 2013).

Armstrong, D.W., Rue, J.-P.H., Wilckens, J.H., et al., 2004. Stress fracture injury in young military men and women. Bone 35 (3), 806–816.

Augustin, J.F., Lin, S.S., Berberian, W.S., et al., 2003. Nonoperative treatment of adult acquired with the Arizona brace. Foot and Ankle Clinics 8 (3), 491.

Aurichio, T.R., Rebelatto, J.R., de Castro, A.P., 2011. The relationship between the body mass index (BMI) and foot posture in elderly people. Archives of Gerontology and Geriatrics 52 (2), e89–e92.

Barske, H., Chimenti, R., Tome, J., et al., 2013. Clinical outcomes and static and dynamic assessment of foot posture after lateral column lengthening procedure. Foot and Ankle International 34 (5), 673–683.

Beck, T.J., Ruff, C.B., Mourtada, F.A., et al., 1996. Dual-energy X-ray absorptiometry derived structural geometry for stress fracture prediction in male U.S. Marine Corps recruits. Journal of Bone and Mineral Research 11 (5), 645–653.

Beck, T.J., Ruff, C.B., Shaffer, R.A., et al., 2000. Stress fracture in military recruits: gender differences in muscle and bone susceptibility factors. Bone 27 (3), 437–444.

Bek, N., Öznur, A., Kavlak, Y., et al., 2003. The effect of orthotic treatment of posterior tibial tendon insufficiency on pain and disability. Pain Clinics 15 (3), 345–350.

Bek, N., Simsek, I.E., Erel, S., et al., 2012. Home-based general versus center-based selective rehabilitation in patients with posterior tibial tendon dysfunction. Acta Orthopaedica et Traumatologica Turcica 46 (4), 286–292.

Bennett, P., Patterson, C., 1998. The Foot Health Status Questionnaire (FHSQ): a new instrument for measuring outcomes of footcare. Australasian Journal of Podiatric Medicine 32 (3), 87–92.

Bennett, P.J., Patterson, C., Wearing, S., et al., 1998. Development and validation of a questionnaire designed to measure foot-health status. Journal of the American Podiatric Medical Association 88 (9), 419–428.

Berger, F.H., de Jonge, M.C., Maas, M., 2007. Stress fractures in the lower extremity. The importance of increasing awareness amongst radiologists. European Journal of Radiology 62 (1), 16–26.

Bluman, E.M., Title, C.I., Myerson, M.S., 2007. Posterior tibial tendon rupture: a refined classification system. Foot and Ankle Clinics 12 (2), 233–249, v.

Boden, B.P., Osbahr, D.C., Jimenez, C., 2001. Low-risk stress fractures. American Journal of Sports Medicine 29 (1), 100–111.

Bodill, C., Concannon, M., 2012. Treatments for posterior tibial tendon dysfunction. Practice Nursing 23 (8), 389–394.

Bolívar, Y.A., Munuera, P.V., Padillo, J.P., 2013. Relationship between tightness of the posterior muscles of the lower limb and plantar fasciitis. Foot and Ankle International 34 (1), 42–48.

Bonanno, D.R., Landorf, K.B., Menz, H.B., 2011. Pressure-relieving properties of various shoe inserts in older people with plantar heel pain. Gait and Posture 33 (3), 385–389.

Bracilovic, A., Nihal, A., Houston, V.L., et al., 2006. Effect of foot and ankle position on tarsal tunnel compartment volume. Foot and Ankle 27 (6), 431–437.

Brilhault, J., Noel, V., 2012. PTT functional recovery in early stage II PTTD after tendon balancing and calcaneal lengthening osteotomy. Foot and Ankle International 33 (10), 813–818.

Brodsky, J.W., Charlick, D.A., Coleman, S.C., et al., 2009. Hindfoot motion following reconstruction for posterior tibial tendon dysfunction. Foot and Ankle International 30 (7), 613–618.

Bruce, J., Sutherland, A., 2013. Surgical versus conservative interventions for displaced intra-articular calcaneal fractures. Cochrane Database Systemic Reviews 1, CD008628.

Budiman-Mak, E., Conrad, K.J., Roach, K.E., 1991. The Foot Function Index: a measure of foot pain and disability. Journal of Clinical Epidemiology 44 (6), 561–570.

Budiman-Mak, E., Conrad, K.J., Mazza, J., et al., 2013. A review of the foot function index and the foot function index – revised. Journal of Foot and Ankle Research 6 (1), 5.

Butterworth, P.A., Landorf, K.B., Smith, S.E., et al., 2012. The association between body mass index and musculoskeletal foot disorders: a systematic review. Obesity Reviews 13 (7), 630–642.

Catley, M.J., Tabor, A., Wand, B.M., et al., 2013. Assessing tactile acuity in rheumatology and musculoskeletal medicine – how reliable are two-point discrimination tests at the neck, hand, back and foot? Rheumatology (Oxford, England) 52 (8), 1454–1461.

Cavazos, G.J., Khan, K.H., D'Antoni, A.V., et al., 2009. Cryosurgery for the treatment of heel pain. Foot and Ankle International 30 (6), 500–505.

Chang, K.-V., Chen, S.-Y., Chen, W.-S., et al., 2012. Comparative effectiveness of focused shock wave therapy of different intensity levels and radial shock wave therapy for treating plantar fasciitis: a systematic review and network meta-analysis. Archives of Physical Medicine and Rehabilitation 93 (7), 1259–1268.

Chang, R., Kent-Braun, J.A., Hamill, J., 2012. Use of MRI for volume estimation of tibialis posterior and plantar intrinsic foot muscles in healthy and chronic plantar fasciitis limbs. Clinical Biomechanics (Bristol, Avon) 27 (5), 500–505.

Chhabra, A., Soldatos, T., Chalian, M., et al., 2011. 3-Tesla magnetic resonance imaging evaluation of posterior tibial tendon dysfunction with relevance to clinical staging. Journal of Foot and Ankle Surgery 50 (3), 320–328.

Cleland, J.A., Abbott, J.H., Kidd, M.O., et al., 2009. Manual physical therapy and exercise versus electrophysical agents and exercise in the management of plantar heel pain: a multicenter randomized clinical trial. Journal of Orthopaedic and Sports Physical Therapy 39 (8), 573–585.

Crawford, F., Thomson, C., 2003. Interventions for treating plantar heel pain. Cochrane Database Systemic Reviews 3, CD000416.

Creighton, D., Olson, V.L., 1987. Evaluation of range of motion of the first metatarsophalangeal joint in runners with plantar fasciitis*. Journal of Orthopaedic and Sports Physical Therapy 8 (7), 357–361.

Daftary, A., Haims, A.H., Baumgaertner, M.R., 2005. Fractures of the calcaneus: a review with emphasis on CT. Radiographics: A Review Publication of the Radiological Society of North America, Inc 25 (5), 1215–1226.

De Garceau, D., Dean, D., Requejo, S.M., et al., 2003. The association between diagnosis of plantar fasciitis and Windlass test results. Foot and Ankle International 24 (3), 251–255.

Dellon, A.L., 2008. The four medial ankle tunnels: a critical review of perceptions of tarsal tunnel syndrome and neuropathy. Neurosurgery Clinics of North America 19 (4), 629–648, vii.

Dellon, E.S., Mourey, R., Dellon, A.L., 1992. Human pressure perception values for constant and moving one- and two-point discrimination. Plastic and Reconstructive Surgery 90 (1), 112–117.

Díaz-Llopis, I.V., Rodríguez-Ruíz, C.M., Mulet-Perry, S., et al., 2012. Randomized controlled study of the efficacy of the injection of botulinum toxin type A versus corticosteroids in chronic plantar fasciitis: results at one and six months. Clinical Rehabilitation 26 (7), 594–606.

DiGiovanni, B.F., Nawoczenski, D.A., Lintal, M.E., et al., 2003. Tissue-specific plantar fascia-stretching exercise enhances outcomes in patients with chronic heel pain. A prospective, randomized study. Journal of Bone and Joint Surgery, American Volume 85-A (7), 1270–1277.

DiGiovanni, B.F., Moore, A.M., Zlotnicki, J.P., et al., 2012. Preferred management of recalcitrant plantar fasciitis among orthopaedic foot and ankle surgeons. Foot and Ankle International 33 (6), 507–512.

Drake, M., Bittenbender, C., Boyles, R.E., 2011. The short-term effects of treating plantar fasciitis with a temporary custom foot orthosis and stretching. Journal of Orthopaedic and Sports Physical Therapy 41 (4), 221–231.

Dugan, S.A., Weber, K.M., 2007. Stress fractures and rehabilitation. Physical Medicine and Rehabilitation Clinics of North America 18 (3), 401–416, viii.

Durrant, B., Chockalingam, N., Hashmi, F., 2011. Posterior tibial tendon dysfunction: a review. Journal of the American Podiatric Medical Association 101 (2), 176–186.

Dye, R.W., 2007. A strapping. 1939. Journal of the American Podiatric Medical Association 97 (4), 282–284.

Eastwood, D.M., Phipp, L., 1997. Intra-articular fractures of the calcaneum: why such controversy? Injury 28 (4), 247–259.

Egol, K.A., Azar, F.M., O'Connor, M.I., 2010. Instructional course lectures, American Academy of Orthopaedic Surgeons, Rosemont IL. Online. Available: <http://ebooks.aaos.org/product/>.

Feibel, J.B., Donley, B.G., 2006. Calcaneal osteotomy and flexor digitorum longus transfer for stage II posterior tibial tendon insufficiency. Operative Techniques in Orthopaedics 16 (1), 53–59.

Gaida, J.E., Ashe, M.C., Bass, S.L., et al., 2009. Is adiposity an under-recognized risk factor for tendinopathy? A systematic review. Arthritis and Rheumatism 61 (6), 840–849.

Goff, J.D., Crawford, R., 2011. Diagnosis and treatment of plantar fasciitis. American Family Physician 84 (6), 676–682.

Gougoulias, N., Khanna, A., McBride, D.J., et al., 2009. Management of calcaneal fractures: systematic review of randomized trials. British Medical Bulletin 92, 153–167.

Greaney, R.B., Gerber, F.H., Laughlin, R.L., et al., 1983. Distribution and natural history of stress fractures in U.S. Marine recruits. Radiology 146 (2), 339–346.

Griffin, D., 2013. UK heel fracture trial: surgical treatment versus non-operative care, Online. Available: <http://www.controlled-trials.com/isrctn/pf/37188541> (accessed 3 Sep 2013).

Guerado, E., Bertrand, M.L., Cano, J.R., 2012. Management of calcaneal fractures: what have we learnt over the years? Injury 43 (10), 1640–1650.

Guyatt, G.H., Oxman, A.D., Vist, G.E., et al., 2008. GRADE: an emerging consensus on rating quality of evidence and strength of recommendations. British Medical Journal 336 (7650), 924–926.

Hawke, F., Burns, J., Radford, J.A., et al., 2008. Custom-made foot orthoses for the treatment of foot pain. Cochrane Database Systemic Reviews 3, CD006801.

Hendrix, C.L., Jolly, G.P., Garbalosa, J.C., et al., 1998. Entrapment neuropathy: the etiology of intractable chronic heel pain syndrome. Journal of Foot and Ankle Surgery 37 (4), 273–279.

Hicks, J.H., 1954. The mechanics of the foot. II. The plantar aponeurosis and the arch. Journal of Anatomy 88 (1), 25–30.

Hiller, L., Pinney, S.J., 2003. Surgical treatment of acquired flatfoot deformity: what is the state of practice among academic foot and ankle surgeons in 2002? Foot and Ankle International 24 (9), 701–705.

Holmes, G.B., Mann, R.A., 1992. Possible epidemiological factors associated with rupture of the posterior tibial tendon. Foot and Ankle International 13 (2), 70–79.

Houck, J.R., Nomides, C., Neville, C.G., et al., 2008. The effect of Stage II posterior tibial tendon dysfunction on deep compartment muscle strength: a new strength test. Foot and Ankle International 29 (9), 895–902.

Houck, J.R., Neville, C., Tome, J., et al., 2009a. Foot kinematics during a bilateral heel rise test in participants with stage II posterior tibial tendon dysfunction. Journal of Orthopaedic and Sports Physical Therapy 39 (8), 593–603.

Houck, J.R., Neville, C.G., Tome, J., et al., 2009b. Ankle and foot kinematics associated with stage II PTTD during stance. Foot and Ankle International 30 (06), 530–539. Online. Available: <http://eutils.ncbi.nlm.nih.gov/entrez/eutils/elink.fcgi?dbfrom=pubmed&id=19486631&retmode=ref&cmd=prlinks>.

Ibrahim, I.K., Medani, S.H., El-Hameed, M.M.A., et al., 2013. Tarsal tunnel syndrome in patients with rheumatoid arthritis, electrophysiological and ultrasound study. Alexandria Journal of Medicine 49 (2), 95–188.

Ibrahim, T., Rowsell, M., Rennie, W., et al., 2007. Displaced intra-articular calcaneal fractures: 15-year follow-up of a randomised controlled trial of conservative versus operative treatment. Injury 38 (7), 848–855.

Irving, D.B., Cook, J.L., Menz, H.B., 2006. Factors associated with chronic plantar heel pain: a systematic review. Journal of Science and Medicine in Sports 9 (1–2), 11–22, discussion 23–24.

Irving, D.B., Cook, J.L., Young, M.A., et al., 2007. Obesity and pronated foot type may increase the risk of chronic plantar heel pain: a matched case-control study. BMC Musculoskeletal Disorders 8, 41.

Irving, D.B., Cook, J.L., Young, M.A., et al., 2008. Impact of chronic plantar heel pain on health-related quality of life. Journal of the American Podiatric Medical Association 98 (4), 283–289.

Jack, E.A., 1953. Naviculo-cuneiform fusion in the treatment of flat foot. Journal of Bone and Joint Surgery, British Volume 35-B (1), 75–82.

Jackson, D.L., Haglund, B., 1991. Tarsal tunnel syndrome in athletes. Case reports and literature review. American Journal of Sports Medicine 19 (1), 61.

Jackson, D.L., Haglund, B.L., 1992. Tarsal tunnel syndrome in runners. Sports Medicine 13 (2), 146–149.

Jain, N.B., Omar, I., Kelikian, A.S., et al., 2011. Prevalence of and factors associated with posterior tibial tendon pathology on sonographic assessment. Physical Medicine and Rehabilitation 3 (11), 998–1004.

Jarvis, H.L., Nester, C.J., Jones, R.K., et al., 2012. Inter-assessor reliability of practice based biomechanical assessment of the foot and ankle. Journal of Foot and Ankle Research 5, 14.

Jerosch, J., Schunck, J., Khoja, A., 2006. Results of surgical treatment of tarsal tunnel syndrome. Foot and Ankle Surgery 12 (4), 205–208.

Jolly, G.P., Zgonis, T., Hendrix, C.L., 2005. Neurogenic heel pain. Clinics in Podiatric Medicine and Surgery 22 (1), 101–113, vii.

Kalaci, A., Cakici, H., Hapa, O., et al., 2009. Treatment of plantar fasciitis using four different local injection modalities: a randomized prospective clinical trial. Journal of the American Podiatric Medical Association 99 (2), 108–113.

Kaux, J.-F., Crielaard, J.-M., 2013. Platelet-rich plasma application in the management of chronic tendinopathies. Acta Orthopaedica Belgica 79 (1), 10–15.

Kavlak, Y., Uygur, F., 2011. Effects of nerve mobilization exercise as an adjunct to the conservative treatment for patients with tarsal tunnel syndrome. Journal of Manipulative and Physiological Therapy 34 (7), 441–448.

Kayhan, A., Gökay, N.S., Alpaslan, R., et al., 2011. Sonographically guided corticosteroid injection for treatment of plantar fasciosis. Journal of Ultrasound Medicine 30 (4), 509–515.

Kennedy, D.M., Stratford, P.W., Wessel, J., et al., 2005. Assessing stability and change of four performance measures: a longitudinal study evaluating outcome following total hip and knee arthroplasty. BMC Musculoskeletal Disorders 6, 3.

Key, J.A., 1953. Partial rupture of the tendon of the posterior tibial muscle. Journal of Bone and Joint Surgery, American Volume 35-A (4), 1006–1008.

Kim, C., Cashdollar, M.R., Mendicino, R.W., et al., 2010. Incidence of plantar fascia ruptures following corticosteroid injection. Foot and Ankle Specialist 3 (6), 335–337.

Kinoshita, M., Okuda, R., Morikawa, J., et al., 2001. The dorsiflexion–eversion test for diagnosis of tarsal tunnel syndrome. Journal of Bone and Joint Surgery, American Volume 83 (12), 1835–1839.

Kinoshita, M., Okuda, R., Yasuda, T., et al., 2006. Tarsal tunnel syndrome in athletes. American Journal of Sports Medicine 34 (8), 1307–1312.

Kohls-Gatzoulis, J., Angel, J., Singh, D., 2004a. Tibialis posterior dysfunction as a cause of flatfeet in elderly patients. The Foot 14 (4), 207–209.

Kohls-Gatzoulis, J., Angel, J.C., Singh, D., et al., 2004b. Tibialis posterior dysfunction: a common and treatable cause of adult acquired flatfoot. British Medical Journal 329 (7478), 1328–1333.

Kohls-Gatzoulis, J., Woods, B., Angel, J.C., et al., 2009. The prevalence of symptomatic posterior tibialis tendon dysfunction in women over the age of 40 in England. Foot and Ankle Surgery 15 (2), 75–81.

Kulig, K., Burnfield, J.M., Requejo, S.M., et al., 2004. Selective activation of tibialis posterior: evaluation by magnetic resonance imaging. Medicine and Science in Sports and Exercise 36 (5), 862–867.

Kulig, K., Burnfield, J.M., Reischl, S., et al., 2005. Effect of foot orthoses on tibialis posterior activation in persons with pes planus. Medicine and Science in Sports and Exercise 37 (1), 24–29.

Kulig, K., Lederhaus, E.S., Reischl, S., et al., 2009a. Effect of eccentric exercise program for early tibialis posterior tendinopathy. Foot and Ankle International 30 (9), 877–885.

Kulig, K., Reischl, S.F., Pomrantz, A.B., et al., 2009b. Nonsurgical management of posterior tibial tendon dysfunction with orthoses and resistive exercise: a randomized controlled trial. Physical Therapy 89 (1), 26–37.

Kulig, K., Popovich, J.M., Noceti-Dewit, L.M., et al., 2011. Women with posterior tibial tendon dysfunction have diminished ankle and hip muscle performance. Journal of Orthopaedic and Sports Physical Therapy 41 (9), 687–694.

Labovitz, J.M., Yu, J., Kim, C., 2011. The role of hamstring tightness in plantar fasciitis. Foot and Ankle Specialist 4 (3), 141–144.

Landorf, B., Menz, B., 2008. Plantar heel pain and fasciitis. Clinical Evidence (Online). BMJ Group Feb 5:2008.

Landorf, K.B., Keenan, A.-M., 2002. An evaluation of two foot-specific, health-related quality-of-life measuring instruments. Foot and Ankle International 23 (6), 538–546.

Landorf, K.B., Radford, J.A., 2008. Minimal important difference: values for the foot health status questionnaire, foot function index and visual analogue scale. The Foot 18 (1), 15–19.

Landorf, K.B., Radford, J.A., Hudson, S., 2010. Minimal Important Difference (MID) of two commonly used outcome measures for foot problems. Journal of Foot and Ankle Research 3, 7.

League, A.C., 2008. Current concepts review: plantar fasciitis. Foot and Ankle International 29 (3), 358–366. Online. Available: <http://www.datatrace.com/e-chemtracts/emailurl.html? http://www.newsletteronline.com/user/user.fas/s=563/fp=20/tp=37?T=open_article,966698&P=article>.

Lee, J.H., Kim, S.B., Lee, K.W., et al., 2011. Biomechanical factors associated with plantar fasciitis in non-obese patients. Korean Journal of Sports Medicine 29 (1), 9–14. Online. Available: <http://dx.doi.org/10.5763/kjsm.2011.29.1.9>.

Lee, S.Y., McKeon, P., Hertel, J., 2009. Does the use of orthoses improve self-reported pain and function measures in patients with plantar fasciitis? A meta-analysis. Physical Therapy in Sport 10 (1), 12–18.

Lemont, H., Ammirati, K.M., Usen, N., 2003. Plantar fasciitis: a degenerative process (fasciosis) without inflammation. Journal of the American Podiatric Medical Association 93 (3), 234–237.

Lentz, T.A., Sutton, Z., Greenberg, S., et al., 2010. Pain-related fear contributes to self-reported disability in patients with foot and ankle pathology. Archives of Physical Medicine and Rehabilitation 91 (4), 557–561.

Li, J., Muehleman, C., 2007. Anatomic relationship of heel spur to surrounding soft tissues: greater variability than previously reported. Clinical Anatomy 20 (8), 950–955.

Lin, J.L., Balbas, J., Richardson, E.G., 2008. Results of non-surgical treatment of stage II posterior tibial tendon dysfunction: a 7- to 10-year followup. Foot and Ankle International 29 (8), 781–786.

Lopes, A.D., Junior, M.L.C.H., Yeung, S.S., et al., 2012. What are the main running-related musculoskeletal injuries? Sports Medicine 42 (10), 891–905.

Lundborg, G., Rosen, B., 2004. The two-point discrimination test – time for a re-appraisal? Journal of Hand Surgery, British and European 29 (5), 418–422.

McCrory, P., Bell, S., Bradshaw, C., 2002. Nerve entrapments of the lower leg, ankle and foot in sport. Sports Medicine 32 (6), 371–391.

McMillan, A.M., Landorf, K.B., Barrett, J.T., et al., 2009. Diagnostic imaging for chronic plantar heel pain: a systematic review and meta-analysis. Journal of Foot and Ankle Research 2, 32.

McMillan, A.M., Landorf, K.B., Gilheany, M.F., et al., 2010. Ultrasound guided injection of dexamethasone versus placebo for treatment of plantar fasciitis: protocol for a randomised controlled trial. Journal of Foot and Ankle Research 3, 15.

McMillan, A.M., Landorf, K.B., Gilheany, M.F., et al., 2012. Ultrasound guided corticosteroid injection for plantar fasciitis: randomised controlled trial. British Medical Journal 344, e3260.

Marie, I., Delafenêtre, H., Massy, N., et al., 2008. Network of the French Pharmacovigilance Centers. Tendinous disorders attributed to statins: a study on ninety-six spontaneous reports in the period 1990–2005 and review of the literature. Arthritis and Rheumatism 59 (3), 367–372.

Martin, R.L., Irrgang, J.J., 2007. A survey of self-reported outcome instruments for the foot and ankle. Journal of Orthopaedic and Sports Physical Therapy 37 (2), 72–84.

Martin, R.L., Irrgang, J.J., Burdett, R.G., et al., 2005. Evidence of validity for the Foot and Ankle Ability Measure (FAAM). Foot and Ankle International 26 (11), 968–983.

Matheson, G.O., Clement, D.B., McKenzie, D.C., et al., 1987. Stress fractures in athletes A study of 320 cases. American Journal of Sports Medicine 15 (1), 46–58.

McPoil, T.G., Martin, R.L., Cornwall, M.W., et al., 2008. Heel pain – plantar fasciitis: clinical practice guidelines linked to the international classification of function, disability, and health from the orthopaedic section of the American Physical Therapy

Association. Journal of Orthopaedic and Sports Physical Therapy 38 (4), A1–A18.

McPoil, T.G., Vicenzino, B., Cornwall, M.W., et al., 2009. Reliability and normative values for the foot mobility magnitude: a composite measure of vertical and medial-lateral mobility of the midfoot. Journal of Foot and Ankle Research 2 (1), 6.

Menz, H.B., Zammit, G.V., Landorf, K.B., et al., 2008. Plantar calcaneal spurs in older people: longitudinal traction or vertical compression? Journal of Foot and Ankle Research 1 (1), 7.

Messier, S.P., Pittala, K.A., 1988. Etiologic factors associated with selected running injuries. Medicine and Science in Sports and Exercise 20 (5), 501–505.

Meyer, J., Kulig, K., Landel, R., 2002. Differential diagnosis and treatment of subcalcaneal heel pain: a case report. Journal of Orthopaedic and Sports Physical Therapy 32 (3), 114–122, discussion 122–124.

Morton, T.N., Zimmerman, J.P., Lee, M., et al., 2013. A review of 105 consecutive uniport endoscopic plantar fascial release procedures for the treatment of chronic plantar fasciitis. Journal of Foot and Ankle Surgery 52 (1), 48–52.

Murley, G.S., Menz, H.B., Landorf, K.B., 2009. Foot posture influences the electromyographic activity of selected lower limb muscles during gait. Journal of Foot and Ankle Research 2, 35.

Murley, G.S., Landorf, K.B., Menz, H.B., 2010. Do foot orthoses change lower limb muscle activity in flat-arched feet towards a pattern observed in normal-arched feet? Clinical Biomechanics (Bristol, Avon) 25 (7), 728–736.

Myerson, M.S., 1996. Instructional course lectures, The American Academy of Orthopaedic Surgeons – adult acquired flatfoot deformity. Treatment of dysfunction of the posterior tibial tendon*†. Journal of Bone and Joint Surgery, America 78 (5), 780–792. Online. Available: <http://www.orthochirurg.com/resources/journals/tib%20post%20dysfunction%20-%20flatfoot.pdf>.

Ness, M.E., Long, J., Marks, R., et al., 2008. Foot and ankle kinematics in patients with posterior tibial tendon dysfunction. Gait and Posture 27 (2), 331–339.

Neville, C.G., Houck, J.R., 2009. Choosing among 3 ankle-foot orthoses for a patient with stage II posterior tibial tendon dysfunction. Journal of Orthopaedic and Sports Physical Therapy 39 (11), 816–824.

Neville, C., Lemley, F.R., 2012. Effect of ankle-foot orthotic devices on foot kinematics in Stage II posterior tibial tendon dysfunction. Foot and Ankle International 33 (5), 406–414.

Neville, C., Flemister, A., Tome, J., et al., 2007. Comparison of changes in posterior tibialis muscle length between subjects with posterior tibial tendon dysfunction and healthy controls during walking. Journal of Orthopaedic and Sports Physical Therapy 37 (11), 661–669.

Neville, C., Flemister, A.S., Houck, J.R., 2010. Deep posterior compartment strength and foot kinematics in subjects with stage II posterior tibial tendon dysfunction. Foot and Ankle International 31 (4), 320–328.

Neville, C., Flemister, A.S., Houck, J., 2013. Total and distributed plantar loading in subjects with stage II tibialis posterior tendon dysfunction during terminal stance. Foot and Ankle International 34 (1), 131–139.

Nolan, M.F., 1983. Limits of two-point discrimination ability in the lower limb in young adult men and women. Physical Therapy 63 (9), 1424–1428.

O'Connor, K., Baumhauer, J., Houck, J.R., 2010. Patient factors in the selection of operative versus nonoperative treatment for posterior tibial tendon dysfunction. Foot and Ankle International 31 (3), 197–202.

Öztuna, V., Özge, A., Eskandari, M.M., et al., 2002. Nerve entrapment in painful heel syndrome. Foot Ankle International 23 (3), 208–211.

Owens, B.D., Wolf, J.M., Seelig, A.D., 2013. Risk factors for lower extremity tendinopathies in military personnel. Orthopaedic Journal of Sports Medicine 1 (1), 2325967113492707.

Padua, L., Aprile, I., Pazzaglia, C., et al., 2007. Contribution of ultrasound in a neurophysiological lab in diagnosing nerve impairment: A one-year systematic assessment. Clinical Neurophysiology 118 (6), 1410–1416.

Page, M.J., O'Connor, D., Pitt, V., et al., 2012. Exercise and mobilisation interventions for carpal tunnel syndrome (Review). Wiley Online Library, Online. Available: <http://onlinelibrary.wiley.com/doi/10.1002/14651858.CD009899/abstract>.

Parker, J., Nester, C.J., Long, A.F., et al., 2003. The problem with measuring patient perceptions of outcome with existing outcome measures in foot and ankle surgery. Foot and Ankle International 24 (1), 56–60.

Patel, A.T., Gaines, K., Malamut, R., et al., 2005. Usefulness of electrodiagnostic techniques in the evaluation of suspected tarsal tunnel syndrome: an evidence-based review. Muscle and Nerve 32 (2), 236–240.

Pelliccioni, A., Bittar, C.K., Zabeu, J., 2012. Surgical treatment of intraarticular calcaneous fractures Sanders II and III. Systematic review. Acta Ortopédica Brasileira 20 (1), 39–42.

Perera, N., Liolitsa, D., Hill, C.S., 2013. Surgical interventions for entrapment and compression of the tibial and deep peroneal nerves including tarsal tunnel syndrome. Cochrane Database Systemic Reviews 7, CD010630.

Pinney, S.J., Van Bergeyk, A., 2003. Controversies in surgical reconstruction of acquired adult deformity. Foot and Ankle Clinics 8 (3), 595–604.

Pohl, M.B., Hamill, J., Davis, I.S., 2009. Biomechanical and anatomic factors associated with a history of plantar fasciitis in female runners. Clinical Journal of Sport Medicine 19 (5), 372–376.

Preston, D.C., Shapiro, B.E., 2013. Tarsal tunnel syndrome. In: Preston, D.C., Shapiro, B.E. (Eds.), Electromyography and neuromuscular disorders, third ed. Elsevier, London, pp. 365–371.

Rabbito, M., Pohl, M.B., Humble, N., et al., 2011. Biomechanical and clinical factors related to stage I posterior tibial tendon dysfunction. Journal of Orthopaedic and Sports Physical Therapy 41 (10), 776–784.

Rammelt, S., Zwipp, H., 2004. Calcaneus fractures: facts, controversies and recent developments. Injury 35 (5), 443–461.

Redmond, A.C., Crane, Y.Z., Menz, H.B., 2008. Normative values for the Foot Posture Index. Journal of Foot and Ankle Research 1 (1), 6.

Ribeiro, A., Trombini-Souza, F., Tessutti, V., 2011. Rearfoot alignment and medial longitudinal arch configurations of runners with symptoms and histories of plantar fasciitis. Clinics (Sao Paulo) 66 (6), 1027–1033.

Riddle, D.L., Pulisic, M., Pidcoe, P., et al., 2003. Risk factors for Plantar fasciitis: a matched case-control study. Journal of Bone and Joint Surgery, America 85 (5), 872–877.

Riddle, D.L., Schappert, S.M., 2004. Volume of ambulatory care visits and patterns of care for patients diagnosed with plantar fasciitis: a national study of medical doctors. Foot and Ankle International 25 (5), 303–310.

Ring, K., Otter, S., 2013. Clinical efficacy and cost-effectiveness of bespoke and prefabricated foot orthoses for plantar heel pain: a prospective cohort study. Musculoskeletal Care Jun 25. Epub ahead of print.

Ringleb, S.I., Kavros, S.J., Kotajarvi, B.R., et al., 2007. Changes in gait associated with acute stage II posterior tibial tendon dysfunction. Gait and Posture 25 (4), 555–564.

Roll, C., Schirmbeck, J., Schreyer, A., et al., 2011. How reliable are CT scans for the evaluation of calcaneal fractures? Archives of Orthopaedic and Traumatic Surgery 131 (10), 1397–1403.

Rome, K., 1997. Anthropometric and biomechanical risk factors in the development of plantar heel pain – a review of the literature. Physical Therapy Reviews 2 (3), 123–134.

Rome, K., Howe, T., Haslock, I., 2001. Risk factors associated with the development of plantar heel pain in athletes. The Foot 11 (3), 119–125.

Ryan, M.B., Wong, A.D., Gillies, J.H., et al., 2009. Sonographically guided intratendinous injections of hyperosmolar dextrose/lidocaine: a pilot study for the treatment of chronic plantar fasciitis. British Journal of Sports Medicine 43 (4), 303–306.

Sahin, N., Oztürk, A., Atici, T., 2010. Foot mobility and plantar fascia elasticity in patients with plantar fasciitis. Acta Orthopaedica et Traumatologica Turcica 44 (5), 385–391.

Sanders, R., 2000. Displaced intra-articular fractures of the calcaneus. Journal of Bone and Joint Surgery, American Volume 82 (2), 225–250.

Sanders, R., Fortin, P., DiPasquale, T., et al., 1993. Operative treatment in 120 displaced intraarticular calcaneal fractures. Results using a prognostic computed tomography scan classification. Clinical Orthopaedics and Related Research 290, 87–95.

Sayed-Noor, A.S., Ågren, P.-H., Wretenberg, P., 2011. Interobserver reliability and intraobserver reproducibility of three radiological classification systems for intra-articular calcaneal fractures. Foot and Ankle International 32 (9), 861–866.

Schepers, T., 2011. The sinus tarsi approach in displaced intra-articular calcaneal fractures: a systematic review. International Orthopaedics 35 (5), 697–703.

Schepers, T., Patka, P., 2008. Calcaneal nonunion: three cases and a review of the literature. Archives of Orthopaedic and Traumatic Surgery 128 (7), 735–738.

Schepers, T., Patka, P., 2009. Treatment of displaced intra-articular calcaneal fractures by ligamentotaxis: current concepts' review. Archives of Orthopaedic and Traumatic Surgery 129 (12), 1677–1683.

Schepers, T., Ginai, A.Z., Van Lieshout, E.M.M., et al., 2008a. Demographics of extra-articular calcaneal fractures: including a review of the literature on treatment and outcome. Archives of Orthopaedic and Traumatic Surgery 128 (10), 1099–1106.

Schepers, T., van Lieshout, E.M.M., van Ginhoven, T.M., et al., 2008b. Current concepts in the treatment of intra-articular calcaneal fractures: results of a nationwide survey. International Orthopaedics 32 (5), 711–715.

Schepers, T., Heetveld, M.J., Mulder, P.G.H., et al., 2008c. Clinical outcome scoring of intra-articular calcaneal fractures. Journal of Foot and Ankle Surgery 47 (3), 213–218.

Schepers, T., van Lieshout, E.M.M., Ginai, A.Z., et al., 2009. Calcaneal fracture classification: a comparative study. Journal of Foot and Ankle Surgery 48 (2), 156–162.

Scher, D.L., Belmont, P.J., Bear, R., et al., 2009. The incidence of plantar fasciitis in the United States military. Journal of Bone and Joint Surgery 91 (12), 2867–2872.

Smith, J.T., Bluman, E.M., 2012. Update on stage IV acquired adult flatfoot disorder: when the deltoid ligament becomes dysfunctional. Foot and Ankle Clinics 17 (2), 351–360.

Sormaala, M., 2006. Bone stress injuries of the foot and ankle. Helsingin Yliopisto. Online. Available: <http://www.doria.fi/handle/10024/2189>.

Sormaala, M.J., Niva, M.H., Kiuru, M.J., et al., 2006. Stress injuries of the calcaneus detected with magnetic resonance imaging in military recruits. Journal of Bone and Joint Surgery, American Volume 88 (10), 2237–2242.

Spitz, D.J., Newberg, A.H., 2002. Imaging of stress fractures in the athlete. Radiologic Clinics of North America 40 (2), 313–331.

Stolwijk, N.M., Louwerens, J.W.K., Nienhuis, B., et al., 2011. Plantar pressure with and without custom insoles in patients with common foot complaints. Foot and Ankle International 32 (1), 57–65.

Stratton, M., McPoil, T.G., Cornwall, M.W., et al., 2009. Use of low-frequency electrical stimulation for the treatment of plantar fasciitis. Journal of the American Podiatric Medical Association 99 (6), 481–488.

Sweeting, D., Parish, B., Hooper, L., et al., 2011. The effectiveness of manual stretching in the treatment of plantar heel pain: a systematic review. Journal of Foot and Ankle Research 4, 19.

Tassler, P.L., Dellon, A.L., 1996. Pressure perception in the normal lower extremity and in the tarsal tunnel syndrome. Muscle and Nerve 19 (3), 285–289.

Taunton, J.E., Ryan, M.B., Clement, D.B., et al., 2002. Plantar fasciitis: a retrospective analysis of 267 cases. Physical Therapy in Sport 3 (2), 57–65.

Therimadasamy, A.K., Seet, R.C., Kagda, Y.H., et al., 2011. Combination of ultrasound and nerve conduction studies in the diagnosis of tarsal tunnel syndrome. Neurology India 59 (2), 296–297.

Thomson, C.E., Crawford, F., Murray, G.D., 2005. The effectiveness of extra corporeal shock wave therapy for plantar heel pain: a systematic review and meta-analysis. BMC Musculoskeletal Disorders 6, 19.

Tong, K.B., Furia, J., 2010. Economic burden of plantar fasciitis treatment in the United States. American Journal of Orthopedics 39 (5), 227–231.

Tornetta, P., Qadir, R., Sanders, R., 2013. Pain dominates summed scores for hindfoot and ankle trauma. Journal of Orthopaedic Trauma 27 (8), 477–482.

Toth, C., McNeil, S., Feasby, T., 2005. Peripheral nervous system injuries in sport and recreation. Sports Medicine 35 (8), 717–738.

Trepman, E., Kadel, N.J., Chisholm, K., et al., 1999. Effect of foot and ankle position on tarsal tunnel compartment pressure. Foot and Ankle International 20 (11), 721–726.

Tu, P., Bytomski, J.R., 2011. Diagnosis of heel pain. American Family Physician 84 (8), 909–916.

Tweed, J.L., Barnes, M.R., Allen, M.J., et al., 2009. Biomechanical consequences of total plantar fasciotomy: a review of the literature. Journal of the American Podiatric Medical Association 99 (5), 422–430.

Vahdatpour, B., Sajadieh, S., Bateni, V., et al., 2012. Extracorporeal shock wave therapy in patients with plantar fasciitis. A randomized, placebo-controlled trial with ultrasonographic and subjective outcome assessments. Journal of Research in Medical Sciences 17 (9), 834–838.

Välimäki, V.-V., Alfthan, H., Lehmuskallio, E., et al., 2005. Risk factors for clinical stress fractures in male military recruits: a prospective cohort study. Bone 37 (2), 267–273.

van de Water, A.T., Speksnijder, C.M., 2010. Efficacy of taping for the treatment of plantar fasciosis a systematic review of controlled trials. Journal of the American Podiatric Medical Association 100 (1), 41–51.

Verdugo, R.J., Salinas, R.A., Castillo, J.L., et al., 2008. Surgical versus non-surgical treatment for carpal tunnel syndrome. Cochrane Database Systemic Reviews 4, CD001552.

Wearing, S., Smeathers, J., Yates, B., et al., 2004. Sagittal movement of the medial longitudinal arch is unchanged in plantar fasciitis. Medicine and Science in Sports and Exercise 36 (10), 1761–1767.

Weinraub, G.M., Heilala, M.A., 2000. Adult flatfoot/posterior tibial tendon dysfunction: outcomes analysis of surgical treatment utilizing an algorithmic approach. Journal of Foot and Ankle Surgery 39 (6), 359–364.

Williams, D.S., McClay, I.S., 2000. Measurements used to characterize the foot and the medial longitudinal arch: reliability and validity. Physical Therapy 80 (9), 864–871.

Yang, Y., Zhao, H., Zhou, J., et al., 2012. Treatment of displaced intraarticular calcaneal fractures with or without bone grafts: A systematic review of the literature. Indian Journal of Orthopaedics 46 (2), 130–137.

Yucel, I., Yazici, B., Degirmenci, E., et al., 2009. Comparison of ultrasound-, palpation-, and scintigraphy-guided steroid injections in the treatment of plantar fasciitis. Archives of Orthopaedic and Traumatic Surgery 129 (5), 695–701.

Yucel, I., Ozturan, K.E., Demiraran, Y., et al., 2010. Comparison of high-dose extracorporeal shockwave therapy and intralesional corticosteroid injection in the treatment of plantar fasciitis. Journal of the American Podiatric Medical Association 100 (2), 105–110.

Yucel, U., Kucuksen, S., Cingoz, H.T., et al., 2013. Full-length silicone insoles versus ultrasound-guided corticosteroid injection in the management of plantar fasciitis: A randomized clinical trial. Prosthetics and Orthotics International 37 (6), 471–476. Epub 2013 Mar 7.

Zaw, H., Calder, J.D.F., 2010. Operative management options for symptomatic flexible adult acquired flatfoot deformity: a review. Knee Surgery, Sports Traumatology, Arthroscopy 18 (2), 135–142.

Zwas, S.T., Elkanovitch, R., Frank, G., 1987. Interpretation and classification of bone scintigraphic findings in stress fractures. Journal of Nuclear Medicine 28 (4), 452.

Chapter 6

Achilles Tendon

Shannon Munteanu

Chapter Outline

INTRODUCTION

PREVALENCE

Achilles tendinopathy is a common musculoskeletal disorder affecting the lower limb. In athletic populations, Achilles tendinopathy has been reported to account for up to 18% of all injuries (Edouard et al. 2011; Johansson 1986; Lysholm and Wiklander 1987; Van Ginckel et al. 2008; Wilson et al. 2011) and has a cumulative lifetime incidence of 24% (Kujala et al. 2005). Achilles tendinopathy is also common in non-athletic people. Recent population-based studies have shown Achilles tendinopathy to be the sixth most common reason for non-traumatic foot and ankle consultations (Menz et al. 2010), and the incidence of Achilles tendinopathy is 1.85 per 1000 patients presenting to their general practitioner (de Jonge et al. 2011). These studies are supported by findings that one-third of those with Achilles tendinopathy are sedentary (Hootman et al. 2002; Rolf et al. 1997). Achilles tendinopathy appears to be more prevalent in males (Hootman et al. 2002) and those above 35 years of age, but this has not been empirically proven (Knobloch et al. 2008).

TERMINOLOGY

There is some confusion within the literature in regards to the terminology used to describe Achilles tendon disorders (Magnussen et al. 2009). The terms 'tendinitis', 'tendonitis' and 'paratenonitis' have been used but are misleading because they imply inflammation is present (Carcia et al. 2010). Although inflammation of the paratenon can occur, Achilles tendon disorders are characterized by tendon degeneration rather than inflammation (Movin et al. 1997). Therefore, the term 'tendinopathy' is a more apt description of Achilles tendon disorders, unless inflammation has been confirmed (Carcia et al. 2010).

Another area of potential confusion relates to the description of the affected structures, with the American Physical Association (Carcia et al. 2010) recommending that the terminology used is tissue-specific. As such, they propose that disorders of the tendon, paratenon, or both be referred to as 'tendinopathy', 'paratendinopathy', or 'pantendinopathy', respectively (Carcia et al. 2010).

Finally, the location of the pathology is an area of potential confusion within the literature. Achilles tendon disorders are commonly described as occurring at two anatomical locations: (i) *mid-portion*, when pain occurs 2 to 6 cm proximal to the calcaneal insertion, or (ii) *insertional*, when symptoms occur at the insertion of the Achilles tendon (Alfredson et al. 2012; Carcia et al. 2010). The risk factors, management, and prognosis for these two disorders are different. Mid-portion Achilles tendinopathy has been reported to be most common (Knobloch et al. 2008; Kvist 1994), and will therefore be the focus of this chapter. As such, cases of mid-portion Achilles tendinopathy will be referred to as 'Achilles tendinopathy' throughout this chapter, unless stated otherwise. Readers with a specific interest in insertional Achilles tendinopathy are referred to the following excellent reviews (Alfredson et al. 2012; Kearney and Costa 2010).

ANATOMICAL CONSIDERATIONS

The Achilles tendon is the thickest and strongest tendon in the human body (Doral et al. 2010). Its length ranges from 110 to 260 mm (average is 150 mm) and its dimensions alter along its length (Doral et al. 2010). Proximally, the Achilles tendon has a broad shape with an average width of 68 mm. However, it becomes progressively thinner so that its mid-portion is more oval-shaped (average width is 18 mm). Just proximal to its insertion, the tendon becomes broader, forming an arcuate shape with an average width of approximately 34 mm (Doral et al. 2010; Lohrer et al. 2008). The tendon is surrounded by a highly vascular paratenon, which is made up of a single layer of cells (Schepsis et al. 2002).

The exact vascularization of the Achilles tendon is not completely understood (Theobald et al. 2005). The posterior tibial artery provides the primary blood supply to the Achilles tendon and the peroneal artery also contributes (Chen et al. 2009; Doral et al. 2010). A significant portion of the blood supply to the tendon comes through the fatty anterior aspect of the Achilles paratenon, which functions as a passageway for blood vessels to reach the tendon (Schepsis et al. 2002). The musculo-tendinous junction and osseous insertion sites also provide tendon vascularization (Theobald et al. 2005). The distribution of the blood supply within the Achilles tendon varies; however, the existence of an area of relative hypovascularity in the mid-zone (2 to 6 cm proximal to the calcaneal insertion) of the Achilles tendon has consistently been shown (Chen et al. 2009; Rompe et al. 2009). This area is a common site for tendinopathy and rupture. Although there is an association between pathology in this region and a relative lack of vascularization, localized tensile forces in this region have been hypothesized as being more important in the development of pathology (Theobald et al. 2005). The sensory innervation is derived from the overlying superficial sural nerve and adjacent deep tibial nerve (Doral et al. 2010).

PATHOLOGY OF ACHILLES TENDINOPATHY

Normal tendon is glistening and white (Khan et al. 1999). Histological analysis of normal tendon shows that it exhibits dense parallel collagen bundles that are slightly wavy. There is an even and sparse distribution of rows of cells, called tenocytes, with slender elongated nuclei between collagen bundles. There is an absence of stainable ground substance. A sparse network of small arterioles is aligned parallel to the collagen fibres in thin, fibrous septa between the bundles (Aström and Rausing 1995; Movin et al. 1997).

Analysis of surgical specimens has provided insights into the macroscopic, histological, and biochemical changes that occur in Achilles tendinopathy (Aström and Rausing 1995). Macroscopically, Achilles tendinopathy is characterized by poorly demarcated dull-greyish discoloration (Aström and Rausing 1995; Movin et al. 1997); histologically, the collagen fibres have reduced bundle formation and demonstrate increased disorganization and metachromatic ground substance. There is an increase in the number of tenocytes and they exhibit a more rounded nuclear appearance; although there is an increase in tendon vascularity, there is an absence of inflammatory cells (Aström and Rausing 1995; Movin et al. 1997). Biochemical changes include an increase in water and ground substance (de Mos et al. 2007; Movin et al. 1997), increased proportion of denatured and immature collagen, as well as increased activity of matrix-degrading enzymes such as matrix metalloproteinase-3 (de Mos et al. 2007).

Together, these findings suggest that Achilles tendinopathy is not an inflammatory disorder, but rather a degenerative process representing the result of a failed tissue-healing response. There is an increased tissue turnover rate as part of an exaggerated repair process, leading to the deposition of a compromised non-physiological tendon matrix (de Mos et al. 2007).

DIAGNOSIS

SYMPTOMS

Patients with Achilles tendinopathy present with pain localized to the posterior leg within the Achilles tendon, 2 to 6 cm proximal to its insertion. Symptoms are usually unilateral, but can present bilaterally. These symptoms generally have an insidious onset but may exist for years. The intensity of the symptoms is usually variable and typically aggravated by weightbearing, particularly high-loading activities such as running and jumping. However, in more severe cases patients may experience pain during daily functional activities such as walking up and down stairs (Galloway et al. 1992). Additionally, patients with Achilles tendinopathy will report stiffness and pain upon weightbearing after prolonged immobility such as sitting or sleeping. In physically active patients, symptoms are more severe at the commencement of activity but lessen as the exercise continues. As the condition worsens a progression of symptoms occurs such that pain is felt throughout the exercise. In some cases it may be necessary to suspend exercise (Carcia et al. 2010). Although these symptoms are typical of Achilles tendinopathy, they are not diagnostic in themselves and a thorough physical examination is required to form an accurate diagnosis (Williams 1993). Other conditions that should be excluded as a cause of pain in the Achilles region are partial tears of the Achilles tendon, insertional Achilles tendinopathy with or with retrocalcaneal bursitis, Sever's disease, Achilles

bursitis, posterior impingement syndrome, referred pain, irritation or neuroma of the sural nerve, accessory soleus muscle, Achilles tendon rupture, and Achilles tendinopathy secondary to inflammatory arthritis (Alfredson et al. 2012; Carcia et al. 2010).

SIGNS

The physical examination should be performed with the patient both weightbearing and non-weightbearing using a standardized approach to assess all structures of the posterior leg, with the following assessments: active movement testing, palpation, passive movement testing, resisted isometric testing, and special tests (Magee 1997).

Active movement testing for posterior leg pain is best assessed with the patient in a weightbearing position and can be performed by asking the patient to perform heel rises, which will cause variable discomfort. Asking the patient to hop on the affected lower limb will often reproduce symptoms.

The Achilles tendon should then be palpated along its entire length from the calcaneal insertion to the musculo-tendinous junction by gently squeezing it between the index finger and thumb. Mid-portion Achilles tendinopathy presents as pain localized 2 to 6 cm from the calcaneal insertion. There may also be associated nodular thickening of the tendon in this region, but this is not always present (Alfredson et al. 2012). The location of a patient's symptoms makes it possible to differentiate mid-portion Achilles tendinopathy from other causes of posterior ankle pain, such as insertional Achilles tendinopathy. However, it can be difficult to distinguish between mid-portion Achilles tendinopathy, partial tears, and paratendinopathy. Further, these conditions may coexist and this can complicate the diagnosis. In such cases, diagnostic imaging may be required.

Passive movement testing is performed on the ankle and subtalar joints to exclude 'non-contractile' causes of the symptoms such as posterior ankle impingement. These assessments are best performed with the patient positioned prone. The assessment of the ankle joint is ideally performed with the knee flexed so as to not have the gastrocnemius muscle interfere with the results of the testing. The magnitude, quality and end-feel of the movement at these joints should be determined. In a person with pathology of the 'contractile tissue-units' such as Achilles tendinopathy, passive movements do not cause symptoms unless the tendinopathy is severe.

Resisted isometric testing should then be performed on all 'contractile tissue-units' that surround the medial, posterior and lateral ankle, to determine whether they are a cause of the symptoms. Owing to the strength of the ankle plantarflexor muscles, it is usually necessary to have the patient standing unilaterally with the weight on the ball of the foot to perform this test. In a patient with Achilles tendinopathy, this test will reproduce a patient's symptoms and may reveal weakness of the ankle plantarflexor muscles of the affected side(s) (Silbernagel et al. 2006).

Special diagnostic tests for Achilles tendinopathy have been described, including the Arc sign test (Williams 1993). The Arc sign test is used to help distinguish between Achilles tendinopathy and paratendinopathy. The patient is asked to dorsiflex and plantarflex the ankle. In Achilles tendinopathy, the area of thickening in the Achilles tendon (determined by palpation) moves with dorsiflexion and plantarflexion of the ankle; in paratendinopathy, the area of thickening does not move with movement of the ankle. When Achilles tendinopathy and paratendinopathy coexist, the area of thickening doubles up, and part of it moves with dorsiflexion and plantarflexion of the ankle while part of the swelling remains fixed (Maffulli et al. 2003; Williams 1993).

There is limited research investigating the reliability and accuracy of clinical diagnostic assessments for Achilles tendinopathy. Silbernagel et al. (2001, 2006) reported that the assessments of the severity of pain [measured using a visual analogue scale (VAS)] with palpation of the mid-portion of the Achilles tendon and during hopping were reliable indicators of Achilles tendinopathy. In another study (Maffulli et al. 2003), the reliability and accuracy of the (i) presence of pain with palpation, and the (ii) Arc sign test were evaluated using orthopaedic surgeons as raters and histology and sonography as the gold standard. Inter-tester reliability was acceptable for both tests, but best for pain on palpation (kappa range 0.72 to 0.86). Both tests displayed equivalent diagnostic accuracy; they displayed poor sensitivity (range=0.53 to 0.58), but high specificity (range=0.83 to 0.85). These findings suggest that if either of these features is present then the diagnosis of Achilles tendinopathy is highly likely. However, the absence of these features in a person presenting with pain within the Achilles tendon does not exclude the diagnosis of Achilles tendinopathy and further assessments may be required. Given that the assessment of pain with palpation demonstrates relative ease of administration, superior reliability, yet equivalent diagnostic accuracy compared with the Arc sign test, this assessment would appear most valid for diagnosing Achilles tendinopathy at present.

In conclusion, a patient with Achilles tendinopathy will present with symptoms of pain within the Achilles tendon localized in the region 2 to 6 cm proximal to the calcaneal insertion. Hopping and resisted isometric testing of the ankle joint plantarflexors will reproduce symptoms. However, there will be no symptoms with passive movement testing of the surrounding joints. A key assessment result is pain with Achilles tendon palpation occurring 2 to 6 cm proximal to the calcaneal insertion.

DIAGNOSTIC IMAGING

The role of diagnostic imaging in clinical practice is primarily to assist with diagnosis when clinical assessment is inconclusive, but it may also be used to help predict and monitor clinical progress (Khan et al. 2003). Musculoskeletal ultrasound (MSUS) and magnetic resonance imaging (MRI) are the imaging modalities of choice for soft-tissue disorders such as Achilles tendon pathology owing to their ability to help differentiate between the various pathologies that may occur within the Achilles tendon and peritendinous tissues. Radiography is used to assess for associated bone abnormalities or exclude these as a source of symptoms (Kader et al. 2002).

Diagnostic Musculoskeletal Ultrasound

Diagnostic MSUS is a convenient, safe, and cost-effective imaging modality for assessment of Achilles tendon pathology. MSUS also allows for functional assessments, and the addition of colour or power Doppler allows for the examination of blood flow within tendons (neovascularization), which is considered a pathognomonic feature of this disorder (Leung and Griffith 2008).

There are several sonographic features that characterize Achilles tendinopathy (Leung and Griffith

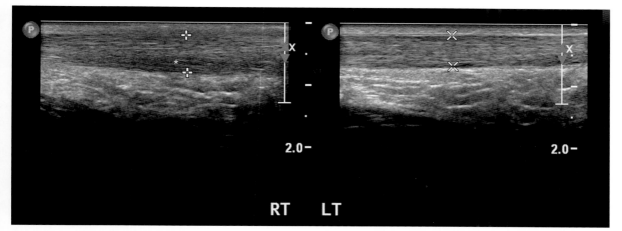

FIGURE 6-1 Musculoskeletal ultrasound of Achilles tendinopathy. Greyscale longitudinal scan of the mid-portion of the Achilles tendon. (Left) Achilles tendinopathy of the right leg showing an increase in tendon thickness, and disruption of the fibrillar pattern of the tendon (hypoechogenicity) (denoted by *). (Right) Normal Achilles tendon of contralateral leg. The letter 'P' on the left side of each image highlights the proximal aspect of the image. Thickness of the Achilles tendons was measured using electronic calipers: 59 mm for Achilles tendinopathy (calipers denoted by +) and 48 mm for the normal contralateral side (calipers denoted by x).

2008). Achilles tendinopathy is associated with an increase in tendon thickness, discrete or generalized disruption of the fibrillar pattern of tendon (hypo-echogenicity), an increase in tendon vascularity, increased Kager's fat pad echogenicity, and paratenon thickening (Leung and Griffith 2008) (Figure 6-1). A study of participants with and without Achilles tendinopathy showed that (i) the mean antero-posterior thickness of the Achilles tendon was significantly greater in those with Achilles tendinopathy [mean (SD) thickness at the mid-portion=0.56 (0.11) versus 0.44 (0.06) cm, $p<0.01$], and that (ii) the most common sonographic features observed in those with Achilles tendinopathy were the presence of focal hypoechoic areas (67%), followed by neovascularization (47%), abnormal Kager's fat pad echogenicity (27%), and diffuse disruption of the fibrillar pattern within the Achilles tendon (20%). Although the presence of fluid with the retrocalcaneal bursa and calcaneal cortical abnormalities were commonly observed in those with Achilles tendinopathy, they were observed just as frequently in asymptomatic controls.

Magnetic Resonance Imaging

MRI is not used as readily as MSUS for the assessment of Achilles tendon pathology owing to its relative expense and inaccessibility. However, a relative advantage of MRI is that its superior detailed images may allow the distinction between various structural abnormalities that may be the cause of symptoms in a patient with complex rearfoot pain. The normal Achilles tendon is normally dark on all MRI sequences. On sagittal sequences, its anterior and posterior margins are parallel and on axial images; its anterior edge is concave for most of its course (Schweitzer and Karasick 2000). In Achilles tendinopathy, the characteristic MRI features are: (i) thickening of the tendon in the antero-posterior diameter causing disruption of the parallel relationship of the anterior and posterior margins, (ii) intratendinous lesions seen as focal or diffuse intermediate or high signal, and (iii) changes within peritendinous tissues. This includes variable paratenon thickening and increased signal around the tendon, as well as increased signal within the Kager's fat pad (Karjalainen et al. 2000; Schweitzer and Karasick 2000).

MRI and MSUS share similar diagnostic accuracy. Both modalities are highly sensitive (sensitivity=80 to 95%) for the detection of Achilles tendon degeneration and symptoms (Karjalainen et al. 2000; Khan et al. 2003). However, tendon degeneration can occur in asymptomatic individuals (Leung and Griffith 2008) and so these modalities lack specificity (50%)

(Khan et al. 2003). Further, MSUS is highly operator-dependent and its ability to differentiate focal degeneration from partial ruptures has been questioned (Kayser et al. 2005). Therefore, the use of imaging for Achilles tendon disorders may complement, but should not replace, a thorough clinical examination with sound clinical judgement.

IMPAIRMENTS

Patients with Achilles tendinopathy may demonstrate deficits in the function of the calf muscle–tendon unit (Carcia et al. 2010). The definition of 'function deficit' is vague, but includes aspects related to flexibility of the plantarflexor muscles (reflected in dorsiflexion range of motion of the ankle), plantarflexor muscle strength, endurance, and the ability to utilize the stretch–shortening cycle (Silbernagel et al. 2007a). As a consequence of this potential spectrum of deficits, a number of tests to assess the various impairments associated with Achilles tendinopathy have been described, and will be reviewed below.

ANKLE JOINT DORSIFLEXION RANGE OF MOTION AND MUSCLE STRENGTH

Clinical guidelines recommend assessing the dorsiflexion range of motion of the ankle joint, as well as the strength and endurance of the ankle joint plantarflexor muscles as part of the examination in Achilles tendinopathy (Carcia et al. 2010). Individuals with Achilles tendinopathy may display reductions in the range of ankle joint dorsiflexion range of motion, or strength and/or endurance of the ankle joint plantarflexor muscles compared with the unaffected (or less affected) side (Carcia et al. 2010).

Ankle Joint Dorsiflexion Range of Motion

Ankle joint dorsiflexion range of motion can be measured with patients positioned in a non-weightbearing position using goniometry, or in a weightbearing position (lunge test) (Gatt and Chockalingam 2011). For both approaches, the assessment can be performed with the knee extended (indicative of gastrocnemius flexibility) and flexed approximately 45° (indicative of soleus flexibility). The weightbearing approach is preferred owing to its superior reliability (Bennell et al. 1998; Munteanu et al. 2009). For the extended-knee

lunge test, the patient is instructed to place both hands on a wall in front of them. The ipsilateral leg to be tested is then positioned behind the contralateral leg as far as possible while ensuring the ipsilateral knee is fully extended. The ipsilateral foot is positioned perpendicular to the wall, in order to attempt to reduce the subtalar joint from pronating during the measurement procedure and therefore falsely elevating the value of ankle joint dorsiflexion. The patient then leans forward until maximum stretch is felt in the ipsilateral posterior leg, while keeping the ipsilateral knee fully extended and the heel in contact with the ground. An inclinometer is then positioned on the midpoint of the anterior tibial border, between the tibial tuberosity and the anterior joint line of the ankle, and the angle the ipsilateral tibia makes to the vertical is then measured (Munteanu et al. 2009). The process is then completed on the contralateral side for comparison.

For the bent-knee lunge test, a similar approach is used. The patient stands in front of a wall, positions the foot perpendicular to the wall and lunges the knee towards the wall (keeping the heel on the ground). The foot is progressively moved away from the wall until the maximum range of ankle joint dorsiflexion is reached without the heel lifting from the ground. An inclinometer is then positioned on the midpoint of the anterior tibial border and the angle the tibia makes to the vertical is then measured (Bennell et al. 1998). Based on analyses of small samples of young asymptomatic adults, the normal values (mean±SD) for the lunge test have been reported to be approximately 35±4° for the straight-leg test (Munteanu et al. 2009), and 51±8° for the bent-knee test (Bennell et al. 1998)

Although the assessment of ankle joint dorsiflexion range of motion is recommended in clinical guidelines (Carcia et al. 2010), the validity of this recommendation can be questioned (Child et al. 2010; Silbernagel et al. 2006). Silbernagel et al. (2006) showed no significant difference in ankle joint dorsiflexion range of motion between the symptomatic and asymptomatic legs of participants with unilateral Achilles tendinopathy [mean (SD) dorsiflexion with knee straight= 34.5° (5) versus 33.7° (5), $p=0.055$]. Supporting this, a recent case–control study of 50 male participants reported that those with Achilles tendinopathy did not demonstrate significantly reduced ankle joint dorsiflexion (Child et al. 2010).

Strength and Endurance of the Ankle Joint Plantarflexor Muscles

Muscle testing through the use of isokinetic dynamometry is considered to be the gold standard approach for the assessment of muscle strength. This approach can be performed to assess the strength of the ankle joint plantarflexor muscles with the knee extended (to isolate gastrocnemius) and flexed (to isolate soleus) (Möller et al. 2005). Patients with Achilles tendinopathy have been shown to display deficits in the strength of their ankle plantarflexor muscles (Alfredson et al. 1998). As most clinics would not have an isokinetic dynamometer, more simple quantitative clinical tests of muscle strength, such as hand-held dynamometry, can be used (Burns et al. 2005; Spink et al. 2010). However, the reliability and validity of this assessment approach in patients with Achilles tendinopathy needs to be determined.

The standing unilateral heel-raise test is reliable and can be performed to determine the endurance of the ankle joint plantarflexor muscles (Silbernagel et al. 2001, 2006). With this test, the patient stands unilaterally facing a wall or beside a table and is allowed to use the fingertips placed on the wall or table for balance. Patients perform unilateral heel raises through the full range of motion with their knee extended. Heel-rises are performed at a rate of one heel-rise every 2 seconds. The test is terminated if the patient leans forward, the ipsilateral knee flexes, or cannot complete a full heel-raise owing to fatigue or pain. At this point, the number of heel-rise repetitions that were performed is documented (Madeley et al. 2007). The process is then completed on the contralateral side for comparison. Despite its simplicity and reliability (Madeley et al. 2007), the validity of this test for Achilles tendinopathy is currently not known and requires further study.

PHYSICAL PERFORMANCE MEASUREMENTS

A battery of measurements to assess the functional capacity of patients with Achilles tendinopathy have been described (Silbernagel et al. 2001, 2006). These measurements include maximum jump height during a one-legged counter-movement jump, one-legged hopping (hopping frequency, hopping height, and flight time/contact time), one-legged drop jump followed by a vertical jump (maximum jump height and contact time), concentric toe-raises (maximum power), and eccentric–concentric toe-raises (maximum power). A patient's level of pain during each of the tests can also be determined using a VAS.

Silbernagel et al. (2001, 2006) have shown that the tests demonstrate fair to excellent reliability (correlation coefficient = 0.61 to 0.93 or Pearson's r = 0.56 to 0.93). They have also shown that patients with Achilles tendinopathy demonstrate deficits in their ability to perform these tests and report more pain than do asymptomatic controls during these tests (Silbernagel et al. 2006). However, one limitation of these tests is that they require the use of sophisticated laboratory equipment so their use in most clinical settings is not practical. Further study is required to develop less-complicated functional tests.

PATIENT-REPORTED OUTCOME MEASUREMENTS

Patient-reported outcome measurements are considered a fundamental measure of the impact of a disease or abnormality on an individual (Landorf and Burns 2008). The clinical severity of Achilles tendinopathy can be determined using the Victorian Institute of Sport Assessment – Achilles (VISA-A) questionnaire (Figure 6-2) (Robinson et al. 2001). The VISA-A questionnaire has been validated (construct validity), and shows good test–retest reliability (Robinson et al. 2001). Other strengths of the VISA-A questionnaire are that it can be self-administered, takes less than 5 minutes to complete, and is sensitive to small changes occurring over a medium duration of time (recommended administration no less than monthly intervals) (Alfredson et al. 2012).

The VISA-A questionnaire contains eight questions that cover three domains of pain (questions one to three), function (questions four to six), and activity (questions seven and eight). Questions one to seven are scored out of 10, and question eight has a maximum score of 30. Scores are summated to give a total score out of 100, and lower scores indicate more severe Achilles tendinopathy. Therefore, theoretically an asymptomatic person would score 100 (Robinson et al. 2001). Previous work has shown that the typical scores for asymptomatic individuals lie between 94

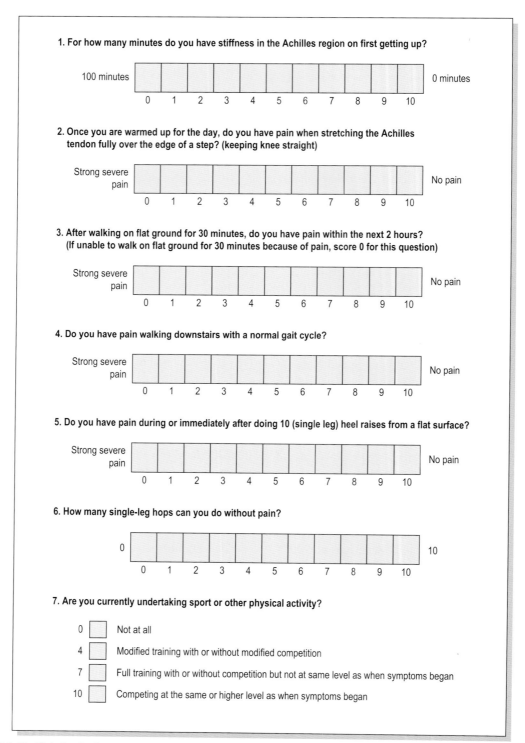

FIGURE 6-2 The Victorian Institute of Sport Assessment – Achilles (VISA-A) questionnaire. (Reproduced from The VISA-A questionnaire: a valid and reliable index of the clinical severity of Achilles tendinopathy, J M Robinson, J L Cook, C Purdam, P J Visentini, J Ross, N Maffulli, J E Taunton, K M Khan, 35(5): 335–341, copyright 2001 with permission from BMJ Publishing Group Ltd.)

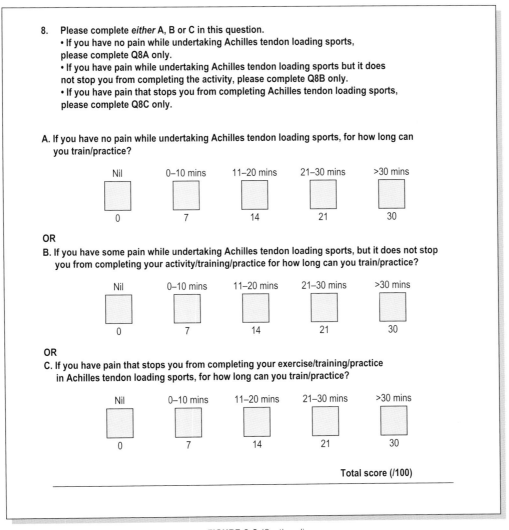

8. Please complete *either* A, B or C in this question.
 • If you have no pain while undertaking Achilles tendon loading sports,
 please complete Q8A only.
 • If you have pain while undertaking Achilles tendon loading sports but it does
 not stop you from completing the activity, please complete Q8B only.
 • If you have pain that stops you from completing Achilles tendon loading sports,
 please complete Q8C only.

A. If you have no pain while undertaking Achilles tendon loading sports, for how long can
 you train/practice?

Nil	0–10 mins	11–20 mins	21–30 mins	>30 mins
0	7	14	21	30

OR

B. If you have some pain while undertaking Achilles tendon loading sports, but it does not stop
 you from completing your activity/training/practice for how long can you train/practice?

Nil	0–10 mins	11–20 mins	21–30 mins	>30 mins
0	7	14	21	30

OR

C. If you have pain that stops you from completing your exercise/training/practice
 in Achilles tendon loading sports, for how long can you train/practice?

Nil	0–10 mins	11–20 mins	21–30 mins	>30 mins
0	7	14	21	30

Total score (/100)

FIGURE 6-2 (Continued)

and 99 (mean=97), whereas scores from patients with Achilles tendinopathy lie between 28 and 69 (mean=54) (Robinson et al. 2001).

One limitation of the VISA-A questionnaire relates to question eight. This question pertains to patients that participate in 'sports', and so cannot be used in sedentary patients. The developers of the VISA-A questionnaire recommend omitting this question and having a maximum score of 70 (Robinson et al. 2001).

Alternatively, this issue may be overcome by replacing the words 'sports' with 'physical activities', and 'train/practice' with 'perform that activity' which avoids changing the maximum possible score. Another limitation of the VISA-A questionnaire is that the minimally important change has not been determined. However, a recent high-quality clinical trial argued that a difference of 12 points is a reasonable estimate (de Vos et al. 2010).

PREDISPOSING FACTORS

The aetiological factors for Achilles tendinopathy are not completely known, mainly because there have been few well-designed prospective cohort studies to identify risk factors for this disorder. Achilles tendinopathy is considered to have a multifactorial aetiology. It is generally agreed that Achilles tendon injury occurs when loading of the Achilles tendon exceeds the ability of the tendon to tolerate the load such as a rapid increase in physical activity, lack of conditioning, and/or reduction in recovery time between bouts of exercise (Alfredson et al. 2012). The presence of both extrinsic and intrinsic risk factors is thought to modulate the susceptibility of a person to develop the condition (Carcia et al. 2010; Clement et al. 1984; Maffulli and Kader 2002). Extrinsic risk factors are defined as those factors external to the body and include inappropriate footwear, type of weightbearing surface, type of activity, and medications. Intrinsic risk factors are factors within the body and include age and sex, co-morbidity, previous injury, pre-existing tendon abnormalities, abnormal lower limb biomechanics, muscle weakness, altered ankle joint dorsiflexion range of motion, as well as genetics (Murphy et al. 2003). Each of these proposed risk factors will be reviewed below.

EXTRINSIC RISK FACTORS

Inappropriate Footwear and Type of Weightbearing Surface

Inappropriate footwear and altered weightbearing surfaces (excessively hard, slippery or uneven) are considered to act as risk factors for Achilles tendinopathy by increasing the tensile load within the Achilles tendon (Clement et al. 1984; Kvist 1994). Two case series studies have attempted to identify the role of footwear or weightbearing surfaces in the development of Achilles tendinopathy (Clement et al. 1984; Longo et al. 2009). Clement et al. reported that 'ineffective footwear' was present in 11 of 109 (10%) cases of Achilles tendinopathy, and 'hill training' was associated with the condition in four cases (4%); from these observations, they proposed footwear with 'inappropriate wedging in the heel' and uphill running act as risk factors for Achilles tendinopathy by demanding increased 'flexibility and force' within the Achilles

tendon. In the second study, Knobloch et al. (2008) conducted a survey of middle-aged elite running athletes; in this study, Achilles tendinopathy was associated with a preference for running surface: asphalt was associated with a reduced relative risk [relative risk (RR)=0.5, 95% CI 0.3 to 0.9], whereas sand was associated with increased risk (RR=10.0, 95% CI 1.1 to 92.8) of Achilles tendon injury.

Type of Activity

Achilles tendon injuries are commonly reported in athletes involved in running and jumping (sports involving the stretch–shorten cycle) suggesting that the type of activity may influence the risk for developing Achilles tendinopathy (Kujala et al. 2005; Kvist 1994). Supporting these findings, a case–control study by Kujala et al. (2005) of male elite ex-athletes and non-athletic controls reported that the cumulative incidence of Achilles tendinopathy before the age of 45 was high for middle- and long-distance runners [42% versus 3%; age- and occupational-group-adjusted odds ratio (OR)=31.2, 95% CI 13.5 to 71.8]. However, a case–control study (Longo et al. 2009) of 178 Masters track and field athletes showed no difference in the prevalence of Achilles tendinopathy between athletes involved in high- and low-impact sport, which challenges this assumption. As tendons show different physical and physiological characteristics as a function of their age and conditioning (Longo et al. 2009), differences in results between these studies could be explained by differences in the age, presence of co-morbidities and/or conditioning of participants.

Medications

The fluoroquinolone class of antibiotics (e.g. ciprofloxacin, levofloxacin, and moxifloxacin) are used widely to treat infection but have been commonly recognized as a cause of tendon injuries including Achilles tendinopathy and rupture, usually during the first weeks of treatment (Khaliq and Zhanel 2003). The mechanism(s) by which fluoroquinolone antibiotics may cause tendon injuries are not completely understood, but speculated mechanisms include ischaemic vascular processes, collagen toxicity leading to necrosis, altered tenocyte viability, altered synthesis of tendon extracellular matrix, and inflammatory-mediated actions within the paratenon (Khaliq and Zhanel 2003).

Numerous case reports have reported fluoroquinolone antibiotic-associated Achilles tendinopathy (Khaliq and Zhanel 2003). The strongest evidence of the association between fluoroquinolone antibiotics and Achilles tendon disorders comes from two large population-based studies by Corrao et al. (2006) and van der Linden et al. (2002). Corrao et al. (2006) showed that current use of fluoroquinolone antibiotics significantly increased the risk of tendon disorders as a whole (OR=1.7, 95% CI 1.4 to 2.0), tendon rupture (OR=1.3, 95% CI 1.0 to 1.8) and rupture of the Achilles tendon (OR=4.1, 95% CI 1.8 to 9.6). Van der Linden et al. (2002) stratified risk by age using 60 years as a cut-off and showed that current use of fluoroquinolone antibiotics was associated with an increased risk of Achilles tendinopathy only in people aged older than 60 years (adjusted RR=3.1, 95% CI 2.1 to 4.9). Individuals with concomitant use of systemic corticosteroid therapy, renal failure, diabetes mellitus, rheumatic disease, hyperparathyroidism, gout, and those that participate in sports appear to be at an increased risk of fluoroquinolone antibiotic-associated tendon disorders (Corrao et al. 2006; Khaliq and Zhanel 2003; van der Linden et al. 2002).

The effect of female sex hormones on tendon health has also received interest. Experimental work showing that oestrogen reduces synthesis of collagen by fibroblasts and also directly affects the tensile properties of connective tissues has led to the theory that sex hormone medication may increase the risk of Achilles tendon disorders (Bryant et al. 2008; Lee et al. 2004). This finding has been supported by one case–control study of 82 patients aged 50 to 74 years with Achilles tendinopathy (Holmes and Lin 2006). In this study, there was a significant association between the use of hormone replacement therapy and oral contraceptives with Achilles tendinopathy (Holmes and Lin 2006); however, these analyses were unadjusted for co-variates such as co-morbidity and should therefore be interpreted with caution. Future prospective studies are required to determine more clearly the role of sex hormones such as oestrogen in the development of Achilles tendinopathy.

INTRINSIC RISK FACTORS

Age and Sex

Achilles tendinopathy is more common in middle-aged individuals (de Jonge et al. 2011; Taunton et al. 2002). Males have commonly been reported to be more likely to develop Achilles tendinopathy, but this has not been proven through prospective studies. Case series of athletes (Kvist 1994; Taunton et al. 2002) suggest that males account for between 58 to 89% of cases. These findings are supported by a large community-based survey of 6315 people (Hootman et al. 2002) showing that Achilles tendon injuries made up 5.7% of all activity-related musculoskeletal injuries in males compared with 0.4% in females. In contrast, a recent population-based study of 57 725 persons visiting their general practitioner showed that the relationship between sex and Achilles tendinopathy was more complex. In this study, the incidence of Achilles tendinopathy was greater in males between the ages of 41 and 60 years only. For the age stratifications of 21 to 40 years, and greater than 61 years, females were more likely to present with the condition (de Jonge et al. 2011). Together, these findings suggest that Achilles tendinopathy is associated with male sex in physically active populations but not in sedentary populations where the involvement of other factors including co-morbidities and hormonal status may play a greater effect.

Co-morbidity

Achilles tendinopathy is associated with obesity, hypertension, hypercholesteraemia, dyslipidaemia, and diabetes in general patient populations (de Jonge et al. 2011; Gaida et al. 2009a; Holmes and Lin 2006), but not in young physically active people (Mahieu et al. 2006). The observed association of lower limb musculoskeletal problems with obesity has historically been attributed to increased loading of these structures. However, recent theories suggest that this may be an oversimplification (Gaida et al. 2009b; Pottie et al. 2006). Systemic metabolic alterations associated with obesity such as dyslipidaemia, hypertension, and insulin resistance, collectively termed 'metabolic syndrome', have been theorized to result in tendon disorders by promoting a systemic chronic low-grade microvascular inflammation (Gaida et al. 2009). Alternatively, the release of cytokines from adipose tissue may directly influence tendon metabolism or response to injury (Gaida et al. 2009). These mechanisms help to explain the prevalence of Achilles tendinopathy in sedentary populations. Patients with systemic inflammatory arthritis are also at an increased risk of Achilles tendon disorders, but the pathology is usually located at the insertion of the Achilles tendon (Moll 1987).

Previous Injury

There is strong evidence from prospective cohort studies that previous injury increases the risk of re-injury to the same location as well as other locations, especially when there has been inadequate rehabilitation (Murphy et al. 2003). This has been attributed to a range of possible factors including proprioceptive deficits, muscle strength and flexibility impairments, ligamentous laxity, and the presence of localized scar tissue. Further, the fear of movement following an injury may play a role by causing altered muscle recruitment strategies (Murphy et al. 2003).

Although previous injury is commonly cited as a risk factor for Achilles tendinopathy, there is limited research (case series studies) investigating the role of this factor for the development of this disorder. Clement et al. (1984) assessed the frequency of previous injury in 109 athletes with Achilles tendinopathy, and observed 'that patients who begin to increase their training levels as soon as they become asymptomatic often experience a total relapse of symptoms' (Clement et al. 1984). In a more recent study (Fredberg et al. 2008) of elite Danish soccer players, 44% of those with Achilles tendon disorders reported a previous history of this complaint.

Pre-existing Tendon Abnormalities

Musculoskeletal ultrasound is a non-invasive, inexpensive and reliable modality commonly used to assess the morphology of tendons. Although it is common for asymptomatic Achilles tendons to show sonographic abnormalities such as focal hypoechoicity (Gibbon et al. 1999; Leung and Griffith 2008), the presence of sonographic tendon abnormalities has been shown to increase the risk of developing tendon pain. Two studies (Fredberg and Bolvig 2002; Fredberg et al. 2008) conducted using elite Danish soccer players have shown that the presence of Achilles tendon sonographic abnormalities (defined as tendon thickening greater than 1 mm or the presence of focal hypoechoicity) during pre-season screening increased the risk of developing Achilles tendon pain during the season (RR=2.8, 95% CI 1.6 to 4.9).

Abnormal Lower Limb Biomechanics

Alterations in lower limb biomechanics, including temporo-spatial parameters, kinematics, dynamic plantar pressures, kinetics (ground reaction forces and joint moments), and muscle activity, are frequently speculated to be important causes of Achilles tendinopathy, although evidence to support their influence is mixed (Kvist 1994; Maffulli and Kader 2002; Rees et al. 2006). One of the most commonly cited biomechanical risk factors for Achilles tendinopathy is the presence of excessive foot pronation (Maffulli and Kader 2002), based on the case series study by Clement et al. (1984), who showed that 61 of the 109 (56%) runners with Achilles tendinopathy demonstrated 'functional overpronation'. Excessive pronation of the foot has been postulate to lead to Achilles tendinopathy through two mechanisms. First, excessive pronation of the foot is speculated to create greater hindfoot eversion motion, resulting in excessive tensile forces on the medial aspect of the tendon and subsequent microtears. Secondly, abnormal pronation of the foot is thought to lead to asynchronous movement between the foot and ankle during the stance phase of gait, resulting in a subsequent 'wringing' effect within the Achilles tendon. This 'wringing' effect is theorized to cause vascular impairment within the tendon and paratenon (Clement et al. 1984) and elevated tensile stress (Williams et al. 2008), leading to subsequent degenerative changes in the Achilles tendon.

However, a recent systematic review of biomechanical risk factors for Achilles tendinopathy questioned this concept (Munteanu and Barton 2011). Although two separate case–control studies (Donoghue et al. 2008b; Ryan et al. 2009) showed greater dynamic eversion range of motion of the ankle in those with Achilles tendinopathy, a large number of other frontal plane rearfoot kinematic variables, which included maximum eversion/pronation, were no different between those with and those without pathology (Munteanu and Barton 2011). Further, two case–control studies (Ryan et al. 2009) showed no differences in transverse plane kinematics of the tibia at the ankle and knee joints in those with and those without Achilles tendinopathy, challenging the theory that torsional stress or 'wringing' of the Achilles tendon was a cause of Achilles tendinopathy (Munteanu and Barton 2011).

The use of dynamic plantar pressure assessment provides an alternative technique to assess foot function. The relationship between abnormal foot biomechanics and Achilles tendinopathy has been investigated in three studies (Baur et al. 2004; Kaufman et al. 1999; Van Ginckel et al. 2008), two of which were of a prospective study design (Kaufman et al. 1999; Van Ginckel et al. 2008). These studies showed that those with Achilles tendinopathy demonstrated a significantly more laterally directed force distribution beneath the forefoot at forefoot flat (Van Ginckel et al. 2008), a significantly more medially directed force distribution during mid-stance (Baur et al. 2004; Van Ginckel et al. 2008), and a significantly reduced total forward progression of the centre of force beneath the foot (Van Ginckel et al. 2008). These findings have been hypothesized to cause the development of Achilles tendinopathy as follows. First, the lateral foot rollover pattern during the contact period of gait in those with Achilles tendinopathy may create diminished shock absorption and exert more stress on the lateral side of the Achilles tendon. Secondly, the more medially directed force distribution during mid-stance phase might represent increased midfoot pronation, unlocking the midtarsal joint. This would increase forefoot mobility and impede the ability of the foot to act as a rigid lever during propulsion. Therefore, higher active tensile forces may need to be transferred through the Achilles tendon to facilitate propulsion, leading to tendon strain and degeneration (Van Ginckel et al. 2008).

In addition to kinematic theories, altered lower limb muscle function (timing, amplitude, or coordination of contractions) has been speculated to be a risk factor for Achilles tendinopathy by increasing tendon loading (Arndt et al. 1998; McCrory et al. 1999; Rees et al. 2006; Williams et al. 2008). Three case–control studies (Azevedo et al. 2009; Baur et al. 2004, 2011) have used electromyography to evaluate the function of a number of lower limb muscles in those with and without Achilles tendinopathy.

Although there were a number of differences in lower limb muscle function between those with and those without pathology, many differences were equivocal. Making inferences concerning the function of lower limb muscles in those with Achilles tendinopathy is therefore difficult. Further, because of the cross-sectional study design used in these studies, it is difficult to determine whether these differences are a cause or an effect of the disorder.

Taken together, the evidence suggests that there are differences in lower limb biomechanics between those with and those without Achilles tendinopathy. However, the findings need to be interpreted with caution owing to the limited quality of some of the included studies, many of which were of a case–control design. Future well-designed prospective studies are required to shed further light on the relationship between lower limb biomechanics and Achilles tendinopathy.

Ankle Joint Dorsiflexion Range of Motion

Limited ankle joint dorsiflexion has been proposed as a cause of Achilles tendinopathy by increasing tensile stress within the Achilles tendon during functional activities such as walking, running, and jumping (Clement et al. 1984). Two prospective studies using military recruits as participants have investigated this, with conflicting findings (Kaufman et al. 1999). Kaufman et al. (1999) showed that participants with limited ankle joint dorsiflexion (defined as less than 11.5° of dorsiflexion measured non-weightbearing with the knee extended) were almost four times more likely to develop 'Achilles tendinitis' during a 25-week training course (RR=3.6, 95% CI=1.0 to 12.7). However, Mahieu et al. (2006) followed 69 cadets during 6 weeks of training and reported opposing results. The authors performed logistic regression analysis to control for confounding factors, and their results showed that increased ankle joint dorsiflexion range of motion (assessed non-weightbearing with the knee extended) was independently associated with the development of Achilles tendinopathy. For every 1° increase in ankle joint dorsiflexion range of motion, there was a corresponding 23% increase (95% CI=3.3 to 46.5%) in the risk of developing Achilles tendinopathy. In both studies, limited ankle joint dorsiflexion with the knee flexed was not a risk factor, which suggests that flexibility of the gastrocnemius muscle was primarily associated with the altered risk for Achilles tendinopathy. Future studies using non-military populations are required to clarify the role of gastrocnemius tightness in the development of Achilles tendinopathy.

Muscle Weakness

Weakness of the plantarflexor muscles of the ankle joint has been speculated to be a cause of Achilles tendinopathy by limiting the ability of the Achilles muscle–tendon unit to absorb high forces associated with weightbearing activities, particularly during exercise (Maffulli and Kader 2002). This hypothesis has been supported by one prospective cohort study of male cadets undergoing a 6-week military training programme (Mahieu et al. 2006). In this study, isokinetic dorsiflexion and plantarflexion strength of the ankle joint muscles was assessed at 30°/s and 120°/s using a Cybex Norm dynamometer. Results showed that altered dorsiflexion strength of the ankle joint was not a risk factor for the development of 'Achilles tendon injury'. However, reduced plantarflexion strength (at 30°/s) of the ankle joint muscles was independently associated with the development of 'Achilles tendon injury'. The authors' statistical modelling indicated that, for every one unit decrease in plantarflexion strength of the ankle joint muscles, there was a corresponding 6% increase (95% CI = 1.3 to 10.5%) in the risk of a participant developing an 'Achilles tendon injury'. Further studies are required to identify whether simple clinical tests of ankle joint muscle strength can also predict the development of this disorder.

Genetics

Several recent studies suggest that there may be a genetic component to tendon injuries. Tendon is a connective tissue consisting of an extracellular matrix made up of different collagen types, proteoglycans, and glycoproteins. Genes encoding for proteins that are either directly or indirectly involved in the synthesis, structure, organization, or catabolism of tendon molecules may all be plausible candidates increasing the risk of developing Achilles tendinopathy. The contribution of genetics to Achilles tendon injuries is most probably the result of (i) complex interactions between a number of proteins encoded by different genes on different chromosomes, and (ii) the interactions of these genetic components with different environmental factors (September et al. 2006).

Since earlier work that showed an association between the ABO blood group (located on chromosome nine) and tendon injuries (September et al. 2006), there has been considerable investigation into the role that variation in genes located on chromosome nine play in the development of Achilles tendinopathy. There are several possible candidate genes for Achilles tendon injuries, which include genes that encode for tenascin-C (*TNC*), type V collagen (*COL5A1*), growth differentiation factor-5 (*GDF5*) and matrix metalloproteinase-3 (*MMP-3*). *TNC* encodes for tenascin-C, which is a glycoprotein located on the surface of collagen fibres within tissues subjected to high tensile forces such as tendons; it is involved in mediating cell–matrix interactions and has been speculated to be involved in mechanical properties of tendon (Järvinen et al. 2000). The *COL5A1* gene encodes type V collagen, which is a fibrillar collagen found in low amounts within tendon, and is involved in regulating assembly of the type I collagen fibres within the extracellular matrix (Birk et al. 1990). Polymorphisms (sequence variations in DNA nucleotides) within the *TNC* (chromosome 9q33) and *COL5A1* (chromosome 9q34.2-q34.3) genes have been shown to be associated with Achilles tendinopathy in active Caucasians (Mokone et al. 2005, 2006). More recent studies have analyzed genes located away from chromosome nine. In one study, individuals who carried a specific polymorphism of the *GDF5* gene (located on chromosome 20) were twice as likely to develop Achilles tendinopathy (OR = 1.8, 95% CI 1.2 to 2.7) (Posthumus et al. 2010), and another study showed that variations within the *MMP-3* gene (located on chromosome 11) was associated with the development of Achilles tendinopathy (OR = 4.9, 95% CI 1.0 to 24.1) (Raleigh et al. 2009).

These findings suggest that there may be a genetic contribution to the development of Achilles tendinopathy. In particular, variations in the *TNC*, *COL5A1*, *GDF5*, and/or *MMP-3* genes may be a risk factor(s) for Achilles tendinopathy. However, the findings from existing studies need to be replicated among larger prospective cohorts, and the exact role of the gene in the pathophysiology of this disorder needs to be elucidated (Gibson 2009). It is possible that other genes are also involved in the pathogenesis of Achilles tendinopathy. Much work is required in this exciting area of research.

MANAGEMENT STRATEGIES

The aims of management are to reduce a patient's symptoms, facilitate healing, promote return to functional activity, and prevent re-injury. Most cases of Achilles tendinopathy can be successfully managed using non-surgical approaches (Schepsis et al. 2002), particularly when treatment is initiated early in the disease (Kader et al. 2002). Although no evidence-based management algorithm for Achilles tendinopathy currently exists, it is generally recommended that a multifaceted treatment approach be used, which includes modification of activity, physical therapy, biomechanical correction, and/or pharmacological therapy (Kader et al. 2002; Schepsis et al. 2002). There is a plethora of research investigating the effectiveness of interventions for Achilles tendinopathy. The purpose of the following section is to review the evidence for the effectiveness of interventions that have commonly been recommended for this disorder, under the categories of lifestyle and education, physical, pharmacological, mechanical, electrotherapeutic, and surgical strategies. The focus will be on randomized controlled trials (RCTs) as such studies are generally considered most likely to provide unbiased estimates of the effects of an intervention.

LIFESTYLE AND EDUCATION STRATEGIES

Rest or modification of activities that provoke symptoms, usually running or jumping, should always be a part of the initial management of Achilles tendinopathy (Schepsis et al. 2002). This is particularly so when training errors have been identified as a likely risk factor. The decision to reduce or cease exercise needs to be individualized to the patient and based on the severity of symptoms. Schepsis et al. (2002) have recommended that, in mild cases of Achilles tendinopathy, patients should reduce exercise volume by at least 25%, then increase it gradually by 10% per week once symptoms are managed. Additionally, fast running, hill running, and hard surfaces should be avoided

during the initial management phases as these activities place an increased demand on the Achilles tendon (Schepsis et al. 2002). Alternative exercises such as cycling, water therapy, and aqua jogging have been recommended to maintain cardiovascular and musculoskeletal fitness during rehabilitation (Schepsis et al. 2002; Silbernagel et al. 2007).

It can often be difficult to advise patients with a sports injury to rest completely from physical activity as these patients are likely to be highly motivated to exercise. A prolonged period of rest or decrease in physical activity may have a negative effect on a patient's sporting performance and quality of life (Silbernagel et al. 2007). To overcome this problem, a pain-monitoring model has been developed (Thomeé 1997) and used as a guideline for the patient and clinician during treatment of Achilles tendinopathy (Silbernagel et al. 2007). This approach allows patients with Achilles tendinopathy to continue with some level of activity during rehabilitation and shows equivalent outcomes to programmes that involve complete rest from the aggravating activity with no negative effects (Silbernagel et al. 2007). Using this approach, patients are advised that they can continue their usual Achilles-loading activities. However, Achilles tendon pain should not be allowed to reach level 5 on a 10 cm VAS during the activity (where 0 is no pain and 10 is the worst pain imaginable). The pain after the activity can reach 5 on the VAS but should have subsided by the following morning. Pain and stiffness in the Achilles tendon should not increase from week to week.

PHYSICAL THERAPY STRATEGIES

Physical therapies are considered the principal management strategy for Achilles tendinopathy (Alfredson and Cook 2007; Sussmilch-Leitch et al. 2012). Physical therapy interventions for Achilles tendinopathy include eccentric calf muscle exercise, calf muscle stretching, and soft-tissue therapies (Carcia et al. 2010; Magnussen et al. 2009; Schepsis et al. 2002).

Eccentric Calf Muscle Exercise

Eccentric calf muscle exercise is considered the primary intervention in the management of Achilles tendinopathy (Alfredson and Cook 2007). The use of eccentric exercise as part of rehabilitation of tendon injuries was originally proposed in 1984 by Curwin

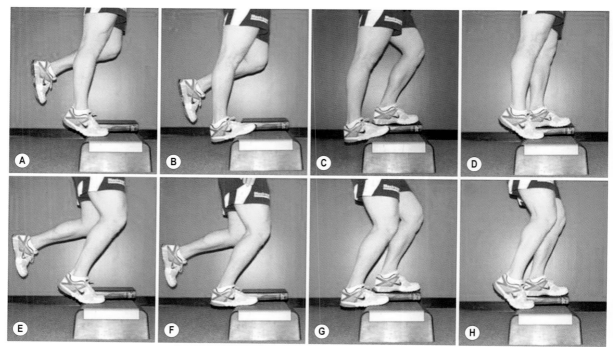

FIGURE 6-3 Alfredson protocol for eccentric calf muscle exercise. Figures A to D show the starting position (A), the lowered position (B), and the use of the contralateral leg to lift the patient back to the starting position for the straight-knee exercise (C and D). Figures E to H show the same technique, but for the bent-knee exercise. Note the use of a block to aid the contralateral leg in lifting the patient.

and Stanish, who showed the effectiveness of a 6-week programme of progressive tendon load (Alfredson et al. 2012). This programme was subsequently modified by Alfredson et al. (1998) for Achilles tendinopathy and is the most commonly used protocol today (Alfredson et al. 2012). The mechanism of action of eccentric muscle exercise has not been fully elucidated. However, this intervention has shown a number of theoretically beneficial effects to tendon, including improved peritendinous microcirculation (Knobloch et al. 2007) and peritendinous type I collagen synthesis (Langberg et al. 2007), as well as the normalization of tendon thickness, structure, and vascularity (Ohberg and Alfredson 2004; Ohberg et al. 2004).

Although variations to the eccentric calf muscle exercise protocol have been described (Meyer et al. 2009), the classic model proposed by Alfredson et al. (1998) is most commonly used and is as follows. Patients are instructed to perform their eccentric exercises twice daily, 7 days per week, for 12 weeks. The

patient stands with the affected foot over the edge of a step. Two types of eccentric exercises are used (Figure 6-3). The calf muscle is eccentrically loaded both with the knee straight (fully extended) and, to maximize the activation of the soleus muscle, also with the knee bent (flexed 45°). For the gastrocnemius drop, the patient begins in a demipointe position with the heel raised and the knee fully extended. From this position, the patient lowers the heel as low as possible. The contralateral leg is then used to lift the patient back to the starting position. The calf of the affected leg contracts eccentrically, no concentric loading is done. For the soleus drop, the patient also begins in a demipointe position with the heel raised, but with the knee flexed 45°. From this position, the patient lowers the heel as low as possible (and usually will be able to achieve the foot being parallel to the ground). Again, the non-injured contralateral leg is used to get back to the start position. In our experience, the use of a block (e.g. telephone book), placed on the step can be used to assist the contralateral leg in lifting the patient. This is especially so when patients have bilateral symptoms as it minimizes concentric contraction of the calf muscle of the contralateral leg.

Each of the two exercises involves 15 repetitions undertaken in three sets. Patients should be advised that muscle soreness during the training is to be expected and is part of the normal recovery process. Further, patients should continue with the exercise even if they experience pain; however, they should stop the exercise if the pain becomes disabling, and resume the following day (Alfredson et al. 2012). When patients can perform the eccentric calf muscle exercise without experiencing any minor pain or discomfort, they should increase the load by adding weight in 5-kg increments. This can be achieved by using a backpack that is successively loaded with weight. If very heavy weight is needed, patients should use a weight machine.

To improve patient compliance with the exercise programme, a detailed instruction sheet or video (see: http://www.youtube.com/watch?v=PwMebcSUdgw) can be provided to patients. Regular review appointments should be made to encourage compliance, monitor progress and ensure that correct technique is being used. A key review is 12 weeks after the eccentric calf muscle exercise programme has started. At this time point, if there has been a marked improvement in a patient's symptoms, a maintenance programme for 6 to 12 months should then be advised. The maintenance programme requires patients to perform the exercises once daily, 3 days per week for up to 9 months. If there has been minimal improvement in a patient's symptoms, then the exercise programme should be continued for a further 12 weeks and adjunctive treatments considered (Alfredson and Cook 2007).

Eccentric calf muscle exercise has been the most frequently investigated intervention for Achilles tendinopathy (Sussmilch-Leitch et al. 2012). Several RCTs have investigated the effectiveness of eccentric calf muscle exercise for Achilles tendinopathy, either as a primary intervention of interest, as a control, or as an adjunct (Sussmilch-Leitch et al. 2012). For a full description of all studies the reader is referred to the reviews by Magnussen et al. (2009) and Sussmilch-Leitch et al. (2012). Some of the key studies investigating eccentric exercise as the primary intervention for Achilles tendinopathy are described below and summarized in Table 6-1.

Eccentric calf muscle exercise has been shown to be superior to a wait-and-see approach or normal activity approach (Mayer et al. 2007; Rompe et al. 2007). Rompe et al. (2007) compared the effectiveness of an eccentric calf muscle exercise programme with a wait-and-see approach for chronic Achilles tendinopathy. In this study, the VISA-A score improved in both groups at 4 months, from 51 to 76 points in the eccentric muscle exercise group, and from 48 to 55 points in the wait-and-see group. Further, 15 of the 25 (60%) participants in the eccentric calf muscle exercise and 6 of 25 (24%) participants in the wait-and-see group reported that they were 'completely recovered' or 'much improved'. However, for all outcome measures, the eccentric calf muscle exercise group showed significantly better results than the wait-and-see group (VISA-A score between group mean difference $=20.6$, 95% CI$=12.3$ to 28.9).

Exercise programmes that consist primarily of eccentric calf muscle contractions have been shown to result in superior outcomes compared with programmes that are focused on concentric calf muscle contractions (Mafi et al. 2001; Niesen-Vertommen et al. 1992; Silbernagel et al. 2001). Mafi et al. (2001) compared the effectiveness of a 12-week eccentric calf muscle exercise programme with a concentric calf muscle exercise programme (both performed twice daily, 7 days per week) in participants with chronic Achilles tendinopathy. Results showed that 82% (18 out of 22) of the participants in the eccentric calf muscle exercise group were satisfied and had resumed activity at their previous level before injury, compared with 36% (8 out of 22) of the participants that were in the concentric calf muscle exercise group (RR success$=2.3$, 95% CI 1.3 to 4.0). In support of this, Niesen-Vertommen et al. (1992) reported a significantly ($p<0.01$) greater decrease in pain ratings at 4, 8, and 12 weeks by participants who performed eccentric-focused calf muscle exercise compared with those who performed concentric-focused calf muscle exercise. Further, the eccentric-focused calf muscle exercise training group produced three times as many pain-free participants at the end of the programme.

TABLE 6-1 **Summary of Major Findings from Clinical Trials Investigating Physical Therapies for Achilles Tendinopathy**

Intervention	Author(s)	Study Primary Intervention(s)	Study Comparator Intervention(s)	Major Finding(s)
Eccentric calf muscle exercise	Rompe et al. (2007)	Eccentric calf muscle exercise ($n=25$)	Wait-and-see approach ($n=25$)	VISA-A score significantly better in the eccentric calf muscle exercise group at 4 months (mean difference= 20.6, 95% CI=12.3 to 28.9)
	Mafi et al. (2001)	Eccentric calf muscle exercise ($n=22$)	Concentric calf muscle exercise ($n=22$)	Risk of satisfaction and resumption of activity to pre-injury levels greater in eccentric calf muscle exercise group at 12 weeks (82% versus 36%, RR=2.3, 95% CI 1.3 to 4.0)
	Niesen-Vertommen et al. (1992)	Eccentric-focused calf muscle exercise ($n=8$)	Concentric-focused calf muscle exercise ($n=9$)	Pain ratings reduced significantly more in the eccentric calf muscle exercise group over 4, 8, and 12 weeks ($p<0.01$)
Calf muscle stretching	Nørregaard et al. (2007)	Calf muscle stretching ($n=17$ at 12 weeks)	Eccentric calf muscle exercise ($n=13$ at 12 weeks)	No significant differences between groups for tenderness with tendon palpation, or symptoms at 3, 6, 9, 12 weeks and at 1 year
	Roos et al. (2004)	(i) Ankle joint dorsiflexion night splint ($n=13$) (ii) Ankle joint dorsiflexion night splint plus eccentric calf muscle exercise ($n=15$)	Eccentric calf muscle exercise programme ($n=16$)	No significant differences between groups for pain (Foot and Ankle Outcome Score pain domain) at 6, 12, 26, and 52 weeks
	De Vos et al. (2007); de Jonge et al. (2010)	Ankle joint dorsiflexion night splint plus eccentric calf muscle exercise ($n=31$ tendons)	Eccentric calf muscle exercise ($n=32$ tendons)	No significant differences in VISA-A score or satisfaction at 12 and 52 weeks
Soft-tissue therapy	Petersen et al. (2007)	(i) AirHeel™ brace alone ($n=35$) (ii) AirHeel™ brace plus eccentric calf muscle exercise ($n=28$)	Eccentric calf muscle exercise programme ($n=37$)	No significant differences between groups for pain (at rest and during activity), function, or health-related quality of life at 6, 12, and 52 weeks
	Knobloch et al. (2008a)	AirHeel™ brace plus eccentric calf muscle exercise ($n=43$)	Eccentric calf muscle exercise programme ($n=49$)	No significant differences between groups for pain, function or other symptoms at 12 weeks

Taken together, these findings suggest that eccentric calf muscle exercise is an effective intervention for Achilles tendinopathy. Eccentric calf muscle exercise gives excellent results in 37 to 90% of patients with Achilles tendinopathy, with a mean reduction in pain of approximately 60% (Kingma et al. 2007). Further, the intervention is inexpensive and can be performed at home by patients. Therefore, in the absence of contraindications, an eccentric calf muscle exercise programme performed twice daily, 7 days per week for

12 weeks, should be considered the primary intervention for Achilles tendinopathy.

Calf Muscle Stretching

Stretching of the gastrocnemius and soleus muscles has been advocated for Achilles tendinopathy, especially in patients who exhibit limited ankle joint dorsiflexion (Carcia et al. 2010; Schepsis et al. 2002). The rationale for the use of stretching as a treatment for this condition is to maintain normal range of motion of the ankle joint, to assist the tendon to regain flexibility, as well as facilitation of tendon healing through the application of controlled traction along normal lines of stress (Paoloni et al. 2004).

Manual Calf Muscle Stretching. One RCT has investigated the effectiveness of an isolated stretching programme as an intervention for Achilles tendinopathy (Nørregaard et al. 2007). In this study (Nørregaard et al. 2007), the effectiveness of a 12-week calf-muscle-stretching programme was compared with a 12-week eccentric calf muscle exercise programme in 45 participants with mid-portion and insertional Achilles tendinopathy. Participants in the calf-muscle-stretching group performed weightbearing soleus and gastrocnemius muscle stretching (five times for a period of 30 seconds for each muscle per session, two sessions per day), whilst participants in the eccentric calf muscle exercise group performed their exercises using the standard Alfredson et al. (1998) protocol. Several outcome measurements were performed and included tenderness with tendon palpation, a questionnaire on pain and other symptoms, as well as participants' global assessment of their improvement. Follow-up was performed at 3, 6, 9, 12 weeks and at 1 year. In both groups, symptoms were significantly improved at 3 weeks and all later time points. However, no significant differences could be observed between the two groups.

Although these results would suggest that a calf-muscle-stretching programme is equivalent to an eccentric exercise programme, the findings should be interpreted with caution. Participants with both insertional and mid-portion Achilles tendinopathy were included in this trial and the Alfredson et al. (1998) protocol of eccentric calf muscle exercise is less effective in those with insertional pathology (Fahlström et al.

2003). Further, it is currently unknown whether there is a differing effect of stretching between these two subpopulations. Further high-quality studies using well-defined participant populations (mid-portion versus insertional Achilles tendinopathy) are necessary to clarify this ambiguity.

Ankle Joint Dorsiflexion Night Splints. Ankle joint dorsiflexion night splints are typically worn at night during sleeping. The rationale for their use in Achilles tendinopathy is to initiate a prolonged stretch on the ankle plantarflexor muscles (de Vos et al. 2007; Paoloni et al. 2004).

Two RCTs, both with a 1-year follow-up, have investigated the effectiveness of ankle joint dorsiflexion night splints for Achilles tendinopathy (de Jonge S et al. 2010; de Vos et al. 2007; Roos et al. 2004). Roos et al. (2004) reported no statistically significant differences in the improvement in pain at 6, 12, 26, and 52 weeks between groups that received: (i) an eccentric calf muscle exercise programme, (ii) an ankle joint dorsiflexion night splint intervention, and (iii) a combined intervention of an eccentric calf muscle exercise programme with an ankle joint dorsiflexion night splint. Similarly, De Vos and colleagues (de Jonge et al. 2010; de Vos et al. 2007) showed that the addition of a dorsiflexion night splint to a 12-week eccentric calf muscle exercise programme did not result in an improved outcome (VISA-A score and satisfaction) at 12 or 52 weeks, despite the finding that compliance with the night splint was excellent or good in the majority (81%) of participants.

Together, these results indicate that a dorsiflexion night splint may be as effective as an eccentric calf muscle exercise programme in improving symptoms of Achilles tendinopathy, but combining an eccentric calf muscle exercise programme with an ankle joint dorsiflexion night splint is unlikely to result in synergistic effects.

Soft-Tissue Therapy

Soft-tissue therapy of the calf muscle and Achilles tendon has been advocated as a treatment for chronic Achilles tendinopathy (Hunter 2000). Chronic Achilles tendinopathy is frequently associated with paratendinopathy (Khan et al. 1999), and manual soft-tissue therapy, such as local massage and mobilization, is regarded as important to loosen adhesions in para-tendinopathy, and to remove metabolites and other waste products via the venous plexus of the paratenon (Knobloch et al. 2008b; Petersen et al. 2007). At present, however, the evidence investigating the effectiveness of manual soft-tissue therapy is limited to only a single case study (Christenson 2007).

An alternative option to manual soft-tissue therapy for Achilles tendinopathy is the AirHeel™ brace (Aircast, USA). The AirHeel™ brace is worn daily and has design features of two interconnected air cells located under the heel and above the calcaneus that apply pulsating compression with every step, with the aim of reducing swelling and enhancing circulation by a local massage effect. Petersen et al. (2007) examined the effectiveness of the AirHeel™ brace in 100 recreational athletes with Achilles tendinopathy who were randomized to three groups: (i) a 12-week eccentric calf muscle exercise programme, (ii) AirHeel™ brace alone, and (iii) a combination of an eccentric calf muscle exercise programme plus AirHeel™ brace. Results showed that pain and function (assessed using the AOFAS Score) improved in all three groups during the study (at 6, 12, and 52 weeks follow-up), and 90% of participants returned to their pre-injury activity level. However, there were no significant differences between groups. Similarly, Knobloch and colleagues (2008a) reported that the addition of the AirHeel™ brace to an eccentric calf muscle exercise programme did not result in better outcomes (pain assessed using a VAS, as well as the Foot and Ankle Outcome Score) relative to an eccentric calf muscle exercise programme alone at 12 weeks.

Taken together, results from these studies suggest that the AirHeel™ brace may be used as an alternative treatment to eccentric calf muscle exercise for Achilles tendinopathy, but there is no synergistic effect.

PHARMACOLOGICAL STRATEGIES
Non-steroidal Anti-inflammatory Drugs and Simple Analgesics

Non-steroidal anti-inflammatory drugs (NSAIDs) have been recommended for the management of soft-tissue injuries including Achilles tendinopathy (Clement et al. 1984; Mazzone and McCue 2002). However, given that Achilles tendinopathy is not an inflammatory

disorder, their use has been questioned (Khan et al. 2002). This has been supported by a small double-blind (participant and assessor) RCT involving 67 participants with mid-portion and insertional Achilles tendinopathy undergoing a stretching and strengthening programme, where there was no benefit of piroxicam (20 mg administered daily for 2 to 4 weeks) over placebo for pain, swelling, ankle joint range of motion, and calf muscle endurance measured across 4 weeks (Aström and Westlin 1992) (Table 6-2). Given the lack of effectiveness of NSAIDs for Achilles tendinopathy, and the increased risk of adverse drug effects from this class of medication (Næsdal and Brown 2006), simple analgesia (paracetamol) should be considered the first line of pain management for Achilles tendinopathy (Hunt et al. 2007).

Local Injection or Application of Corticosteroids

Corticosteroid injections have been used for many years for the treatment of chronic tendon disorders such as Achilles tendinopathy (Andres and Murrell 2008). Corticosteroids are potent anti-inflammatory agents, so the rationale for their use in the management of Achilles tendinopathy is questionable as the condition is primarily degenerative rather than inflammatory (Khan et al. 1999). However, it has been hypothesized that local application of corticosteroids, via injections or iontophoresis, may offer other potentially beneficial effects including lysis of any tendon–paratenon adhesions, alteration of the function of pain-generating nociceptors in the region, and/or normalization of tendon morphology (Cook and Purdam 2009; Fredberg et al. 2004; Magnussen et al. 2009). There is a question of safety with using these agents for this condition (Coombes et al. 2010). The most common adverse effect associated with corticosteroid injections is reversible subcutaneous atrophy (incidence of 9%) (Coombes et al. 2010). Rupture of the Achilles tendon is rare (incidence less than 1%), and its risk can be minimized by using sonographic guidance to inject the corticosteroid peritendinously, and not within the tendon substance (Andres and Murrell 2008; Coombes et al. 2010).

Two double-blind (participant and assessor) RCTs (DaCruz et al. 1988; Neeter et al. 2003) have evaluated the effectiveness of local corticosteroids for Achilles tendinopathy, with both studies suggesting that

TABLE 6-2 Summary of Major Findings from Clinical Trials Investigating Pharmacological Interventions for Achilles Tendinopathy

Intervention	Author(s)	Study Primary Intervention(s)	Study Comparator Intervention(s)	Major Finding(s)
NSAIDs	Aström and Westlin (1995)	Piroxicam (40 mg for 2 days, then 20 mg for a minimum of 2 weeks but maximum 4 weeks) plus physical therapy (strengthening and stretching) ($n=34$)	Placebo plus physical therapy (strengthening and stretching) ($n=33$)	No significant differences between groups for pain, swelling, ankle joint range of motion, and calf muscle endurance at 3, 7, 14, and 28 days
Local injection or application of corticosteroids	Da Cruz et al. (1988)	Single injection of 40 mg methyl prednisolone acetate in 1 mL 0.25% marcaine plus 4 weeks' physiotherapy ($n=19$ tendons)	Single 2 mL 0.25% marcaine injection plus 4 weeks' physiotherapy ($n=15$ tendons)	No significant differences between groups in pain or return to full function at 12 weeks
	Neeter et al. (2003)	Iontophoresis with 3 mL dexamethasone (four sessions over 2 weeks) plus progressive exercise programme for 10 weeks ($n=14$)	Iontophoresis with 3 mL saline (four sessions over 2 weeks) plus progressive exercise programme ($n=11$)	No significant differences between groups in pain or function at 2 or 6 weeks, and 3 and 12 months
Autologous growth factor injections	De Vos et al. (2010a)	Single PRP injection plus eccentric calf muscle exercise ($n=27$)	Single saline injection plus eccentric calf muscle exercise ($n=27$)	No significant differences between groups in VISA-A scores at 6, 12, or 24 weeks
Sclerosing agents	Alfredson and Öhberg (2005)	Up to two 5 mg/mL polidocanol injections ($n=10$)	Up to two 5 μg/mL lidocaine and epinephrine injections ($n=10$)	Mean improvement for pain during Achilles tendon loading activities significantly greater for the polidocanol group at 3 months (mean change in VAS=36 versus 2 mm, $p<0.005$)
Transdermal glyceryl trinitrate (GTN)	Paoloni et al. (2004)	Continuous GTN (1.25 mg/24 h) plus rehabilitation (relative rest, stretching, eccentric exercise, and heel raises) ($n=41$ tendons)	Placebo patch plus rehabilitation ($n=33$ tendons)	Significant reductions in: pain with activity in the GTN group at 12 weeks (mean VAS score=0.9 versus 1.6 cm; $p=0.02$), and at 24 weeks (mean VAS score= 0.4 versus 1.0 cm, $p=0.03$); pain after hopping (mean VAS score=0.5 versus 1.6 cm, $p<0.01$)
	Kane et al. (2008)	GTN (2.5 mg/24 h) plus eccentric calf muscle exercise ($n=20$)	Eccentric calf muscle exercise alone ($n=20$)	No significant differences between groups for pain or disability at 6 months

this intervention is not effective (see Table 6-2). In a study of 34 tendons (36 participants) by Da Cruz et al. (1988), a single peritendinous injection of 40 mg methylprednisolone acetate in 1 mL 0.25% marcaine (19 tendons) was no more effective than a 2 mL marcaine injection alone (15 tendons) in relieving pain or enabling return to full function at 12 weeks [estimated number needed to treat (NNT) for full return to activity =7, 95% CI −6 to 2]. There were no reports of rupture in this study, suggesting the treatment protocol used was safe, albeit ineffective. In another placebo-controlled study, Neeter et al. (2003) evaluated the effectiveness of iontophoresis (four treatments over 2 weeks) with 3 mL dexamethasone ($n=14$) versus 3 mL saline ($n=11$) on pain and function over 1 year in athletes with Achilles tendinopathy undergoing a 10-week progressive exercise programme. Large improvements in pain and function were observed in both groups during the course of the study. However, there were few between-group differences, suggesting that dexamethasone iontophoresis was no more effective than placebo.

Autologous Growth Factor Injections (Autologous Whole Blood and Platelet-rich Plasma)

Autologous growth factor injections are becoming an increasingly popular intervention for musculoskeletal soft-tissue injuries including Achilles tendinopathy (de Vos et al. 2010b; Paoloni et al. 2011; Taylor et al. 2011). Patients who have not responded to multiple non-surgical interventions have been suggested to be candidates for this treatment (Foster et al. 2009). Growth factors include transforming growth factor-β, insulin-like growth factors, vascular endothelial growth factor, basic fibroblast growth factor, hepatocytic growth factor, and epithelial growth factor (de Vos et al. 2010b; Foster et al. 2009; Paoloni et al. 2011). The provision of such endogenous growth factors directly to the injury site is theorized to lead to tendon healing through stimulation of collagen synthesis and well-ordered angiogenesis (de Vos et al. 2010b; Foster et al. 2009). These growth factors are administered via the injection of autologous whole blood or platelet-rich plasma (PRP).

One high-quality RCT has investigated the effectiveness of autologous blood injections for Achilles tendinopathy and the results were disappointing (see Table 6-2) (de Vos et al. 2010a). In this study, 54 participants were randomized to receive a single PRP or saline (placebo) injection (administered as five small depots at three injection sites) into their Achilles tendon as an adjunctive treatment to a 12-week eccentric calf muscle exercise programme. At 6, 12, and 24 weeks there was a progressive improvement in the VISA-A score of both groups [mean (SD) VISA-A score improvement from baseline at 24 weeks=21.7 (22.1) versus 20.5 (22.5) for the PRP and placebo groups respectively]. However, there were no significant differences between groups at any time point. Further, at 24 weeks approximately 60% of participants in the PRP group and 70% of participants in the placebo group were satisfied with treatment and had returned to their desired sport, respectively. However, there were no significant differences between the groups. A follow-up study by these authors also showed that there was no significant difference between the two groups in the improvement in the sonographic characteristics of the Achilles tendons at 24 weeks (de Vos et al. 2011).

These findings suggest that a single PRP injection is not an effective intervention for Achilles tendinopathy in patients undergoing an eccentric calf muscle exercise programme. However, future studies in this area are required to determine: (i) the optimum volume, number, and frequency of injections and optimum treatment regimen if multiple injections are used, (ii) the optimum injection technique (one depot versus multiple depots), (iii) the optimum preparation of PRP, and (iv) whether treatment is effective in head-to-head comparisons of physical therapy versus autologous blood injections (for those people who are non-compliant with rehabilitation or where it is contraindicated) (de Vos et al. 2010b; Paoloni et al. 2011; Taylor et al. 2011).

Sclerosing Injections

Neovascularization arising from the paratenon on the ventral side of the Achilles tendon has been associated with painful Achilles tendinopathy. It has been suggested that the sensory and sympathetic nerves within these blood vessels are responsible for pain, and therefore it follows that destruction of the vessels and nerves may lead to pain relief (van Sterkenburg and van Dijk 2011). Polidocanol (ethoxysclerol) is a sclerosing agent that is frequently used to treat varicose veins. It is injected into blood vessels to shrink or cause localized thrombosis, fibrosis, and obliteration of the vessels. It has also been suggested to have extravascular anaesthetic effects (Alfredson and Öhberg 2005). Given these biological actions, polidocanol injections have been recommended for the management of Achilles tendinopathy. Following sclerosing injection treatment, a period of rest for 1 to 3 days, followed by a gradual increase in tendon loading activity (but no maximum loading such as jumping, fast running, or heavy strength training during the first 2 weeks) is recommended. After 2 weeks, maximal tendon loading is allowed (Alfredson and Cook 2007).

Only one small RCT has investigated the effectiveness of sclerosing agents for Achilles tendinopathy and the findings were promising (see Table 6-2) (Alfredson and Öhberg 2005). In this double-blind (participant and injector) study, 20 middle-aged active participants with chronic Achilles tendinopathy were randomized to receive an injection of 5 mg/mL polidocanol or 5 µg/mL lidocaine and epinephrine (adrenaline) (control). All injections were performed using greyscale and colour Doppler to ensure accurate deposition of the agents into the areas of neovascularization outside the ventral aspect of the Achilles tendon. Participants were given a maximum of two treatments at 3- to 6-week intervals. At 3 months (range 6 to 20 weeks), the mean improvement for pain during Achilles tendon loading activities was significantly greater for the polidocanol treatment group relative to the control group (mean change in VAS=36 versus 2 mm for the polidocanol and control groups respectively, $p<0.005$). Clinical improvement correlated with elimination of the colour Doppler appearance of neovascularization. Further, there were no adverse events in either group, suggesting that the protocol was safe.

Although these findings are promising, they should be interpreted with caution as the study sample size was small and there were differences in the baseline characteristics of participants (sex and duration of symptoms) which may have biased the results (van Sterkenburg et al. 2010). In addition, only approximately half of patients with Achilles tendinopathy will display neovascularization of their affected tendon(s)

and be candidates for this treatment (van Sterkenburg et al. 2010). Further, a recent large case-series study suggested that sclerosing therapy was successful in less than 50% of participants in the short and long term (6 weeks and approximately 3 years, respectively). Well-designed RCTs using larger sample sizes, robust randomization techniques, validated outcome measurements, and longer follow-ups are required to further evaluate this therapy.

Glyceryl Trinitrate Patches

Glyceryl trinitrate (GTN) transdermal patches are traditionally used for the management of ischaemic heart disease owing to their effect of relaxing smooth muscle and consequent dilation of peripheral arteries and veins. However, GTN transdermal patches have also been recommended for Achilles tendinopathy that has been unresponsive to a 12-week calf muscle eccentric exercise programme (Alfredson and Cook 2007). The rationale for the use of GTN patches in Achilles tendinopathy is that GTN is a nitric oxide donor, which stimulates collagen synthesis and remodelling by tenocytes in degenerative tendon thereby leading to improved tendon healing (Langberg et al. 2007; Murrell et al. 1997; Schäffer et al. 1997).

Two RCTs have investigated the effectiveness of GTN patches for Achilles tendinopathy with conflicting results (see Table 6-2) (Kane et al. 2008; Paoloni et al. 2004). Paoloni et al. (2004) compared continuous application of transdermal GTN (1.25 mg/24 hours) plus rehabilitation (relative rest, stretching, eccentric exercise, and heel raises) versus placebo patch plus rehabilitation (control) in a double-blind trial of 65 participants (84 Achilles tendons). Compared with the control group, there was a statistically significant reduction in Achilles tendon pain with activity in the GTN group at 12 weeks (mean VAS score=0.9 versus 1.6 cm; $p=0.02$). At 24 weeks, results also favoured GTN treatment with significant reductions in Achilles tendon pain with activity (mean VAS score=0.4 versus 1.0 cm, $p=0.03$), and after a hop test (mean VAS score=0.5 versus 1.6 cm, $p<0.01$). Further, at 24 weeks, 78% of tendons in the GTN group were rated as excellent (indicating that the tendon was asymptomatic with activities of daily living) as opposed to 49% in the control group. Additionally, there was no significant difference between the two groups with regard to the number of days on which participants were affected by headache, suggesting that the use of GTN patches was safe. In the GTN group, 17 participants experienced at least one headache for a total of 85 days. In the placebo group, 15 participants experienced at least one headache for a total of 101 days.

The findings of Paoloni et al. (2004) are in contrast to a more recent study by Kane et al. (2008), who randomized 40 participants with Achilles tendinopathy to continuous transdermal GTN (2.5 mg/24 hours) plus daily physical therapy (eccentric calf muscle exercise), or daily physical therapy alone (control). Participants were assessed using the pain and disability VAS domains of the Ankle Osteoarthritis Scale at 6 months. Results showed that there was a significant improvement in pain and disability scores for both groups. However, there was no significant difference in scores between the groups for pain (mean VAS=3.0 versus 3.1 cm, p=0.42) or disability (mean VAS=2.2 versus 2.3 cm, p=0.38). In addition, histological examination of Achilles tendons of participants that did not respond to treatment and required surgery showed no difference in neovascularization, collagen synthesis, or tenocyte stimulation between the two groups. Further, there was no evidence of modulation of nitric oxide synthase, a marker of nitric oxide production, in those tendons treated with GTN. Four of the 20 participants (20%) had to stop using the GTN patches due to 'unacceptable' side effects (versus none in the control group).

Taken together, the effectiveness and safety of GTN patches for Achilles tendinopathy are currently equivocal. Further, clinicians should be cautious in recommending this treatment owing to the increased risk of adverse events and interactions with other medications (Paoloni et al. 2004).

ELECTROTHERAPEUTIC STRATEGIES

Extracorporeal Shock Wave Therapy

Extracorporeal shock wave therapy (ECSWT) was originally developed for use as a non-invasive treatment for kidney, gallbladder or liver stones, but in the past 15 years has become a popular, albeit controversial, treatment for soft-tissue disorders. The mechanism of action of ECSWT was not completely known, but the rationale for its use is stimulation of soft-tissue

healing and inhibition of pain receptors (Rompe et al. 2007, 2009).

Four RCTs have investigated the effectiveness of low-level ECSWT for chronic (symptoms greater than 3 months) Achilles tendinopathy (Costa et al. 2005; Rasmussen et al. 2008; Rompe et al. 2007, 2009). There is no consensus regarding its use (Rompe et al. 2009). The treatment regimen has been three to four treatments at weekly intervals (Rasmussen et al. 2008; Rompe et al. 2007, 2009). However, one trial (Costa et al. 2005) treated patients at monthly intervals for 3 months. The dose per session used was 1500 pulses (up to 0.2 mJ/mm²) (Costa et al. 2005) or 2000 pulses (0.10 to 0.51 mJ/mm²) (Rasmussen et al. 2008; Rompe et al. 2007, 2009).

In these trials, the comparator intervention has varied from a no-treatment approach (Rompe et al. 2007) to sham ECSWT (Costa et al. 2005; Rasmussen et al. 2008), to eccentric calf muscle exercise (Rompe et al. 2007). An additional study has compared a combined treatment of ECSWT plus eccentric calf muscle exercise with eccentric calf muscle exercise alone (Rompe et al. 2009). The outcome measurements have been performed at 7 to 16 weeks post-treatment in these studies.

The results of these studies have produced equivocal results as the findings differ as a function of the comparator intervention (Table 6-3). When the comparator intervention has been a sham, there are conflicting results. Rasmussen et al. (2008) compared ECSWT with sham and showed that ECSWT significantly reduced symptoms of Achilles tendinopathy at 12 weeks (American Orthopedic Foot and Ankle Society Score between group mean difference =10.0, 95% CI 3.2 to 15.8). However, Costa et al. (2005) did not report any significant differences between participants (with mid-portion and insertional complaints) for self-reported pain during walking, at rest, or during sport at 12 weeks in the real and sham ECSWT groups. One explanation for the difference in findings between these two studies is that the monthly (rather than weekly) treatment regimen used by Costa et al. (2005) may have resulted in an underdosing of the ECSWT.

ECSWT has been shown to be an effective intervention for Achilles tendinopathy, when compared with a no-treatment approach or when combined in a multimodal treatment approach. Rompe et al. (2007)

TABLE 6-3 **Summary of Major Findings from Clinical Trials Investigating Electrotherapeutic Strategies for Achilles Tendinopathy**

Intervention	Author(s)	Study Primary Intervention(s)	Study Comparator Intervention(s)	Major Finding(s)
Extracorporeal shock wave therapy (ECSWT)	Rasmussen et al. (2008)	ECSWT (n=24)	Sham ECSWT (n=24)	Significant differences between groups in AOFAS score at 12 weeks favouring ECSWT (mean difference=10.0, 95% CI 3.2 to 15.8)
	Costa et al. (2005)	ECSWT (n=22)	Sham ECSWT (n=27)	No significant differences between groups for pain during walking, at rest, or during sport at 12 weeks
	Rompe et al. (2007)	ECSWT (n=25)	(i) Wait-and-see approach (n=25) (ii) Eccentric calf muscle exercise alone (n=25)	(i) Significantly better VISA-A scores in ECSWT versus wait-and-see group at 4 months (mean difference 15.4, 95% CI 7.8 to 23.0) (ii) No significant differences between ECSWT group versus eccentric calf muscle exercise group in VISA-A score at 4 months
	Rompe et al. (2009)	ECSWT plus eccentric calf muscle exercise (n=34)	Eccentric calf muscle exercise alone (n=34)	VISA-A score significantly better in combined treatment group at 4 months (mean difference=13.5, 95% CI=5.5 to 22.5); significant difference between groups in proportion of participants being 'completely recovered' or 'much improved' at 4 months favouring primary intervention (82 versus 56%); no significant differences between groups at 1 year
Low-level laser therapy (LLLT)	Stergioulas et al. (2008)	LLLT plus eccentric calf muscle exercise (n=20)	Sham LLLT plus eccentric calf muscle exercise (n=20)	Significantly less pain during physical activity (VAS mm) in LLLT plus eccentric calf muscle exercise group compared with sham LLLT plus eccentric calf muscle exercise at 4 (mean difference=−17.9, 95% CI −28.4 to −7.4), 8 (mean difference=−25.5, 95% CI=−39.5 to −11.5), and 12 (mean difference=−20.0, 95% CI −36.1 to −3.9) weeks
	Tumilty et al. (2012)	LLLT plus eccentric calf muscle exercise (n=20)	Sham LLLT plus eccentric calf muscle exercise (n=20)	No significant differences between groups in VISA-A scores at 12 and 52 weeks. Significantly worse VISA-A scores in active LLLT plus eccentric calf muscle exercise group at 4 weeks (mean difference=−9.3, 95% CI=−16.0 to −1.9)

compared ECSWT with a wait-and-see approach, and an eccentric calf muscle exercise programme. Participants treated with ECSWT reported better improvements in pain and function compared with those in the wait-and-see group at 4 months (VISA-A score between group mean difference=15.4, 95% CI 7.8 to 23.0). In the same trial (Rompe et al. 2007), ECSWT showed equivalent effectiveness to an eccentric calf muscle exercise programme (VISA-A score mean difference=5.2, 95% CI −3.9 to 14.3).

In another study (Rompe et al. 2009), a multimodal treatment of ECSWT combined with eccentric calf muscle exercise showed superior effectiveness relative to an eccentric calf muscle exercise programme alone; in this trial the VISA-A score was significantly better in the combined treatment group at 4 months (mean difference=13.5, 95% CI=5.5 to 22.5). Further, 82% (28 of 34) of participants who had received the combined treatment reported being 'completely recovered' or 'much improved' at 4 months as opposed to 56% (19 out of 34) of participants who performed the eccentric calf muscle exercise alone (RR success=1.5, 95% CI=1.1 to 2.1). However, at 1 year there was no difference between the groups.

Taken together, these studies suggest that low-level ECSWT is an effective intervention for chronic Achilles tendinopathy. ECSWT is more effective than no treatment and shows comparable effectiveness to an eccentric calf muscle exercise programme, suggesting that it may be indicated as an alternative treatment for Achilles tendinopathy in patients who are unable to perform eccentric calf muscle exercise. Further, adding ECSWT to an eccentric calf muscle exercise programme results in improved patient outcomes. However, further research is required to determine the optimum dosage of ECSWT for Achilles tendinopathy, and to clarify its effectiveness against a sham treatment.

Low-level Laser Therapy

Low-level laser therapy (LLLT) has been recommended as a treatment for Achilles tendinopathy in the clinical practice guidelines of the American Physical Therapy Association (Carcia et al. 2010). The rationale for the use of LLLT as a treatment for Achilles tendinopathy is the reduction of inflammation within peritendinous tissues (Bjordal et al. 2006), increased angiogenesis, increased tenocyte activity leading to increased collagen synthesis, increased tensile strength, and reduced pain (Tumilty et al. 2012).

Two adequately powered RCTs have investigated the effectiveness of LLLT when used as an adjunctive treatment to an eccentric calf muscle exercise programme for Achilles tendinopathy, with conflicting results (see Table 6-3) (Stergioulas et al. 2008; Tumilty et al. 2012). Stergioulas et al. (2008) reported that the addition of LLLT (two times per week over 4 weeks, then one treatment for 4 weeks) to an eccentric calf muscle exercise programme resulted in less pain during physical activity compared with an eccentric exercise group alone [mean VAS between group difference (mm) at 4 weeks=−17.9 (95% CI −28.4 to −7.4), at 8 weeks=−25.5, (95% CI =−39.5

to −11.5), and at 12 weeks=−20.0 (95% CI −36.1 to −3.9)]. In contrast, Tumilty et al. (2012) showed that the addition of LLLT (three times per week over 4 weeks) to an eccentric calf muscle exercise programme did not result in improved patient outcomes at 4, 12, and 52 weeks (mean VISA-A score between-group difference at week 12=−6.4, 95% CI −13.7 to 0.9).

Differences in findings between these two studies (Stergioulas et al. 2008; Tumilty et al. 2012) are likely to have occurred as a result of differences in the participant characteristics, LLLT protocols used, and/or eccentric calf muscle exercise protocols. In this regard, the intensity of the eccentric calf muscle exercise protocol used by Stergioulas et al. (2008) was notably less than Tumilty et al. (2012) (i.e. 144 repetitions per day, 4 days per week over 8 weeks versus 180 repetitions per day, 7 days per week for 12 weeks), and this underdosing may have led to a relative increase in the effect provided by the LLT treatment. Further work is required to determine the optimum dosage of LLLT for Achilles tendinopathy, and to ascertain whether LLLT is effective when used alone rather than in a multimodal approach.

MECHANICAL STRATEGIES

Taping, foot orthoses, heel lifts, and footwear modifications are commonly recommended interventions for Achilles tendinopathy (Alfredson et al. 2012; Hunter 2000; Kountouris and Cook 2007; Mazzone and McCue 2002; Schepsis et al. 2002).

Taping

Taping techniques that limit either dorsiflexion excursion of the ankle joint (such as 'offloading' methods), or abnormal frontal plane movement of the rearfoot (such as 'anti-pronation' methods) (Smith et al. 2004) may be able to reduce strain on the Achilles tendon and alleviate symptoms of Achilles tendinopathy during weightbearing activities (Carcia et al. 2010). However, there are currently no RCTs that have evaluated this intervention for Achilles tendinopathy, so its effectiveness is unknown.

Foot Orthoses

The biomechanical rationale for the use of foot orthoses is not fully established (Donoghue et al. 2008c; Maffulli and Kader 2002; Mayer et al. 2007). The traditional rationale is that foot orthoses reduce bending stress within the Achilles tendon by the correction of abnormal eversion of the calcaneus in the presence of excessive pronation (Maffulli and Kader 2002; Ryan et al. 2009). However, the validity of this hypothesis is questionable as Donoghue et al. (2008b) have shown that foot orthoses slightly increase rearfoot eversion in people with Achilles tendinopathy. More recently, alternative biomechanical hypotheses have been proposed, including increasing variability of rearfoot movement to reduce repetitive Achilles tendon stress (Donoghue et al. 2008a), and improved function of lower limb musculature including the triceps surae (Hertel et al. 2005; Wyndow et al. 2010).

Although there are case reports showing beneficial effects of custom foot orthoses and anti-pronation foot strapping on pain in people with Achilles tendon symptoms (Donoghue et al. 2008c; Smith et al. 2004), at present only one small short-term RCT has investigated the effectiveness of foot orthoses for Achilles tendinopathy (Table 6-4) (Mayer et al. 2007). In this study, participants were randomized to one of three groups; physiotherapy, foot orthoses or control. The physiotherapy group received 10 sessions of a multimodal physical therapy programme that included eccentric calf muscle exercise over 4 weeks. Participants in the foot orthoses group were prescribed customized semi-rigid moulded foot orthoses, which

included 'bowl-shaped heels, moulded, longitudinal arch support and detorsion wedge'. Dynamic plantar pressure measurements were used to prescribe the foot orthoses, but the prescription protocol was not stated. The control group did not receive any treatment. At 4 weeks, there was a significant improvement in pain for both the foot orthoses and physiotherapy groups relative to the control group.

Heel Lifts

Heel lifts are a simple and inexpensive intervention that has been advocated for Achilles tendinopathy by reducing the rate and/or magnitude of tensile load within the Achilles tendon (Hunter 2000; Mazzone and McCue 2002; Schepsis et al. 2002). There is no consensus on the optimum height of the heel lift, but heights of 7.5 to 15.0 mm have been suggested (Schepsis et al. 2002). At present, no high-quality RCTs have evaluated the effectiveness of heel lifts for Achilles tendinopathy, although two studies [one low-quality RCT (Lowdon et al. 1984) and one case series study (Maclellan and Vyvyan 1981)] have demonstrated equivocal findings as to their ability to reduce symptoms (see Table 6-4). Interestingly, biomechanical analyses have shown that the effects of heel lifts on peak Achilles tendon force and average rate of loading are subject-specific (Dixon and Kerwin 1998, 2002; Reinschmidt and Nigg 1995). Unfortunately, there are

TABLE 6-4 Summary of Major Findings from Clinical Trials Investigating Mechanical Therapies for Achilles Tendinopathy

Intervention	Author(s)	Study Primary Intervention(s)	Study Comparator Intervention(s)	Major Finding(s)
Foot orthoses	Mayer et al. (2007)	Foot orthoses (custom semi-rigid) (n=9)	(i) Physiotherapy (10 sessions of physical therapy that included eccentric calf muscle exercise for 4 weeks) (n=11) (ii) Control (no treatment) (n=8)	Significant improvement in pain for both the foot orthoses and physiotherapy groups relative to the control group; no significant differences between foot orthoses and physiotherapy groups at 4 weeks
Heel lifts	Lowdon et al. (1984)	(i) Sorbothane heel pad plus strengthening and stretching (n=11) (ii) Molefoam plus strengthening and stretching (n=10)	No pad (control) plus strengthening and stretching	No between group analyses; trends for pain (assessed using VAS), swelling, and activity levels to be more improved in the control group at 2 months

currently no clinical tests that predict an individual's biomechanical response to this intervention.

Footwear

There are currently no RCTs that have investigated the role of footwear modifications as a treatment for Achilles tendinopathy, although footwear with 'inappropriate wedging in the heel' has been proposed as a risk factor for this condition (Clement et al. 1984). Therefore, in the absence of evidence, clinicians should use a logical approach in assessing the general characteristics of all footwear (sports and everyday activities) worn by patients with Achilles tendon pathology, recommending footwear that is less likely to increase strain within the Achilles tendon. Such an approach would include recommendations to avoid wearing flat shoes, and ensuring that any athletic footwear worn by patients is appropriate for their foot type and sport.

SURGICAL STRATEGIES

Non-surgical treatment for Achilles tendinopathy has been estimated to be ineffective in approximately 25 to 46% of patients. Factors adversely influencing the likelihood of success of non-surgical treatment include increasing patient age, female sex, increasing duration of symptoms, and more severe pathological tendon changes (Clement et al. 1984; de Vos et al. 2007; Kvist 1994; Nørregaard et al. 2007; Paavola et al. 2002; Sayana and Maffulli 2007; van Sterkenburg et al. 2010). Surgery is considered the final option in the management of Achilles tendinopathy that is persistent despite 3 to 6 months of non-surgical therapy (Andres and Murrell 2008; Maffulli et al. 2009).

Several surgical techniques for Achilles tendinopathy have been described. The most commonly described technique is open surgical debridement of the tendon and/or peritendinous tissue (with repair or augmentation of the tendon, generally when greater than 50% of the tendon requires debridement) (Andres and Murrell 2008; Maffulli et al. 2009). Open surgery involves a longitudinal incision being made along the medial or lateral side of the Achilles tendon. Any fibrotic lesions or areas of failed healing are excised, and multiple longitudinal incisions are made in the Achilles tendon to detect intratendinous lesions and stimulate remaining viable tenocytes to initiate healing

(Maffulli et al. 2009). Depending on the extent of surgical repair, patients are placed in a non-weightbearing cast or cam-walker for up to 8 weeks and light jogging can be resumed from 2 to 4 months (Schepsis et al. 2002). Apart from the significant recovery time with this technique, there is also a relatively high risk of complications (11%) associated with wound healing (Paavola et al. 2000).

Percutaneous longitudinal tenotomy (with or without ultrasound guidance) is an alternative less invasive surgical technique for Achilles tendinopathy that can be performed on an outpatient basis and requires less post-operative care (Testa et al. 2002). This technique involves tenotomy (single or multiple) incisions of approximately 3 to 4 cm length being performed in the main body of the Achilles tendon (Maffulli et al. 1997; Testa et al. 2002). Positive effects associated with this technique are speculated to result from improvements to localized circulation, which allows better tendon nourishment and normalization of tendon biochemistry (Maffulli et al. 1997). Full weightbearing occurs after 3 days and limited jogging is permitted as early as 2 weeks. However, a major limitation of this technique is that it is less effective in cases of coexisting paratendinopathy as it does not allow stripping of any adhesions between the paratenon and the Achilles tendon (Maffulli et al. 1997).

A novel surgical technique for Achilles tendinopathy is minimally invasive stripping, which can be used in isolation or in conjunction with other surgical techniques (Mokone et al. 2006). Minimally invasive stripping aims to strip neovessels and the accompanying nerve supply of the Achilles tendon from the Kager's fat pad, thereby reducing pain (Longo et al. 2008). Four incisions are made on the medial and lateral side of the Achilles tendon at its proximal and distal aspects. A surgical instrument is then inserted into the incisions and the proximal and distal portions of Achilles tendon are freed from any peritendinous adhesions. A suture thread is then inserted proximally, passing through the two proximal incisions over the anterior aspect of the Achilles tendon. The suture is retrieved from the distal incisions, over the anterior aspect of the Achilles tendon. The suture is slid on the tendon, which strips it free from any adhesions. The procedure is repeated for the posterior aspect of the Achilles tendon (Longo et al. 2008). This technique is considered relatively inexpensive, easy to perform, and low risk in terms of developing infection (Longo et al. 2008).

Following surgery for Achilles tendinopathy, early post-operative rehabilitation that continues for 6 to 12 months is required to return strength and functional capacity to the affected lower limb (Schepsis et al. 2002). Athletic patients should be advised that a period of 6 months will be required before they can return to their sports activities (Maffulli et al. 2009). A recent systematic review of effectiveness of surgical interventions for Achilles tendinopathy concluded that the results of surgery vary from 67 to 86% (Andres and Murrell 2008). Further, a retrospective analysis of athletes surgically treated for Achilles tendinopathy demonstrated that the average (range) time to return to running was 7 (3–12) months and competitive sport was 11 (6–18) months (Bohu et al. 2009). The likelihood of success is inversely associated with the extent of tendon damage and the activity levels of the patient (Andres and Murrell 2008; Maffulli et al. 2006). Importantly, all surgical studies for Achilles tendinopathy are case-series study designs, which lack a control group (Andres and Murrell 2008). Therefore, delineating the intervention effects from any non-intervention effects from existing studies in this area is not possible.

FUTURE DIRECTIONS

Achilles tendinopathy is a common overuse injury that occurs in active and sedentary populations, particularly those that are middle-aged. The condition is not an inflammatory disorder, but rather a degenerative process representing the result of a failed tissue healing response. The condition can usually be diagnosed with a structured physical exam that includes pain with palpation of the tendon 2 to 6 cm proximal to the calcaneal insertion. However, MSUS and MRI may be beneficial to aid diagnosis in a patient with equivocal findings or complex rearfoot pain.

Identification and addressing modifiable risk factors for Achilles tendinopathy are key components of effective management. Given that the primary inciting factor for this disorder is excessive Achilles tendon loading, clinicians should evaluate patients' physical activity relative to their conditioning. Other factors that can increase the risk of developing Achilles tendinopathy requiring evaluation are a patient's footwear, biomechanics, calf muscle strength and flexibility, presence of certain medical conditions particularly obesity, as well as medication use. In athletes, the running surface and rehabilitation from any previous injuries should also be determined.

Management of Achilles tendinopathy is aimed at reducing a patient's symptoms, facilitating tendon healing, promoting return to functional activity, and preventing re-injury. Most cases of Achilles tendinopathy can be successfully managed using a multifaceted non-surgical approach that includes modification of activity, and physical therapy. Based on the existing evidence, a 12-week eccentric calf muscle exercise programme should be the first line of treatment for this disorder. However, where an eccentric calf muscle exercise programme is contraindicated or in non-compliant patients, the AirHeel brace and/or ECSWT may be used. Interventions with equivocal effectiveness that could be considered second-line treatments for this disorder are simple analgesics, local injections of corticosteroids (peritendinous) or sclerosing agents, GTN patches, calf muscle stretching, soft-tissue mobilization, mechanical therapies (taping, foot orthoses, and heel lifts), and LLLT. Surgical management is recommended for cases that are resistant to at least 3 months of non-surgical intervention.

Despite the significant body of evidence that currently exists as to the aetiology and management of Achilles tendinopathy, numerous gaps still exist. Although a number of potential risk factors for Achilles tendinopathy have been identified, there is currently little research evaluating preventative strategies for this condition. Further work is therefore required to develop effective preventative interventions for those identified at risk of Achilles tendinopathy. In addition, more research is required to evaluate rigorously the effectiveness of many of the proposed interventions for Achilles tendinopathy. Such research should evaluate these interventions when used alone and as part of a multimodal approach. Finally, the identification of parameters that predict outcome to specific interventions is also required. Such parameters include participant characteristics, disease characteristics, as well as the timing of the intervention(s).

INVITED COMMENTARY

We congratulate the author for the effort to produce such a chapter. There are many key points outlined that clarify the key issues of Achilles tendinopathy, and we now add some further points that may be of interest.

The clinical criteria to diagnose Achilles tendinopathy are indeed tendon pain, tenderness, and thickening on tendon palpation. In addition to those described, another clinical test favoured is the Royal London Hospital test. This test is positive when sharp pain is present on tendon palpation; on the other hand, pain and discomfort disappear or are reduced when the tendon is palpated with the ankle flexed.

The importance of neovascularization associated with tendinopathy is becoming more questionable. Recent work suggests that its prognostic value is limited, its relationship to clinical symptoms is not strong, and that vessel presence is influenced by recent physical activity. Neovascularization could therefore be regarded as a 'red herring' (Tol et al. 2012).

The distinction between partial and complete tears of the Achilles tendon is really only theoretical. Partial tears, though frequently reported by radiologists at MRI and ultrasound scans, do not exist from a practical viewpoint. This is the reason why they have to be considered as total ruptures. In regard to risk factors, genetic predisposition to Achilles tendinopathy seems likely, with COL5A1 and TNC amongst others being possible markers (Magra and Maffulli 2007). Furthermore, obesity and diabetes can limit immune responses, produce a low-grade inflammation and impaired insulin sensitivity that act as risk factors for a failed healing response after an acute tendon insult, and predispose to the development of chronic overuse tendinopathies (Del Buono et al. 2011)

The role of eccentric training is still controversial. In reality, the success rate after eccentric exercises is modest, accounting for just above 60% at best. Therefore, other therapies should be considered. There are some promising options. For instance, high-volume image-guided injection therapy for resistant tendinopathy. These involve 10 mL of 0.5% bupivacaine hydrochloride, 25 mg of hydrocortisone acetate, and 40 mL of 0.9% NaCl saline solution and can reduce neovascularization, decrease maximal tendon thickness, and improve VISA-A scores at short-term follow-up (Humphrey et al. 2010). Also, platelet-rich plasma therapies have potential but require further critical research (Maffulli and Del Buono 2012). In addition, when using autologous stem cells, the price to pay after their application should be considered (Maffulli, 2013).

Nicola Maffulli MD, MS, PhD, FRCP, FRCS, FFSEM
Professor of Musculoskeletal Disorders, Consultant
Orthopaedic Surgeon, University of Salerno, Salerno, Italy;
Honorary Professor of Sport and Exercise Medicine,
Queen Mary University of London, London, UK

REFERENCES

Alfredson, H., Öhberg, L., 2005. Sclerosing injections to areas of neo-vascularisation reduce pain in chronic Achilles tendinopathy: a double-blind randomised controlled trial. Knee Surgery, Sports Traumatology, Arthroscopy 13 (4), 338–344.

Alfredson, H., Cook, J., 2007. A treatment algorithm for managing Achilles tendinopathy: new treatment options. British Journal of Sports Medicine 41 (4), 211–216.

Alfredson, H., Pietila, T., Jonsson, P., et al., 1998. Heavy-load eccentric calf muscle training for the treatment of chronic Achilles tendinosis. American Journal of Sports Medicine 26 (3), 360–366.

Alfredson, H., Cook, J., Silbernagel, K., et al., 2012. Pain in the Achilles region. In: Brukner, P., Khan, K. (Eds.), Brukner and Khan's clinical sports medicine, fourth ed. North Rhyde NSW, McGraw-Hill Australia Pty, pp. 776–805.

Andres, B.M., Murrell, G.A., 2008. Treatment of tendinopathy: what works, what does not, and what is on the horizon. Clinical Orthopaedics and Related Research 466 (7), 1539–1554.

Arndt, A.N., Komi, P.V., Bruggemann, G.P., et al., 1998. Individual muscle contributions to the in vivo Achilles tendon force. Clinical Biomechanics (Bristol, Avon) 13 (7), 532–541.

Aström, M., Rausing, A., 1995. Chronic Achilles tendinopathy. A survey of surgical and histopathologic findings. Clinical Orthopaedics and Related Research 316, 151–164.

Aström, M., Westlin, N., 1992. No effect of piroxicam on achilles tendinopathy. A randomized study of 70 patients. Acta Orthopaedica Scandinavica 63 (6), 631–634.

Azevedo, L.B., Lambert, M.I., Vaughan, C.L., et al., 2009. Biomechanical variables associated with Achilles tendinopathy in runners. British Journal of Sports Medicine 43 (4), 288–292.

Baur, H., Divert, C., Hirschmuller, A., et al., 2004. Analysis of gait differences in healthy runners and runners with chronic Achilles tendon complaints. Isokinetics and Exercise Science 12 (2), 111–116.

Baur, H., Müller, S., Hirschmüller, A., et al., 2011. Comparison in lower leg neuromuscular activity between runners with unilateral mid-portion Achilles tendinopathy and healthy individuals. Journal of Electromyography and Kinesiology 21 (3), 499–505.

Bennell, K., Talbot, R.C., Wajswelner, H., et al., 1998. Intra-rater and inter-rater reliability of a weight-bearing lunge measure of ankle dorsiflexion. Australian Journal of Physiotherapy 44 (3), 175–180.

Birk, D.E., Fitch, J.M., Babiarz, J.P., et al., 1990. Collagen fibrillogenesis in vitro: interaction of types I and V collagen regulates fibril diameter. Journal of Cell Science 95 (4), 649–657.

Bjordal, J.M., Lopes-Martins, R.A.B., Iversen, V.V., 2006. A randomised, placebo controlled trial of low level laser therapy for activated Achilles tendinitis with microdialysis measurement of peritendinous prostaglandin E2 concentrations. British Journal of Sports Medicine 40 (1), 76–80.

Bohu, Y., Lefèvre, N., Bauer, T., et al., 2009. Surgical treatment of Achilles tendinopathies in athletes. Multicenter retrospective series of open surgery and endoscopic techniques. Orthopaedics and Traumatology: Surgery and Research 95 (Suppl. 8), 72–77.

Bryant, A.L., Clark, R.A., Bartold, S., et al., 2008. Effects of estrogen on the mechanical behavior of the human Achilles tendon in vivo. Journal of Applied Physiology 105 (4), 1035–1043.

Burns, J., Redmond, A., Ouvrier, R., et al., 2005. Quantification of muscle strength and imbalance in neurogenic pes cavus, compared with health controls, using hand-held dynamometry. Foot and Ankle International 26 (7), 540–544.

Carcia, C.R., Martin, R.L., Houck, J., et al., 2010. Achilles pain, stiffness, and muscle power deficits: achilles tendinitis. Journal of Orthopaedic and Sports Physical Therapy 40 (9), A1–A26.

Chen, T.M., Rozen, W.M., Pan, W.-R., et al., 2009. The arterial anatomy of the Achilles tendon: anatomical study and clinical implications. Clinical Anatomy 22 (3), 377–385.

Child, S., Bryant, A., Clark, R., et al. (Eds.), 2010. Clinical measures in athletes with and without Achilles tendinopathy and their relationship to tendon-aponeurosis strain. 2010 Asics Conference of Science and Medicine in Sport; The Sheraton Mirage Port Douglas, Elsevier, Chatswood NSW. Journal of Science and Medicine in Sport (Suppl.), 79. Online. Available: <http://www.docstoc.com/?docId=152661348&download=1>.

Christenson, R.E., 2007. Effectiveness of specific soft tissue mobilizations for the management of Achilles tendinosis: Single case study – experimental design. Manual Therapy 12 (1), 63–71.

Clement, D.B., Taunton, J.E., Smart, G.W., 1984. Achilles tendinitis and peritendinitis: etiology and treatment. American Journal of Sports Medicine 12 (3), 179–184.

Cook, J.L., Purdam, C.R., 2009. Is tendon pathology a continuum? A pathology model to explain the clinical presentation of load-induced tendinopathy. British Journal of Sports Medicine 43 (6), 409–416.

Coombes, B.K., Bisset, L., Vicenzino, B., 2010. Efficacy and safety of corticosteroid injections and other injections for management of tendinopathy: a systematic review of randomised controlled trials. The Lancet 376 (9754), 1751–1767.

Corrao, G., Zambon, A., Bertu, L., et al., 2006. Evidence of tendinitis provoked by fluoroquinolone treatment: a case-control study. Drug Safety 29 (10), 889–896.

Costa, M.L., Shepstone, L., Donell, S.T., et al., 2005. Shock wave therapy for chronic Achilles tendon pain: a randomized placebo-controlled trial. Clinical Orthopaedics and Related Research 440, 199–204.

DaCruz, D.J., Geeson, M., Allen, M.J., et al., 1988. Achilles paratendonitis: an evaluation of steroid injection. British Journal of Sports Medicine 22 (2), 64–65.

de Jonge, S., de Vos, R.J., van Schie, H.T., et al., 2010. One-year follow-up of a randomised controlled trial on added splinting to eccentric exercises in chronic midportion Achilles tendinopathy. British Journal of Sports Medicine 44 (9), 673–677.

de Jonge, S., van den Berg, C., de Vos, R.J., et al., 2011. Incidence of midportion Achilles tendinopathy in the general population. British Journal of Sports Medicine 45 (13), 1026–1028.

Del Buono, A., Battery, L., Denaro, V., et al., 2011. Tendinopathy and inflammation: some truths. International Journal of Immunopathology and Pharmacology 24 (1 Suppl. 2), 45–50.

de Mos, M., van El, B., DeGroot, J., et al., 2007. Achilles tendinosis: changes in biochemical composition and collagen turnover rate. American Journal of Sports Medicine 35 (9), 1549–1556.

de Vos, R.J., Weir, A., Visser, R.J.A., et al., 2007. The additional value of a night splint to eccentric exercises in chronic midportion Achilles tendinopathy: a randomised controlled trial. British Journal of Sports Medicine 41 (7), e5.

de Vos, R.J., Weir, A., van Schie, H.T.M., et al., 2010a. Platelet-rich plasma injection for chronic Achilles tendinopathy: a randomized controlled trial. Journal of the American Medical Association 303 (2), 144–149.

de Vos, R.J., van Veldhoven, P.L.J., Moen, M.H., et al., 2010b. Autologous growth factor injections in chronic tendinopathy: a systematic review. British Medical Bulletin 95 (1), 63–77.

de Vos, R.J., Weir, A., Tol, J.L., et al., 2011. No effects of PRP on ultrasonographic tendon structure and neovascularisation in chronic midportion Achilles tendinopathy. British Journal of Sports Medicine 45 (5), 387–392.

Dixon, S.J., Kerwin, D.G., 1998. The influence of heel lift manipulation on Achilles tendon loading in running. Journal of Applied Biomechanics 14 (4), 374–389.

Dixon, S.J., Kerwin, D.G., 2002. Variations in Achilles tendon loading with heel lift intervention in heel-toe runners. Journal of Applied Biomechanics 18, 321–331.

Donoghue, O.A., Harrison, A.J., Coffey, N., et al., 2008a. Functional data analysis of running kinematics in chronic Achilles tendon injury. Medicine and Science in Sports and Exercise 40 (7), 1323–1335.

Donoghue, O.A., Harrison, A.J., Laxton, P., et al., 2008b. Lower limb kinematics of subjects with chronic Achilles tendon injury during running. Research in Sports Medicine 16 (1), 23–38.

Donoghue, O.A., Harrison, A.J., Laxton, P., et al., 2008c. Orthotic control of rear foot and lower limb motion during running in participants with chronic Achilles tendon injury. Sports Biomechanics 7 (2), 194–205.

Doral, M.N., Alam, M., Bozkurt, M., et al., 2010. Functional anatomy of the Achilles tendon. Knee Surgery, Sports Traumatology, Arthroscopy 18 (5), 638–643.

Edouard, P., Morin, J.-B., Pruvost, J., et al., 2011. Injuries in high-level heptathlon and decathlon. British Journal of Sports Medicine 45 (4), 346.

Fahlström, M., Jonsson, P., Lorentzon, R., et al., 2003. Chronic Achilles tendon pain treated with eccentric calf-muscle training. Knee Surgery, Sports Traumatology, Arthroscopy 11 (5), 327–333.

Foster, T.E., Puskas, B.L., Mandelbaum, B.R., et al., 2009. Platelet-rich plasma: from basic science to clinical applications. American Journal of Sports Medicine 37 (11), 2259–2272.

Fredberg, U., Bolvig, L., 2002. Significance of ultrasonographically detected asymptomatic tendinosis in the patellar and Achilles tendons of elite soccer players: a longitudinal study. American Journal of Sports Medicine 30 (4), 488–491.

Fredberg, U., Bolvig, L., Pfeiffer-Jensen, M., et al., 2004. Ultrasonography as a tool for diagnosis, guidance of local steroid injection and, together with pressure algometry, monitoring of the treatment of athletes with chronic jumper's knee and Achilles tendinitis: a randomized, double-blind, placebo-controlled study. Scandinavian Journal of Rheumatology 33 (2), 94–101.

Fredberg, U., Bolvig, L., Andersen, N.T., 2008. Prophylactic training in asymptomatic soccer players with ultrasonographic abnormalities in Achilles and patellar tendons: the Danish Super League Study. American Journal of Sports Medicine 36 (3), 451–460.

Gaida, J.E., Alfredson, L., Kiss, Z.S., et al., 2009a. Dyslipidemia in Achilles tendinopathy is characteristic of insulin resistance. Medicine and Science in Sports and Exercise 41 (6), 1194–1197.

Gaida, J.E., Ashe, M.C., Bass, S.L., et al., 2009b. Is adiposity an under-recognized risk factor for tendinopathy? A systematic review. Arthritis and Rheumatism 61 (6), 840–849.

Galloway, M.T., Jokl, P., Dayton, O.W., 1992. Achilles tendon overuse injuries. Clinics in Sports Medicine 11 (4), 771–782.

Gatt, A., Chockalingam, N., 2011. Clinical assessment of ankle joint dorsiflexion: a review of measurement techniques. Journal of the American Podiatric Medical Association 101 (1), 59–69.

Gibbon, W.W., Cooper, J.R., Radcliffe, G.S., 1999. Sonographic incidence of tendon microtears in athletes with chronic Achilles tendinosis. British Journal of Sports Medicine 33 (2), 129–130.

Gibson, W.T., 2009. Genetic association studies for complex traits: relevance for the sports medicine practitioner. British Journal of Sports Medicine 43 (5), 314–316.

Hertel, J., Sloss, B.R., Earl, J.E., 2005. Effect of foot orthotics on quadriceps and gluteus medius electromyographic activity during selected exercises. Archives of Physical Medicine and Rehabilitation 86 (1), 26–30.

Holmes, G.B., Lin, J., 2006. Etiologic factors associated with symptomatic achilles tendinopathy. Foot and Ankle International 27 (11), 952–959.

Hootman, J.M., Macera, C.A., Ainsworth, B.E., et al., 2002. Epidemiology of musculoskeletal injuries among sedentary and physically active adults. Medicine and Science in Sports and Exercise 34 (5), 838–844.

Humphrey, J., Chan, O., Crisp, T., et al., 2010. The short-term effects of high volume image guided injections in resistant non-insertional Achilles tendinopathy. Journal of Science and Medicine in Sport 13 (3), 295–298.

Hunt, R.H., Choquette, D., Craig, B.N., et al., 2007. Approach to managing musculoskeletal pain: acetaminophen, cyclooxygenase-2 inhibitors, or traditional NSAIDs? Canadian Family Physician 53 (7), 1177–1184.

Hunter, G., 2000. The conservative management of Achilles tendinopathy. Physical Therapy in Sport 1 (1), 6–14.

Järvinen, T.A.H., Kannus, P., Järvinen, T.L.N., et al., 2000. Tenascin-C in the pathobiology and healing process of musculoskeletal tissue injury. Scandinavian Journal of Medicine and Science in Sports 10 (6), 376–382.

Johansson, C., 1986. Injuries in elite orienteers. American Journal of Sports Medicine 14 (5), 410–415.

Kader, D., Saxena, A., Movin, T., et al., 2002. Achilles tendinopathy: some aspects of basic science and clinical management. British Journal of Sports Medicine 36 (4), 239–249.

Kane, T.P.C., Ismail, M., Calder, J.D.F., 2008. Topical glyceryl trinitrate and noninsertional Achilles tendinopathy. American Journal of Sports Medicine 36 (6), 1160–1163.

Karjalainen, P.T., Soila, K., Aronen, H.J., et al., 2000. MR imaging of overuse injuries of the Achilles tendon. American Journal of Roentgenology 175 (1), 251–260.

Kaufman, K.R., Brodine, S.K., Shaffer, R.A., et al., 1999. The effect of foot structure and range of motion on musculoskeletal overuse injuries. American Journal of Sports Medicine 27 (5), 585–593.

Kayser, R., Mahlfeld, K., Heyde, C.E., 2005. Partial rupture of the proximal Achilles tendon: a differential diagnostic problem in ultrasound imaging. British Journal of Sports Medicine 39 (11), 838–842.

Kearney, R., Costa, M.L., 2010. Insertional achilles tendinopathy management: a systematic review. Foot and Ankle International 31 (8), 689–694.

Khaliq, Y., Zhanel, G.G., 2003. Fluoroquinolone-associated tendinopathy: a critical review of the literature. Clinical Infectious Diseases 36 (11), 1404–1410.

Khan, K.M., Cook, J.L., Bonar, F., et al., 1999. Histopathology of common tendinopathies. Update and implications for clinical management. Sports Medicine 27 (6), 393–408.

Khan, K.M., Cook, J.L., Kannus, P., et al., 2002. Time to abandon the 'tendinitis' myth. British Medical Journal 324 (7338), 626–627.

Khan, K.M., Forster, B.B., Robinson, J., et al., 2003. Are ultrasound and magnetic resonance imaging of value in assessment of Achilles tendon disorders? A two year prospective study. British Journal of Sports Medicine 37 (2), 149–153.

Kingma, J.J., de Knikker, R., Wittink, H.M., et al., 2007. Eccentric overload training in patients with chronic Achilles tendinopathy: a systematic review. British Journal of Sports Medicine 41 (6), e3.

Knobloch, K., Kraemer, R., Jagodzinski, M., et al., 2007. Eccentric training decreases paratendon capillary blood flow and preserves paratendon oxygen saturation in chronic achilles tendinopathy. Journal of Orthopaedic and Sports Physical Therapy 37 (5), 269–276.

Knobloch, K., Schreibmueller, L., Longo, U.G., et al., 2008a. Eccentric exercises for the management of tendinopathy of the main body of the Achilles tendon with or without the AirHeel™ Brace. A randomized controlled trial. A: Effects on pain and microcirculation. Disability and Rehabilitation 30 (20–22), 1685–1691.

Knobloch, K., Yoon, U., Vogt, P.M., 2008b. Acute and overuse injuries correlated to hours of training in master running athletes. Foot and Ankle International 29 (7), 671–676.

Kountouris, A., Cook, J., 2007. Rehabilitation of Achilles and patellar tendinopathies. Best Practice and Research in Clinical Rheumatology 21 (2), 295–316.

Kujala, U., Sarna, S., Kaprio, J., 2005. Cumulative incidence of Achilles tendon rupture and tendinopathy in male former elite athletes. Clinical Journal of Sport Medicine 15 (3), 133–135.

Kvist, M., 1994. Achilles tendon injuries in athletes. Sports Medicine 18 (3), 173–201.

Landorf, K.B., Burns, J., 2008. Health outcome assessment. In: Yates, B. (Ed.), Merriman's assessment of the lower limb, third ed. Elsevier/Churchill Livingstone, Edinburgh, pp. 33–51.

Langberg, H., Ellingsgaard, H., Madsen, T., et al., 2007. Eccentric rehabilitation exercise increases peritendinous type I collagen synthesis in humans with Achilles tendinosis. Scandinavian Journal of Medicine and Science in Sports 17 (1), 61–66.

Lee, C.Y., Liu, X., Smith, C.L., et al., 2004. The combined regulation of estrogen and cyclic tension on fibroblast biosynthesis derived from anterior cruciate ligament. Matrix Biology 23 (5), 323–329.

Leung, J.L., Griffith, J.F., 2008. Sonography of chronic Achilles tendinopathy: a case-control study. Journal of Clinical Ultrasound 36 (1), 27–32.

Lohrer, H., Arentz, S., Nauck, T., et al., 2008. The Achilles tendon insertion is crescent-shaped: an in vitro anatomic investigation. Clinical Orthopaedics and Related Research 466 (9), 2230–2237.

Longo, U.G., Ramamurthy, C., Denaro, V., et al., 2008. Minimally invasive stripping for chronic Achilles tendinopathy. Disability and Rehabilitation 30 (20–22), 1709–1713.

Longo, U., Rittweger, J., Garau, G., et al., 2009. No influence of age, gender, weight, height, and impact profile in Achilles tendinopathy in masters track and field athletes. American Journal of Sports Medicine 37 (7), 1400–1405.

Lowdon, A., Bader, D.L., Mowat, A.G., 1984. The effect of heel pads on the treatment of Achilles tendinitis: A double blind trial. American Journal of Sports Medicine 12 (6), 431–435.

Lysholm, J., Wiklander, J., 1987. Injuries in runners. American Journal of Sports Medicine 15 (2), 168–171.

Maclellan, G.E., Vyvyan, B., 1981. Management of pain beneath the heel and Achilles tendonitis with visco-elastic heel inserts. British Journal of Sports Medicine 15 (2), 117–121.

Madeley, L.T., Munteanu, S.E., Bonanno, D.R., 2007. Endurance of the ankle joint plantar flexor muscles in athletes with medial tibial stress syndrome: a case–control study. Journal of Science and Medicine in Sport 10 (6), 356–362.

McCrory, J.L., Martin, D.F., Lowery, R.B., et al., 1999. Etiologic factors associated with Achilles tendinitis in runners. Medicine and Science in Sports and Exercise 31 (10), 1374–1381.

Maffulli, N., 2013. Haematopoietic stem cell transplantation and the price to pay for. Translational Medicine@UniSa 5, 4.

Maffulli, N., Kader, D., 2002. Tendinopathy of the tendo achillis. Journal of Bone and Joint Surgery British Volume 84 (1), 1–8.

Maffulli, N., Del Buono, A., 2012. Platelet plasma rich products in musculoskeletal medicine: any evidence? The Surgeon 10 (3), 148–150.

Maffulli, N., Testa, V., Capasso, G., et al., 1997. Results of percutaneous longitudinal tenotomy for Achilles tendinopathy in middle- and long-distance runners. American Journal of Sports Medicine 25 (6), 835–840.

Maffulli, N., Kenward, M.G., Testa, V., et al., 2003. Clinical diagnosis of Achilles tendinopathy with tendinosis. Clinical Journal of Sport Medicine 13 (1), 11–15.

Maffulli, N., Testa, V., Capasso, G., et al., 2006. Surgery for chronic Achilles tendinopathy yields worse results in nonathletic patients. Clinical Journal of Sport Medicine 16 (2), 123–128.

Maffulli, N., Longo, U.G., Denaro, V., 2009. Achilles tendinopathy: recent advances. Advances in Orthopaedics 1 (4), 143–150.

Mafi, N., Lorentzon, R., Alfredson, H., 2001. Superior short-term results with eccentric calf muscle training compared with concentric training in a randomized prospective multicenter study on patients with chronic Achilles tendinosis. Knee Surgery, Sports Traumatology, Arthroscopy 9 (1), 42–47.

Magee, D.J., 1997. Orthopaedic physical assessment, third ed. WB Saunders, Philadelphia.

Magnussen, R.A., Dunn, W.R., Thomson, A.B., 2009. Nonoperative treatment of midportion Achilles tendinopathy: a systematic review. Clinical Journal of Sport Medicine 19 (1), 54–64.

Magra, M., Maffulli, N., 2007. Genetics: does it play a role in tendinopathy? Clinical Journal of Sport Medicine 17 (4), 231–233.

Mahieu, N.N., Witvrouw, E., Stevens, V., et al., 2006. Intrinsic risk factors for the development of achilles tendon overuse injury: a prospective study. American Journal of Sports Medicine 34 (2), 226–235.

Mayer, F., Hirschmuller, A., Muller, S., et al., 2007. Effects of short-term treatment strategies over 4 weeks in Achilles tendinopathy. British Journal of Sports Medicine 41 (7), e6.

Mazzone, M.F., McCue, T., 2002. Common conditions of the Achilles tendon. American Family Physician 65 (9), 1805–1810.

Menz, H.B., Jordan, K.P., Roddy, E., et al., 2010. Characteristics of primary care consultations for musculoskeletal foot and ankle problems in the UK. Rheumatology (Oxford, England) 49 (7), 1391–1398.

Meyer, A., Tumilty, S., Baxter, G., 2009. Eccentric exercise protocols for chronic non-insertional Achilles tendinopathy: how much is enough? Scandinavian Journal of Medicine and Science in Sports 19 (5), 609–615.

Mokone, G.G., Gajjar, M., September, A.V., et al., 2005. The guanine–thymine dinucleotide repeat polymorphism within the tenascin-C gene is associated with achilles tendon injuries. American Journal of Sports Medicine 33 (7), 1016–1021.

Mokone, G.G., Schwellnus, M.P., Noakes, T.D., et al., 2006. The COL5A1 gene and Achilles tendon pathology. Scandinavian Journal of Medicine and Science in Sports 16 (1), 19–26.

Moll, J.M.H., 1987. Seronegative arthropathies in the foot. Baillière's Clinical Rheumatology 1 (2), 289–314.

Möller, M., Lind, K., Styf, J., et al., 2005. The reliability of isokinetic testing of the ankle joint and a heel-raise test for endurance. Knee Surgery, Sports Traumatology, Arthroscopy 13 (1), 60–71.

Movin, T., Gad, A., Reinholt, F.P., et al., 1997. Tendon pathology in long-standing achillodynia. Biopsy findings in 40 patients. Acta Orthopaedica Scandinavica 68 (2), 170–175.

Munteanu, S., Barton, C., 2011. Lower limb biomechanics during running in individuals with achilles tendinopathy: a systematic review. Journal of Foot and Ankle Research 4 (1), 15.

Munteanu, S.E., Strawhorn, A.B., Landorf, K.B., et al., 2009. A weightbearing technique for the measurement of ankle joint dorsiflexion with the knee extended is reliable. Journal of Science and Medicine in Sport 12 (1), 54–59.

Murphy, D.F., Connolly, D.A.J., Beynnon, B.D., 2003. Risk factors for lower extremity injury: a review of the literature. British Journal of Sports Medicine 37 (1), 13–29.

Murrell, G.A., Szabo, C., Hannafin, J.A., et al., 1997. Modulation of tendon healing by nitric oxide. Inflammation Research 46 (1), 19–27.

Næsdal, J., Brown, K., 2006. NSAID-associated adverse effects and acid control aids to prevent them: a review of current treatment options. Drug Safety 29 (2), 119–132.

Neeter, C., Thomeé, R., Silbernagel, K.G., et al., 2003. Iontophoresis with or without dexamethazone in the treatment of acute Achilles tendon pain. Scandinavian Journal of Medicine and Science in Sports 13 (6), 376–382.

Niesen-Vertommen, S.L., Taunton, J.E., Clement, D.B., et al., 1992. The effect of eccentric versus concentric exercise in the management of Achilles tendonitis. Clinical Journal of Sport Medicine 2 (2), 109–113.

Nørregaard, J., Larsen, C.C., Bieler, T., et al., 2007. Eccentric exercise in treatment of Achilles tendinopathy. Scandinavian Journal of Medicine and Science in Sports 17 (2), 133–138.

Ohberg, L., Alfredson, H., 2004. Effects on neovascularisation behind the good results with eccentric training in chronic midportion Achilles tendinosis? Knee Surgery, Sports Traumatology, Arthroscopy 12 (5), 465–470.

Ohberg, L., Lorentzon, R., Alfredson, H., 2004. Eccentric training in patients with chronic Achilles tendinosis: normalised tendon structure and decreased thickness at follow up. British Journal of Sports Medicine 38 (1), 8–11.

Paavola, M., Orava, S., Leppilahti, J., et al., 2000. Chronic Achilles tendon overuse injury: complications after surgical treatment. An analysis of 432 consecutive patients. American Journal of Sports Medicine 28 (1), 77–82.

Paavola, M., Kannus, P., Järvinen, T., et al., 2002. Achilles tendinopathy. Journal of Bone and Joint Surgery, American Volume 84-A (11), 2062–2076.

Paoloni, J.A., Appleyard, R.C., Nelson, J., et al., 2004. Topical glyceryl trinitrate treatment of chronic noninsertional Achilles tendinopathy: a randomized, double-blind, placebo-controlled trial. Journal of Bone and Joint Surgery, American Volume 86 (5), 916–922.

Paoloni, J., De Vos, R.J., Hamilton, B., et al., 2011. Platelet-rich plasma treatment for ligament and tendon injuries. Clinical Journal of Sport Medicine 21 (1), 37–45.

Petersen, W., Welp, R., Rosenbaum, D., 2007. Chronic Achilles tendinopathy. American Journal of Sports Medicine 35 (10), 1659–1667.

Posthumus, M., Collins, M., Cook, J., et al., 2010. Components of the transforming growth factor-β family and the pathogenesis of human Achilles tendon pathology – a genetic association study. Rheumatology (Oxford, England) 49 (11), 2090–2097.

Pottie, P., Presle, N., Terlain, B., et al., 2006. Obesity and osteoarthritis: more complex than predicted! Annals of the Rheumatic Diseases 65 (11), 1403–1405.

Raleigh, S.M., van der Merwe, L., Ribbans, W.J., et al., 2009. Variants within the MMP3 gene are associated with Achilles tendinopathy: possible interaction with the COL5A1 gene. British Journal of Sports Medicine 43 (7), 514–520.

Rasmussen, S., Christensen, M., Mathiesen, I., et al., 2008. Shockwave therapy for chronic Achilles tendinopathy: a double-blind, randomized clinical trial of efficacy. Acta Orthopaedica 79 (2), 249–256.

Rees, J.D., Wilson, A.M., Wolman, R.L., 2006. Current concepts in the management of tendon disorders. Rheumatology (Oxford, England) 45 (5), 508–521.

Reinschmidt, C., Nigg, B.M., 1995. Influence of heel height on ankle joint moments in running. Medicine and Science in Sports and Exercise 27 (3), 410–416.

Robinson, J.M., Cook, J.L., Purdam, C., et al., 2001. The VISA-A questionnaire: a valid and reliable index of the clinical severity of Achilles tendinopathy. British Journal of Sports Medicine 35 (5), 335–341.

Rolf, C., Movin, T., 1997. Etiology, histopathology, and outcome of surgery in achillodynia. Foot and Ankle International 18 (9), 565–569.

Rompe, J.D., Nafe, B., Furia, J.P., et al., 2007. Eccentric loading, shock-wave treatment, or a wait-and-see policy for tendinopathy of the main body of tendo Achillis: a randomized controlled trial. American Journal of Sports Medicine 35 (3), 374–383.

Rompe, J.D., Furia, J., Maffulli, N., 2009. Eccentric loading versus eccentric loading plus shock-wave treatment for midportion Achilles tendinopathy. American Journal of Sports Medicine 37 (3), 463–470.

Roos, E.M., Engström, M., Lagerquist, A., et al., 2004. Clinical improvement after 6 weeks of eccentric exercise in patients with mid-portion Achilles tendinopathy: a randomized trial with 1-year follow-up. Scandinavian Journal of Medicine and Science in Sports 14 (5), 286–295.

Ryan, M., Grau, S., Krauss, I., et al., 2009. Kinematic analysis of runners with Achilles mid-portion tendinopathy. Foot and Ankle International 30 (12), 1190–1195.

Sayana, M.K., Maffulli, N., 2007. Eccentric calf muscle training in non-athletic patients with Achilles tendinopathy. Journal of Science and Medicine in Sport 10 (1), 52–58.

Schäffer, M.R., Efron, P.A., Thornton, F.J., et al., 1997. Nitric oxide, an autocrine regulator of wound fibroblast synthetic function. Journal of Immunology 158 (5), 2375–2381.

Schepsis, A.A., Jones, H., Haas, A.L., 2002. Achilles tendon disorders in athletes. American Journal of Sports Medicine 30 (2), 287–305.

Schweitzer, M.E., Karasick, D., 2000. MR imaging of disorders of the Achilles tendon. American Journal of Roentgenology 175 (3), 613–625.

September, A., Mokone, G.G., Schwellnus, M.P., et al., 2006. Genetic risk factors for Achilles tendon injuries. International SportMed Journal 7 (3), 201–215.

Silbernagel, K.G., Thomeé, R., Thomeé, P., et al., 2001. Eccentric overload training for patients with chronic Achilles tendon pain – a randomised controlled study with reliability testing of the evaluation methods. Scandinavian Journal of Medicine and Science in Sports 11 (4), 197–206.

Silbernagel, K., Gustavsson, A., Thomeé, R., et al., 2006. Evaluation of lower leg function in patients with Achilles tendinopathy. Knee Surgery, Sports Traumatology, Arthroscopy 14 (11), 1207–1217.

Silbernagel, K.G., Thomeé, R., Eriksson, B.I., et al., 2007a. Full symptomatic recovery does not ensure full recovery of muscle-tendon function in patients with Achilles tendinopathy. British Journal of Sports Medicine 41 (4), 276–280, discussion 280. Epub 2007 Jan 29.

Silbernagel, K.G., Thomeé, R., Eriksson, B.I., et al., 2007b. Continued sports activity, using a pain-monitoring model, during rehabilitation in patients with Achilles tendinopathy: a randomized controlled study. American Journal of Sports Medicine 35 (6), 897–906.

Smith, M., Brooker, S., Vicenzino, B., et al., 2004. Use of anti-pronation taping to assess suitability of orthotic prescription: case report. Australian Journal of Physiotherapy 50 (2), 111–113.

Spink, M.J., Fotoohabadi, M.R., Menz, H.B., 2010. Foot and ankle strength assessment using hand-held dynamometry: reliability and age-related differences. Gerontology 56 (6), 525–532.

Stergioulas, A., Stergioula, M., Aarskog, R., et al., 2008. Effects of low-level laser therapy and eccentric exercises in the treatment of recreational athletes with chronic Achilles tendinopathy. American Journal of Sports Medicine 36 (5), 881–887.

Sussmilch-Leitch, S.P., Collins, N.J., Bialocerkowski, A.E., et al., 2012. Physical therapies for Achilles tendinopathy: systematic review and meta-analysis. Journal of Foot and Ankle Research 5 (1), 15.

Taunton, J.E., Ryan, M.B., Clement, D.B., et al., 2002. A retrospective case–control analysis of 2002 running injuries. British Journal of Sports Medicine 36 (2), 95–101.

Taylor, D.W., Petrera, M., Hendry, M., et al., 2011. A systematic review of the use of platelet-rich plasma in sports medicine as a new treatment for tendon and ligament injuries. Clinical Journal of Sport Medicine 21 (4), 344–352.

Testa, V., Capasso, G., Benazzo, F., et al., 2002. Management of Achilles tendinopathy by ultrasound-guided percutaneous tenotomy. Medicine and Science in Sports and Exercise 34 (4), 573–580.

Theobald, P., Benjamin, M., Nokes, L., et al., 2005. Review of the vascularisation of the human Achilles tendon. Injury 36 (11), 1267–1272.

Thomeé, R., 1997. A comprehensive treatment approach for patellofemoral pain syndrome in young women. Physical Therapy 77 (12), 1690–1703.

Tol, J.L., Spiezia, F., Maffulli, N., 2012. Neovascularization in Achilles tendinopathy: have we been chasing a red herring? Knee Surgery, Sports Traumatology, Arthroscopy 20 (10), 1891–1894.

Tumilty, S., McDonough, S., Hurley, D.A., et al., 2012. Clinical effectiveness of low-level laser therapy as an adjunct to eccentric exercise for the treatment of Achilles' tendinopathy: a randomized controlled trial. Archives of Physical Medicine and Rehabilitation 93 (5), 733–739.

van der Linden, P.D., Sturkenboom, M.C., Herings, R.M., et al., 2002. Fluoroquinolones and risk of Achilles tendon disorders: case-control study. British Medical Journal 324 (7349), 1306–1307.

Van Ginckel, A., Thijs, Y., Hesar, N.G.Z., et al., 2008. Intrinsic gait-related risk factors for Achilles tendinopathy in novice runners: a prospective study. Gait and Posture 29 (3), 387–391.

van Sterkenburg, M., van Dijk, C., 2011. Mid-portion Achilles tendinopathy: why painful? An evidence-based philosophy. Knee Surgery, Sports Traumatology, Arthroscopy 19 (8), 1367–1375.

van Sterkenburg, M.N., de Jonge, M.C., Sierevelt, I.N., et al., 2010. Less promising results with sclerosing ethoxysclerol injections for midportion Achilles tendinopathy: a retrospective study. American Journal of Sports Medicine 38 (11), 2226–2232.

Williams, D.S.B., Zambardino, J.A., Banning, V.A., 2008. Transverse-plane mechanics at the knee and tibia in runners with and without a history of Achilles tendonopathy. Journal of Orthopaedic and Sports Physical Therapy 38 (12), 761–767.

Williams, J.G., 1993. Achilles tendon lesions in sport. Sports Medicine 16, 216–220.

Wilson, F., Byrne, A., Gissane, C., 2011. A prospective study of injury and activity profile in elite soccer referees and assistant referees. Irish Medical Journal 104 (10), 295–297.

Wyndow, N., Cowan, S.M., Wrigley, T.V., et al., 2010. Neuromotor control of the lower limb in Achilles tendinopathy: implications for foot orthotic therapy. Sports Medicine 40 (9), 715–727.

Chapter 7

Stress Fracture/Stress Reaction of the Lower Leg and Foot

Mark W. Creaby, Peter D. Brukner, and Kim L. Bennell

Chapter Outline

INTRODUCTION

Stress fractures and stress reactions of the lower leg and foot typically present as localized pain and tenderness of insidious onset that is aggravated by weight-bearing activity. They are most commonly observed in individuals participating in heavy physical training that involves repetitive impacts to the lower leg, such as that associated with the footstrike during running. This repetitive loading leads to microfractures in the bone, and it is the propagation of these microfractures that is ultimately thought to lead to the development of a stress fracture. Stress fracture represents the endpoint failure along a continuum of stress responses that may be observed in bone, and collectively can be described as bone stress injuries. These injuries range from mild, and often asymptomatic, 'bone strains', through to stress reactions and painful stress fractures that require an extended period of non-weightbearing and subsequent rehabilitation. Although most of these injuries have a good prognosis, stress fractures at some specific anatomical sites are associated with a high risk of delayed healing and/or lengthy rehabilitation periods.

In this chapter we outline the pathological mechanisms at play along the stress fracture continuum, and how these pathological mechanisms link with the populations most commonly affected by the injury. We then discuss specific predisposing factors for these injuries, and how these factors relate to the underlying pathomechanics of the injury. In diagnosing and treating the injury, there are various factors that must be considered, including appropriate use of medical imaging through to the choice of pharmacological, physical, and/or surgical options for treatment. Each of these factors requires careful consideration to ensure a successful outcome for the patient, and the best available evidence will be used to outline the benefits and limitations associated with the current diagnostic and management options. We conclude with the anticipated advances in the prevention, diagnosis, and management of stress fractures over the next 10 years, which will contribute to a reduction in the incidence of these injuries and improvements in treatment outcomes.

Much of the research evidence in this area has focused upon full stress fractures, and not the milder forms of the injury (bone strains and stress reactions). For this reason, we use the term 'stress fracture' when referring to the spectrum of injury. As the stress fracture represents the end point on a continuum, it is considered that the factors associated with the injury are consistent across this continuum.

AETIOLOGY

Two of the primary functions of the bones of the lower leg are (i) to bear the mechanical load of body weight during stance and ambulation, and (ii) to provide rigid mechanical levers to transmit the forces developed through muscular contraction. As such, these bones are exposed to repeated mechanical loading during activities of daily living such as standing and walking, as well as during more physically demanding tasks such as running and jumping. These loads translate to strain within the bone; that is, these applied loads cause the bone tissue to deform. This may be in the form of compressive, tensile, bending, twisting, and shear loads, or any combination of these. Bone is generally well adapted to resist deformation, and can typically absorb compressive strain of up to 1% of its length before acute failure (Warden et al. 2006). The magnitude of strain acting upon the bones of the lower limb during different activities is in the order of 0.1–0.3% (Burr et al. 1996; Milgrom et al. 2003) (Figure 7-1). Although normal physical activity is not associated with the magnitude of strain required to invoke acute failure of bone, small fractures in the bone tissue at a macroscopic level frequently occur with a moderately high magnitude or rate of strain. When associated with appropriate rest between loading bouts, these 'microfractures' will contribute towards the maintenance of bone health, via damage-related remodelling to repair and strengthen the bone (via alterations in bone geometry and bone material

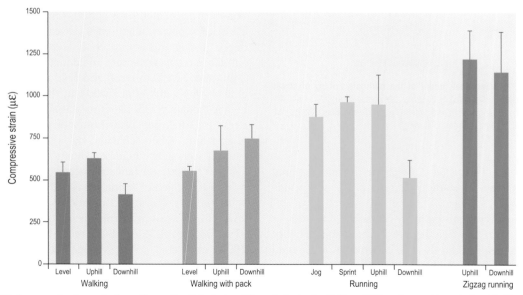

FIGURE 7-1 Compressive bone strains acting on the tibia during different physical activities. 1000 $\mu\varepsilon$ is equal to a strain of 0.1%. (Reprinted from Burr DB, Milgrom C, Fyhrie D, et al. In vivo measurement of human tibial strains during vigorous activity, Bone, 18(5), 405-410 © 1996, with permission from Elsevier.)

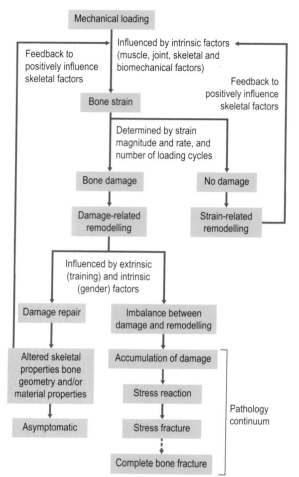

FIGURE 7-2 Theoretical model of the pathophysiology of stress fracture injury. (Reprinted from Magee JD, Zachazewski JE, Quillen WS, eds. (2001), Pathology and Intervention in Musculoskeletal Rehabilitation, WB Saunders, with permission from Elsevier.)

properties). This leaves the bone better prepared to resist future loading at a similar magnitude (Figure 7-2).

The pathological pathway of stress fractures is believed to ensue when the rate at which bony damage occurs is greater than the rate at which it is repaired (see Figure 7-2). If this situation continues, bony damage will accrue, resulting in stress fracture. The longer this continues, the more severe the injury is likely to become. Moreover, with the accrual of damage, bone becomes mechanically weaker and thus

the injury can deteriorate as the bone becomes less able to resist the mechanical loading associated with continued activity.

EPIDEMIOLOGY

Given the involvement of repeated bone loading in the aetiology of stress fractures, it is not surprising that stress fractures to the lower leg and foot are most common in populations participating in sports or activities involving running. In particular, distance-running athletes and military recruits sustain a high incidence of stress fractures. Stress fractures have also been reported in a wide variety of other competitive and recreational sporting groups. In these groups, the incidence of lower limb stress fractures varies dramatically and this is likely to be related to the varying nature of bone loading and exposure to other predisposing factors for stress fractures between these groups, together with methodological differences in terms of stress fracture diagnosis. For example, over a 2-year period, 15 of 139 elite male and female tennis players reported stress fractures (10.7%) (Maquirriain and Ghisi 2006). In female soccer players, however, the annual incidence is reported to be just 0.8% (Giza et al. 2005).

Prospective studies – those that observe a population over a specified time period – represent the most statistically powerful approach to establish injury incidence. Using this approach it is reported that the annualized stress fracture incidence varies between 2.9% and 21.1% in track and field athletes (Bennell et al. 1996; Nattiv et al. 2000). In the study with the higher incidence (21.1%), this was equivalent to 0.70 stress fractures per 1000 hours of training (Bennell et al. 1996). When separated by event, long-distance runners were at the highest risk of stress fracture, followed by middle-distance runners, then sprinters and field event athletes (Bennell et al. 1996).

In military training populations the incidence of lower limb stress fractures varies between 1% and 31% (Beck et al. 2000; Bijur et al. 1997; Gam et al. 2005; Jones et al. 1993; Milgrom et al. 1985; Pester and Smith 1992; Protzman and Griffis 1977; Shaffer et al. 2006). Care must be taken however, in the interpretation of these data, as the observation period varies between studies (6 to 12 weeks), and is much shorter than in the athletic studies reported above.

Moreover, the observation period typically covers the duration of specific military training courses involving heavy physical activity, and thus the reported incidence is likely to be higher than that observed in military service personnel as a whole.

There is some evidence that lower limb stress fracture incidence is marginally higher in females, compared with males. A recent systematic review by Wentz and colleagues (2011) reports that the average incidence of lower limb stress fractures in female athletes was 9.7%, but only 6.5% in male athletes. In military populations this difference between the genders was more marked, with an average incidence of 9.2% in females and 3% in males. It is important to note that direct comparisons between the genders are difficult given differences in training volumes and intensities. In the one known study to control for training volume, there was no difference in stress fracture incidence between the genders (Bennell et al. 1996); however, this study was not statistically powered to detect a difference in fracture incidence between the genders. In military populations where females have been exposed to the same training volume and intensity as their male counterparts, incidence is generally much higher in females (Brudvig et al. 1983; Protzman and Griffis 1977). (The mechanisms that contribute to the different incidence between the genders is discussed in the Gender section of Predisposing factors.)

The distribution of stress fractures between the bones of the lower limb appears to be largely consistent across studies in athletic populations, whereas there is some variation in the pattern of fracture distribution between studies in military populations (Wentz et al. 2011). Across nine studies of stress fracture distribution in athletes, Wentz and colleagues (2011), report that the tibia was by far the most common site of fracture, accounting for between 16% and 48.2% of all stress fractures (Korpelainen et al. 2001; Myburgh et al. 1990). This is followed by metatarsal (8–34.7%) and navicular (11.8–18.3%) fractures (Wentz et al. 2011). In military populations, the most common fracture site varies between the tibia (14–74%) and metatarsals (9–52.5%) (Armstrong et al. 2004; Pester and Smith 1992; Wentz et al. 2011). The relative distribution of lower leg and foot stress fractures will be influenced by numerous factors, including the type of sporting activities undertaken,

bone strength, and also ease of diagnosis at the particular site.

PREDISPOSING FACTORS

A fundamental aspect in the prevention of stress fractures is the identification of 'at-risk' individuals. Risk factors are markers that can be used to identify such individuals, and specific strategies may then be employed to reduce an individual's risk. Importantly, the risk factors themselves may not be involved in a stress fracture's pathogenesis; rather, they directly or indirectly increase the chance of a stress fracture developing. This may be by their influence on either the mechanical environment of bone or the remodelling process.

Risk factors can be separated into two distinct categories: (i) intrinsic and (ii) extrinsic. Intrinsic risk factors refer to factors within the individual that affect risk, for example bone density. Extrinsic risk factors refer to factors external to the individual that affect risk, for example training surface.

INTRINSIC FACTORS

Injury History

Previous history of stress fracture injury has been identified as a strong risk factor for subsequent stress fracture development. In a study of 127 female cross-country runners, stress fracture risk was 6.7 times higher (95% CI: 1.80, 22.87) in those with a previous history of stress fractures (Kelsey et al. 2007). This elevated risk of stress fracture was above and beyond its association with bone mineral content and density, suggesting that either a history of stress fracture in itself elevates the risk of subsequent fracture, or that it is indicative of risk factors other than bone content and density. Thus, it is particularly important that individuals with a history of stress fractures and their coaches are mindful of this increased risk and take appropriate steps to minimize the individual's exposure to risk factors.

Bone Strength

The ability of bone to resist the mechanical loads applied upon it is termed 'bone strength'. This is of particular importance in stress fracture injury as an inability to resist mechanical load results in microfracture within the bone, which over time may propagate to a full stress fracture injury. The main factors that determine bone strength are its density and geometry. Generally, a stronger bone is one with higher density and a larger cross-sectional size relative to its length. Consistent with this, it is widely reported that runners with a history of stress fracture injuries have lower bone density (Bennell et al. 1996; Carbon et al. 1990; Myburgh et al. 1990) and a smaller cross-sectional size (Crossley et al. 1999; Franklyn et al. 2008; Popp et al. 2009) than runners with no history of stress fractures. From these density and geometry data, Popp and colleagues (2009) estimated the bending strength of the tibia, and indeed found it to be weaker in female runners with a history of tibial stress fracture compared with uninjured female runners.

More powerful evidence for the role of bone strength in the development of stress fractures comes from longitudinal cohort studies in runners and also in military recruits. In a study of competitive female cross-country runners (aged 18–26 years), Kelsey et al. (2007) identified low whole-body bone mineral density at entry to the study as a substantial risk factor for stress fracture development over the following 2 years; for every 293.2 g decrease in whole-body bone content the risk of lower limb stress fracture increased by 2.70 times (95% CI: 1.26, 5.88). Lower bone density measured at specific sites, such as the hip and the spine, were also significant risk factors for stress fracture development. Similarly, Bennell et al. (1996) identified low lumbar spine bone density as a risk factor for stress fracture in female track and field athletes, but low bone density was not a risk factor in their male counterparts. Data from military recruits show a similar pattern. A large prospective study of 1288 recruits (Beck et al. 2000) mirrors the findings of Bennell et al. (1996), in that low bone density is a risk factor for stress fracture in females but not in males.

Aspects of bone cross-sectional geometry play an important role in determining the bone strength with respect not only to compressive loads, but also to bending and torsional loads. Given the combination of loads acting upon the long bones of the leg, it is not surprising that a smaller cross-sectional bone geometry has been linked with increased fracture risk.

Prospective studies in military populations (Beck et al. 1996, 2000; Giladi et al. 1987; Milgrom et al. 1988, 1989) indicate that smaller anterior–posterior tibial width, medial–lateral tibial width, and the distribution of bone closer to its neutral axis are likely to increase the risk of tibial and femoral stress fracture development. Although not investigated prospectively, cross-sectional data in runners indicate a similar pattern of smaller cross-sectional tibial geometry in individuals with a history of tibial stress fracture (Crossley et al. 1999; Popp et al. 2009).

To date, our understanding of the role of bone structural and material properties in stress fracture injuries of the lower leg is limited to measurements taken of the tibia. It is not known whether site-specific bone properties are an important risk factor for the development of stress fractures in the fibula, or the bones of the foot. Although the structural and material properties of the metatarsals are known to influence bone strength in older individuals (Courtney et al. 1997; Muehleman et al. 2000), their influence upon stress fracture risk in young and otherwise healthy individuals is considered to be minimal in comparison to other risk factors.

Genetic and Nutritional Factors

There is growing evidence that genetic factors may play a role in predisposing an individual to lower leg stress fractures. A family history (parents, grandparents, or siblings) of osteoporosis or osteopenia has been shown to triple the risk of stress fractures in female adolescents participating in impact sports (OR: 2.96; 95% CI: 1.36, 6.45) (Loud et al. 2007). This is supported by similar findings in female and male military recruits (Friedl et al. 1992; Yanovich et al. 2012). Genetic factors play a significant role in determining bone strength (Nguyen and Eisman 2000) via their direct influence upon structural factors such as collagen distribution (Uitterlinden et al. 1998), or indirect effects upon the endocrine and digestive systems (Morrison et al. 1994; Langdahl et al. 2000). It is proposed that, through this relationship with bone strength, genetic factors affect stress fracture risk.

The primary gene that has been studied to date in relation to stress fracture risk is the vitamin D receptor gene (*VDR*). Vitamin D binds to *VDR* with high affinity, and this aids in the efficient absorption of calcium from the intestine (Achermann and Jameson 2003; Norman 1990). This mechanism enables the adequate supply of calcium for the maintenance of bone density, such that vitamin D is positively associated with bone density (Cranney et al. 2008). Polymorphisms in the VDR gene (that affect gene expression) have been associated with an increased risk of stress fractures in military recruits (Chatzipapas et al. 2009; Yanovich et al. 2012), and may similarly influence stress fracture risk in athletes. It is also for their role in this pathway that low calcium (RR: 0.53; 95% CI: 0.29, 0.97) and vitamin D intake in the diet are associated with increased stress fracture risk (Nieves et al. 2010; Välimäki et al. 2005). In a similar light, calcium and vitamin D supplementation may be marginally beneficial in protecting against the incidence of stress fractures in female military recruits (OR: 0.789; 95% CI: 0.616, 1.01) (Lappe et al. 2008). Based on this most recent data, it is recommended that female athletes ensure their daily calcium intake is upwards of 1500 mg (Tenforde et al. 2010).

Muscle

Muscle plays an important role in modulating bone load during activity, and has therefore been linked with stress fracture development. Typically, external forces act at an angle to the long axis of bones, thus imparting bending and torsional loads upon the bone in addition to compressive loads. Muscle contraction can act to minimize these off-axis loads, whilst increasing compressive bone load (Haris Phuah et al. 2010; Sasimontonkul et al. 2007; Scott and Winter 1990). Importantly, as bone strength in compression is generally much greater than that in bending or torsion, muscle contraction is considered to protect bone against stress fractures (Radin 1986). Consistent with this, a prospective clinical study demonstrated a protective effect of greater strength during a 1RM leg press in male military recruits (Hoffman et al. 1999). Recruits who were able to press 1.11 kg/kg of body weight or less were more likely to develop a lower limb stress fracture than their stronger counterparts who were able to press more than 1.72 kg/kg of body weight (RR: 5.2, 95% CI: 1.8, 14.7). Others have reported no differences in knee extension (Schnackenburg et al. 2011; Välimäki et al. 2005), or ankle plantarflexion, inversion, and eversion strength

(Schnackenburg et al. 2011), between those with compared with those without stress fractures. However, limitations in study design (Schnackenburg et al. 2011), and measurement setup (Välimäki et al. 2005), limit confidence in these findings. Supporting the findings of Hoffman and colleagues (1999), measurements of thigh and calf muscle size indices indicate that a larger thigh and calf may be protective against lower limb stress fractures (Beck et al. 2000; Bennell et al. 1996). However, global indices of muscle strength (including upper body strength measurements) were not predictive of stress fracture development in military recruits after adjusting for covariates (Mattila et al. 2007).

Local muscular endurance may also be important in protecting against stress fractures. Studies of calf muscle fatigue have demonstrated that with the onset of fatigue the magnitude and rate of strain upon the tibia increases (Fyhrie et al. 1998; Milgrom et al. 2007). The implication of this is that poor calf muscle endurance will subject the individual to detrimental bone loads increasing the risk of stress fracture development. Evidence of this relationship from prospective studies is required.

Biomechanics

The intrinsic risk factors discussed above are largely considered to influence stress fracture risk via their effect upon bone strength. Of import, the external loads applied to bone will play an important role in determining bone health. One's biomechanics plays a central role in determining the rate, magnitude, and direction of the external loads applied to the bones of the body during every single running step. In this respect, both structural biomechanical factors, such as foot type, and functional biomechanical factors, such as stride length, can play an important role in stress fracture risk.

Structure. In female track and field athletes, a difference in leg length of greater than 0.5 cm was associated with increased risk of stress fracture development (Bennell et al. 1996). This is thought to be related to poor skeletal alignment in these individuals; however, fractures did not appear to occur predominantly in the shorter or longer limb (Bennell et al. 1996). A longer tibia relative to body size, however, was associated with increased risk of stress fracture in males during military training (Beck et al. 2000). With a longer bone there is an increase in the leverage of the forces applied upon the bone, such that higher bending loads – which may contribute to fracture development – are likely to be observed (Haris Phuah et al. 2010).

The sit-and-reach flexibility test, hip internal and external range of motion, foot type, lower limb alignment, calf flexibility, and ankle dorsiflexion range of motion have been shown not to relate to stress fracture risk in male and female track and field athletes (Bennell et al. 1996). In systematically reviewing the literature with regards to foot type and tibial stress injuries, Barnes and colleagues (2008) found only limited evidence supporting a link between high- and low-arched foot structures and increased risk of tibial stress fractures. There is however, a degree of consistency across the literature with respect to forefoot alignment. Compared with a neutral or valgus forefoot alignment, a varus alignment of the forefoot appears to increase the risk of stress fracture (Hughes 1985; Korpelainen et al. 2001; Matheson et al. 1987). Given the ease with which many of the structural biomechanical factors can be measured in the clinical setting, further investigation is merited to establish with greater certainty their relationship with stress fracture development.

Function. Measurement of the movement of the body (kinematics), and forces that drive that movement (kinetics), during activity can provide an indication of the rate, magnitude, and frequency of the loads that are acting on the bones of the lower leg during that particular activity. As these mechanical loads play a central role in determining bone strain, and ultimately any resulting microfracture to the bone, an individual's kinematics and kinetics have the potential to influence their risk of stress fracture development. Given that straight-line running is a common component of many sporting and military training activities, much of our understanding of the role of functional biomechanics in lower leg stress fracture comes from investigations of this fundamental skill.

Ground reaction forces provide valuable information regarding the rate, magnitude, and direction of external loads acting upon the body during contact with the ground. The vertical component of the ground reaction force is by far the largest component

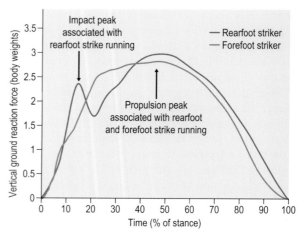

FIGURE 7-3 Typical vertical ground reaction forces for rearfoot- and forefoot-striking runners.

of this force during running and walking, but also during other movements such as kicking, jumping, landing, and changes of direction. During straight-line running, for a typical rearfoot striker, the vertical ground reaction force rapidly increases upon heel-strike, exhibits a sharp 'impact' peak, lowers somewhat before a larger 'propulsion' peak around mid-stance, and then gradually reduces to toe-off (Figure 7-3). Midfoot and forefoot strikers on the other hand do not typically exhibit the first 'impact' peak, and thus are generally associated with a lower rate of loading during the impact phase (see Figure 7-3).

Over the last 20 years several research groups have reported on the relationship between stress fracture history and characteristics of the ground reaction force. In order to provide some clarity around the conflicting findings of different studies in this area, Zadpoor and Nikooyan (2011) pooled data across all eligible studies in runners and military recruits. They found that vertical loading rate was 0.55 BW/s; (95% CI: 0.251, 0.840) higher with a history of tibial stress fracture, but the peak magnitude of the vertical ground reaction force was not different (mean difference: 0.10 BW; 95% CI: −0.159, 0.369). Vertical ground reaction forces did not appear to be related to stress fractures of the metatarsals; peak vertical ground reaction force was lower, but not significantly so in those with a metatarsal stress fracture history (mean difference:

−0.120 BW; 95% CI: −0.701, 0.461) (Zadpoor and Nikooyan 2011). There is also some evidence that the free moment of ground reaction force (the torsional moment between the foot and the ground) is higher in female runners with tibial stress fracture history (Milner et al. 2006a; Pohl et al. 2008). For every unit increase in the free moment, the odds of having a history of tibial stress fracture increased by 1.37 times (95% CI not provided). Whilst these factors may represent risk factors for injury development, we cannot be certain of this without evidence from a prospective study. To date, only one small study (10 subjects, 5 of which sustained a fracture) has examined the role of ground reaction forces in tibial stress fracture development. Consistent with the retrospective data, a higher loading rate of ground reaction force but not peak force magnitude appears to be a risk factor for tibial stress fracture development (Davis et al. 2004). Although limited to rearfoot strikers, these data suggest that midfoot and forefoot strikers are likely to be at lower risk of tibial stress fracture given the lower vertical loading rates exhibited by these groups (Nilsson and Thorstensson 1989). On the flipside of this, given the longer time period spent loading the forefoot, midfoot and forefoot strikers may be at increased risk of metatarsal stress fracture development.

In addition to ground reaction forces, many studies have investigated the role of running gait kinematics in tibial stress fracture injury, including hip, knee, and rearfoot motion (Milner et al. 2007, 2010; Pohl et al. 2008). Our ability to draw conclusions with respect to injury risk is, however, limited by the retrospective design of these studies (i.e. it is not possible to determine whether these differences are a cause or an effect of the stress fracture). With the more powerful prospective study design, Hetsroni et al. (2008) examined military recruits during barefoot treadmill walking prior to basic training. They reported that the less time the rearfoot spends in pronation the greater is the risk of tibial and femoral stress fracture during training; the odds ratio for stress fracture was 0.29 (95% CI: 0.09, 0.95) for the right leg, and 0.09 (95% CI: 0.02, 0.40) for the left leg if peak pronation was reached after 40% of stance, compared with those reaching peak pronation before 20% of stance. The magnitude and range of rearfoot pronation were not related to

stress fracture risk. Theoretically, it may be possible to alter the time the rearfoot spends in pronation by retraining gait patterns or using alternative footwear. It is not clear whether such alterations will affect stress fracture risk, however.

Physical Fitness

Poor physical fitness at the commencement of training is a well-established risk factor for stress fracture development in the military (Beck et al. 2000; Lappe et al. 2005). Female recruits who participated in weightbearing exercise at least three times a week prior to enrolment in military training were protected against stress fractures during training (RR: 0.65; 95% CI: 0.51, 0.82) (Lappe et al. 2005). Consistent with this, increased frequency of aerobic training prior to enrolment was protective in male military recruits (OR: 0.220; 95% CI: 0.082, 0.592) (Moran et al. 2012). The factors underlying this protective effect are unknown, but are probably related to the positive effects of prior exercise upon bone and muscle factors, amongst others. In sporting populations – who, unlike military recruits, generally spend many years gradually increasing their training load alongside increases in physical fitness – little is known about the role of physical fitness in stress fracture development. However, contrary to the findings in military, some recent evidence indicates that a longer history of participation in running increases the risk of stress fracture in females (OR: 1.288; 95% CI: 1.000, 1.658) (Wentz et al. 2012).

Gender

As discussed earlier, the incidence of lower limb stress fractures is typically higher in females than males. This may relate to a number of the other intrinsic risk factors discussed above that tend to place females at greater risk; for example, the cross-sectional geometry of the lower limb bones tends to be much smaller in females than males (Beck et al. 2000), which leaves the bone weaker, increasing the risk of stress fracture development.

The female athlete triad is also believed to play a substantial role in stress fracture development in females. The triad is described as a complex series of interrelationships between energy availability, menstrual status, and bone health (Manore et al. 2007).

Both restricted energy availability (Loucks 2007) and disrupted menstrual patterns (Drinkwater et al. 1984) have been associated with weaker bones, and this may in turn dispose to stress fracture development. Moreover, amenorrhoea (absent menstruation) and oligomenorrhoea (infrequent menstruation) have been associated with stress fracture in retrospective and prospective studies (Barrow and Saha 1988; Bennell et al. 1996; Lloyd et al. 1986; Myburgh et al. 1990). The precise pathways underlying this relationship between menstrual status and stress fracture are still not entirely clear. Whilst menstrual disturbance influences bone density, female athletes in this category are also likely to exhibit an impaired bone remodelling response (Zanker and Swaine 1998a, 1998b) such that bony damage sustained during training takes longer to repair and thus microfractures in the bone are more likely to propagate towards stress fracture injury.

Use of the oral contraceptive pill (OCP) may also have the potential to influence stress fracture risk. Several studies have examined the effect of OCP use upon bone material properties, with some promising findings. In synthesizing this literature, Liu and Lebrun (2006) concluded there was good evidence of bone density gains – indicating increased bone strength – with OCP use in peri-menopausal women, and fair evidence from bone density gains in pre-menopausal women with oligomenorrhoea or amenorrhoea. However, there was limited evidence of any benefits to pre-menopausal eumenorrhoeic women (Liu and Lebrun 2006). Supporting this, a recent study of female runners demonstrated a non-significant effect of OCP use protecting against stress fractures, alongside small increases in bone density (Cobb et al. 2007). However, as there is some evidence of OCP use inhibiting exercise-induced bone density gains (Weaver et al. 2001), caution should be exercised when considering OCP use to improve bone health.

EXTRINSIC FACTORS
Training Load

Repetitive mechanical loading arising from physical training can contribute to stress fracture development. However, the relative contribution of training volume, frequency, and intensity upon stress fracture development is not clearly understood. As discussed in the Aetiology section, with each footstrike external loads cause bone strains, which if large enough result in 'microfractures' within the bone tissue. Under normal conditions, and with the provision of adequate recovery, these fractures will resolve through the natural remodelling process. Although this remodelling process generally leads to increases in, or at least the maintenance of, bone strength in the longer term, bone resorption during the initial phases of remodelling may weaken the bone for up to 8 weeks following heavy loading. It is for this reason that some military training institutions employ so-called 'orthopaedic holidays' of 2 to 4 days rest at 6- to 8-week intervals during basic training (Ross and Allsopp 2002). Similar rest periods may be beneficial for athletic populations, particularly those with a high exposure to other risk factors for the injury. Other aspects of training load and recovery are also of vital importance in protecting against stress fracture, as nicely demonstrated in a recent military study. Finestone and Milgrom (2008) mandated a minimum nightly sleep requirement of 6 hours alongside a reduction in total marching hours, and observed a 62% reduction in the incidence of stress fractures. High training volume also increases the risk of lower limb stress fractures in runners. In a study of competitive and recreational runners, running greater than 30 miles per week, compared with running less than 20 miles per week, increased the risk of stress fracture by 5.9 times in females but only 1.8 times in males (Brunet et al. 1990).

There are many reports across the literature that stress fracture is typically preceded by a *change* in training load. This may come in a variety of forms, including an increase in training volume, frequency, and running speed, and the onset of interval training or hill running. These factors will either contribute to greater bone damage via increased magnitude or frequency of bone strain (e.g. increased running speed or training volume) or leave the bone less time to remodel and repair the damage incurred (e.g. shorter recovery periods due to increased training frequency). Consistent with this, up to 86% of athletes who sustain injuries report a change in training prior to injury development (Goldberg and Pecora 1994; Sullivan et al. 1984). However, it is not known whether this percentage of training changes is different from athletes that do not sustain stress fracture. Further study is required to establish the extent to which change in training affects stress fracture risk, and whether thresholds exist with respect to the magnitude of increases in training that can safely be applied.

Footwear

Both the type of footwear worn and use of shoe inserts or orthotics can influence stress fracture risk. Alterations in the mechanical properties of the shoe or insert will influence its ability to attenuate external loads, and thus the loads translated to bone. This is supported by findings from a study in Israeli military recruits that indicates the use of a modified basketball shoe – instead of the standard issue military boot – may protect against stress fractures of the metatarsals (RR: 0.07; 95% CI: 0.00, 1.26) (Milgrom et al. 1992; Rome et al. 2005), presumably due to the load attenuation properties of the shoe. This modified shoe, however, did not affect the incidence of tibial stress fractures (RR: 1.12; 95% CI: 0.72, 1.73) (Milgrom et al. 1992; Rome et al. 2000). Although the effect of shoe type upon stress fracture incidence in athletes has not been evaluated, measurement of ground reaction forces and plantar pressures indicate that running in racing flats may increase the risk of stress fractures in the foot compared with more mechanically compliant training shoes (Wiegerinck et al. 2009).

Modifying the attenuation of ground reaction forces may also be achieved with the use of shoe inserts of differing mechanical properties. Many varieties are available, some of the more well known are Neoprene, Sorbothane® and Poron®. Although there is some evidence of their effectiveness in reducing ground reaction forces (Dixon et al. 2003; Nigg et al. 1988) and plantar pressures (Windle et al. 1999), they do not appear to influence injury rates in military training (Andrish et al. 1974; Milgrom et al. 1985; Schwellnus et al. 1990; Snyder et al. 2009; Withnall et al. 2006). For example, Rome and colleagues (2000) reported on the findings of an earlier US military study (Bensel and Kaplan 1986) of urethane foam insoles that were shown to have no protective effect upon tibial (RR: 0.30; 95% CI: 0.05, 1.76), calcaneal (RR: 1.15; 95% CI: 0.61, 2.19) or metatarsal stress reactions (RR: 0.76; 95% CI: 0.31, 1.91). Although this suggests that shock-absorbing inserts are unlikely to reduce stress fracture risk in other populations, there is no research evidence currently available to substantiate this thought.

Rigid, or semi-rigid, orthotic shoe inserts may also be beneficial in reducing the risk of stress fracture development. These devices typically incorporate either a medial/lateral wedge-shaped top surface or contouring to provide additional support to the plantar surface of the foot, or both of these features. During running, this type of insert design has been demonstrated to alter the motion of the lower limb and the loads acting upon it (Mündermann et al. 2003; Nigg et al. 2003; Williams et al. 2003). It is not clear, however, whether the specific changes observed during running gait translate to a reduction in bone loading and stress fracture risk. In one small study, Ekenman et al. (2002) inserted strain gauges into the medial aspect of the tibia to quantify tibial bone strain during running with and without two orthotic devices. Semi-rigid orthotics (contoured to the shape of the foot, but with no wedging) did not influence the magnitude of peak strain, or strain range during running (Ekenman et al. 2002). It is not clear how these orthotics may influence bone strain at other sites. Moreover, there is currently no direct evidence of the influence of rigid or semi-rigid orthotic use upon stress fracture incidence in runners. Data are available from military populations, but again, these should be interpreted with caution given the differences in training activities and also the different footwear in which the orthotics are worn. These data suggest that there is a moderate protective effect of semi-rigid orthotics moulded to the shape of the individual's foot upon tibial (RR: 0.46; 95% CI: 0.22, 0.93) but not metatarsal (RR: 0.14; 95% CI: 0.01, 3.42) stress fractures (Finestone et al. 1999; Rome et al. 2000). The effect of orthotic use may also depend upon an individual's biomechanics. For example, orthotic use in military recruits with a low foot arch demonstrate a reduction in metatarsal stress fractures, whereas those with high arches demonstrate a reduction in femoral stress fractures (Simkin et al. 1989).

Running Surface

In the same manner that shock-absorbing insoles may attenuate load, different running surfaces may aid in reducing bone loads and thus stress fracture risk. Whereas some studies illustrate no reduction in peak loads and loading rates with softer, more compliant surfaces (Karamanidis et al. 2006), reductions in loading rate have been demonstrated (Dixon et al. 2000). There is also some evidence that reductions in loading rate may be subject-specific, such that only some individuals experience reduced loading when running on softer surfaces (Wheat et al. 2003). Recent evidence from a small retrospective study of female runners indicates a marginal association between stress fracture history and spending a larger percentage of training time on hard surfaces (OR: 1.032; 95% CI: 0.999, 1.066) (Wentz et al. 2012). Large epidemiological studies, however, have failed to demonstrate a relationship between running surface and injuries (Marti et al. 1988; Walter et al. 1989).

In addition to surface, running on uneven or cambered surfaces may accentuate intrinsic biomechanical risk factors or lead to increases in ground reaction forces and higher bone load. Similarly, running on a sharply curved track has been shown to elevate tibial loads over running on a track with a more gentle curvature (Kawamoto et al. 2002).

DIAGNOSIS

In the assessment of a patient presenting with a possible diagnosis of stress fracture, three questions need to be answered:

1. Is the pain bony in origin?
2. If so, which bone is involved?
3. At what stage in the continuum of bone stress is this injury?

To obtain an answer to these three questions, a thorough history, precise examination, and appropriate use of imaging techniques are used. In many cases the diagnosis of a leg or foot stress fracture will be relatively simple. In others, especially when the pattern of pain may be non-specific (e.g. navicular), the diagnosis can present a challenge for the physician. In addition to diagnosing the injury, the assessment needs to identify potential predisposing factors for the injury.

DIFFERENTIAL DIAGNOSIS

In the differential diagnosis of stress fracture, the causes can be non-bony or bony. Non-bony causes in particular relate to muscle or tendon injury (either muscle strain, haematoma, or delayed-onset muscle soreness or tendon inflammation) or degenerative change. Compartment syndrome, especially in the anterior and deep posterior compartments of the lower leg, may mimic a stress fracture as it also presents with exercise-related pain. Traction periostitis, such as that previously termed shin splints or medial tibial stress syndrome, may also mimic stress fractures, although the relationship of pain to exercise is different. Bone scan appearances of both compartment syndrome and periostitis differ from that of stress fracture.

Bony pathologies that can mimic stress fracture include tumour and infection. Osteoid osteoma is commonly mistaken for a stress fracture as it presents with pain at a discrete focal area with increased uptake on isotope bone scan. Two distinguishing features of osteoid osteoma are the presence of night pain and the relief of pain with the use of aspirin.

HISTORY

The history of the patient with a stress fracture is typically one of insidious onset of activity-related pain. Initially the pain will usually be described as a mild ache occurring after a specific amount of exercise. If the patient continues to exercise, the pain may well become more severe or occur at an earlier stage of exercise. The pain may increase, eventually limiting the quality or quantity of the exercise performed or occasionally forcing cessation of all activity. In the early stages, pain will usually cease soon after exercise. However, with continued exercise and increased severity of symptoms, the pain may persist after exercise. Night pain may occasionally occur.

The location of the pain may be ill-defined for some stress fractures, particularly in the early stages of the injury. For example, for the navicular, the pain typically radiates along the medial aspect of the longitudinal arch or along the dorsum of the foot but may also radiate distally along the first or second ray or laterally toward the cuboid.

It is also important to determine the presence of predisposing factors to the injury. Therefore a training or activity history is essential. In particular, note should be taken of recent changes in activity level such as increased quantity of training, increased intensity of training, and changes in surface, equipment (especially shoes), and technique. It may be necessary to obtain information from the patient's coach or trainer. A full dietary history should be taken with estimation of energy availability and particular attention should be paid to the possible presence of eating disorders. In females a menstrual history should be taken, including age of menarche and subsequent menstrual status.

A history of previous similar injury or any other musculoskeletal injury should be obtained. It is essential to obtain a brief history of the patient's general health, medications, and personal habits to gain an understanding of other factors that may be influencing bone health. It is also important to obtain from the history an understanding of the patient's work and sporting commitments. In particular, it is important to know the level, how serious the patient is about his or her sport, and what significant sporting commitments are ahead in the short and medium term.

PHYSICAL EXAMINATION

On physical examination the most obvious feature is localized bony tenderness. Palpable periosteal thickening may also be found, especially in a long-standing fracture of the tibia or fibula. Obviously tenderness is easier to determine in bones that are relatively superficial. It is important to be precise in the palpation of the affected areas, particularly in regions such as the foot where a number of bones and joints in a relatively small area may be affected. For stress fractures of the posteromedial tibia, palpation usually elicits specific point tenderness. This differs from medial tibial stress syndrome where the tenderness along the posteromedial tibial border extends along a greater length. Examination of the navicular bone requires precise knowledge of the anatomy of the midfoot and skilful palpation of the talonavicular joint. Having located this joint while inverting and everting the foot, the examiner palpates the proximal dorsal portion of the navicular bone. This has been described as the 'N-spot' and is typically the site of tenderness in the presence of navicular stress fracture (Khan et al. 1994).

There is often little else to find on physical examination. Occasionally, redness and swelling may be present at the site of the stress fracture. In the case of a medial malleolar stress fracture, an ankle effusion may be present. Joint range of motion is usually unaffected. Weightbearing can be difficult, particularly

shortly after exercise and for foot stress fractures. For a sesamoid stress fracture, the patient will often walk with the weight laterally to compensate.

It has been suggested that the presence of pain when either therapeutic continuous ultrasound or a vibrating tuning fork is applied over the area of the stress fracture is of potential use in diagnosis. A recent systematic review and meta-analysis identified nine articles assessing the diagnostic accuracy of ultrasound (seven articles) and tuning fork (two articles) for lower limb stress fractures (Schneiders et al. 2012). For ultrasound there was a pooled sensitivity, specificity, positive likelihood ratio (+LR), and negative likelihood ratio (−LR) of 64% (95% CI: 55, 73), 63% (95% CI: 54, 71), 2.1 (95% CI: 1.1, 3.5), and 0.3 (95% CI: 0.1, 0.9), respectively. Although tuning fork data could not be pooled, sensitivity, specificity, +LR, and −LR ranged from 35 to 92%, 19 to 83%, 0.6 to 3.0, and 0.4 to 1.6 respectively. These results do not support the use of ultrasound or tuning forks as standalone diagnostic tests for lower limb stress fractures.

The physical examination must also take into account the potential predisposing factors. In all stress fractures involving the lower limb, a full biomechanical examination must be performed. Any evidence of leg-length discrepancy, malalignment (especially excessive subtalar pronation), muscle imbalance, weakness, or lack of flexibility should be noted.

IMAGING

Imaging plays an important role in supplementing clinical examination to determine the answers to the three questions mentioned above. In many cases a clinical diagnosis of stress fracture is sufficient. The classic history of exercise-associated bone pain and typical examination findings of localized bony tenderness have a high correlation with the diagnosis of stress fracture. However, if the diagnosis is uncertain, or in the case of the serious or elite athlete who wishes to continue training if at all possible and requires more specific knowledge of his or her condition, various imaging techniques are available. Summaries comparing the imaging features and utility of the different techniques are shown respectively in Tables 7-1 and 7-2.

Attempts have been made to classify the stress fracture continuum into 'bone strain', 'stress reaction' and

TABLE 7-1   Image Characteristics, Advantages and Disadvantages of Tools Available to Detect Stress Reactions and Stress Fractures of the Lower Extremities

	Image Characteristics of Bone Stress Changes	Advantage	Disadvantage
Conventional radiography	Cortical bone: radiolucency at fracture line: callus formation at periosteal and endosteal surfaces; periosteal reaction; trabecular bone: line of sclerosis	Assess healing in late phase	Exposure to ionizing radiation, insensitive in detecting early stress changes
Bone scintigraphy	Non-specific tracer uptake in soft tissues and skeleton; degree of uptake depends on rate of bone turnover and blood flow	Detects early-stage bone stress, which may prevent progression to stress fracture; can differentiate between soft-tissue and bone injury	Repeat scanning prohibitive due to whole-body radiation exposure; diffuse, non-specific uptake; scan may be positive but patient asymptomatic; abnormal uptake may persist for several months
CT	Osteopenia as discrete lucent area; sclerotic fracture line; periosteal reaction; callus formation	Detects osteopenia; allows for differential diagnosis of bone pathology	Does not detect lesion activity; information obtained only for specific scan site; limited value for assessing soft tissue
MR imaging	Early changes: bone marrow, periosteal and muscle oedema. Later changes: low-signal fracture line surrounded by zone of oedema	High sensitivity and specificity for detecting early osseous changes; can localize injury site; no ionizing radiation; best for suspected femoral neck fractures	Cost; inferior imaging of cortical bone
Ultrasonography	Cortex appears linear and echogenic; periosteal elevation; fluid collection and soft-tissue oedema; increased vascularity at fracture area	No ionizing radiation; easy to perform	Further studies needed to confirm value of sonography as a diagnostic tool

CT=computed tomography; MR=magnetic resonance.
Reprinted from Moran DS, Evans RK, Hadad E. Imaging of Lower Extremity Stress Fracture Injuries, Sports Med 2008: 38(4), 345–356, with permission from Springer Science+Business Media.

'full stress fracture'. Many of the features associated with each stage of the continuum can be identified with imaging technologies. As the imaging characteristics differ between different imaging tools (Table 7-1), the choice of imaging tool will affect the clinicians' ability to determine the presence or severity of stress fracture injury. For example, although X-ray and CT imaging can be used to identify a fracture line associated with a full stress fracture, they cannot capture the changes in bone remodelling that occur with bone strains or stress reactions. Thus, imaging of a bone strain or stress reaction will appear normal with X-ray or CT. Contrary to this, radioisotopic bone scan is sensitive enough to image the increased remodelling associated with a bone strain or stress reaction, but cannot differentiate between these and a full stress fracture. MRI is currently the best available imaging technology to differentiate between the different severities of injury on the stress fracture continuum. With bone strain, increased high signal may be apparent and becomes clearly apparent with a stress reaction. With a stress fracture, increased high signal is apparent, and is often accompanied with evidence of a cortical defect. The sensitivity and specificity of each imaging tool is discussed in the following section.

TABLE 7-2 Utility of Methods Used to Detect Stress Reactions and Stress Fractures of the Lower Extremity

	Exposure to Ionizing Radiation	Early Detection of Bone Stress	Detects Bone Marrow Abnormalities	Detects Soft-tissue Abnormalities	Detects Cortical Changes	Differential Diagnosis	Ability to Localize Lesion Site	Follow-up to Assess Healing
Conventional radiography	Yes	+	+	+	+++	+++	+	++
Bone scintigraphy	Yes	+++	+++	+	++	+	++	+
CT	Yes	+	+	+	+++	++	+++	++
MR imaging	No	+++	+++	+++	++	+++	+++	+++
Ultrasonography	No	+	—	—	+	+	—	—

CT=computed tomography; MR=magnetic resonance; + indicates low utility; ++ indicates moderate utility; +++ indicates high utility; — indicates utility not known.
Reprinted from Moran DS, Evans RK, Hadad E. Imaging of Lower Extremity Stress Fracture Injuries, Sports Med 2008: 38(4), 345–356 with permission from Springer Science+Business Media.

Radiography

Radiography has poor sensitivity but high specificity in the diagnosis of stress fractures. The classic radiographic abnormalities seen in a stress fracture are new periosteal bone formation, a visible area of sclerosis, the presence of callus, or a visible fracture line. Stress fractures present differently in cortical and trabecular bone. Trabecular bone is characterized by a predictable pattern manifested by a line of sclerosis perpendicular to the trabeculae; cortical bone demonstrates periosteal reaction or a cortical fracture line (Moran et al. 2008).

Unfortunately, in most stress fractures there is no obvious radiographic abnormality. The abnormalities on radiography are unlikely to be seen unless symptoms have been present for at least 2 to 3 weeks. In certain cases they may not become evident for up to 3 months and in a percentage of cases never become abnormal.

Isotopic Bone Scan (Scintigraphy)

The triple-phase bone scan has long been recommended for the diagnosis of stress fractures but is increasingly being supplanted by MRI because of its greater specificity and lack of ionizing radiation (Moran et al. 2008). The bone scan is highly sensitive but has low specificity (Leffers and Collins 2009), and while false-negative scans are relatively rare they have been reported (Gaeta et al. 2005).

Technetium-99 methylene disphosphonate (MDP) is the usual radionuclide substance. Other possibilities include gallium citrate (Ga-67) and indium-111-labelled leukocytes. The advantage of technetium-99 MDP is its short half-life (6 hours), allowing a higher dose to be administered with improved resolution.

In the first phase of the bone scan, flow images are obtained immediately after intravenous injection of the tracer. These initial images are usually taken every 2 seconds and correspond roughly to contrast angiography, albeit with much lower spatial and temporal resolution. This first phase of the bone scan evaluates perfusion to bone and soft tissues from the arterial to the venous circulation.

The second phase of the bone scan consists of a static blood pool image taken 1 minute after the injection and reflects the degree of hyperaemia and capillary permeability of bone and soft tissue. Generally speaking, the more acute and severe the injury, the greater is the degree of increased perfusion and blood pool activity.

The third phase of the bone scan is the delayed image, taken 3 to 4 hours after injection when approximately 50% of the tracer has concentrated in the bone matrix through the mechanism of chemisorption to the hydroxyl-apatite crystals. On the 3-hour delayed image, the uptake of the tracer is proportional to the rate of osteoblastic activity, extraction, efficiency, and amount of tracer delivered per unit of time or blood flow. The inclusion of the first and second phases of the bone scan permits estimation of the age of stress-induced focal bony lesions and the severity of bony injuries, and helps to differentiate soft-tissue inflammation from bony injury. As the bony lesion heals, the perfusion returns to normal first, followed by normalization of the blood pool image a few weeks later. Focal increased uptake on the delayed scan resolves last because of ongoing bony remodelling and generally lags well behind the disappearance of pain. As healing continues, the intensity of the uptake diminishes gradually over a 3- to 6-month period following an uncomplicated stress fracture, with a minimal degree of uptake persisting for up to 10 months or even longer.

In the appropriate clinical setting, the scintigraphic diagnosis of a stress fracture is defined as focal increased uptake in the third phase of the bone scan. However, bone scintigraphy lacks specificity because other non-traumatic lesions such as tumour (especially osteoid osteoma), osteomyelitis, bony infarct, and bony dysplasias can also produce localized increased uptake (Kiuru et al. 2002; Prather et al. 1977). It is therefore vitally important to correlate the bone-scan appearance with the clinical features.

The radionuclide scan will detect evolving stress fractures at the stage of accelerated remodelling (Moran et al. 2008). At that stage, which may be asymptomatic, the uptake is usually of mild intensity, progressing to more intense and better-defined uptake as microfractures develop.

In stress fractures all three phases of the triple-phase bone scan are positive. Other bony abnormalities such as periostitis (shin splints/medial tibial stress syndrome) are only positive on delayed images, whereas certain other overuse soft-tissue injuries would be positive only in the angiogram and blood pool phase, thus allowing one to differentiate between bony and soft-tissue pathology (Moran et al. 2008). The characteristic bone-scan appearance of a stress fracture is of a sharply marginated or fusiform area of increased uptake involving one cortex or occasionally extending the width of the bone (Figure 7-4). Radio-isotope bone scan is also effective in demonstrating

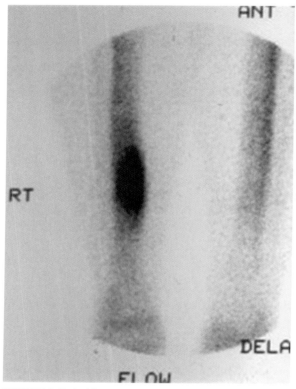

FIGURE 7-4 Typical bone-scan appearance of a stress fracture of the tibia. (Reprinted with permission from Bruckner P and Khan K (eds) (2012) Clinical Sports Medicine (4th Ed.) North Ryde, NSW, Australia: McGraw-Hill Publishing, p 743.)

increased bony stress in the navicular. Plantar views have been more useful than the standard frontal, medial, and lateral views (Pavlov et al. 1983). The characteristic appearance of a positive radioisotope scan outlines the entire navicular bone.

Increased radionuclide uptake is frequently found in asymptomatic sites (Nielsen et al. 1991). Originally the presence of increased tracer uptake at non-painful sites in athletes was interpreted as unrecognized stress fractures; other authors postulated that this may be non-specific stress changes related to bone remodelling, a false-positive finding, or an uncertain finding (Matheson et al. 1987b; Nielsen et al. 1991).

The sensitivity of bone scintigraphy can be further increased by the use of single-photon emission computed tomography (SPECT). Bone SPECT is most helpful in complex areas of the skeleton with overlapping structures that may obscure pathology such as the foot, pelvis, and spine.

Computed Tomography

CT provides detailed bone anatomy in multiple planes, often demonstrating the endosteal remodelling or fracture line in stress fractures (Sofka 2006). However, CT should not be used as a routine initial investigation in stress fracture detection given its lower sensitivity (even using newer multidetector CT) compared with bone scans and MRI (Gaeta et al. 2005; Groves et al. 2005). Instead its use is reserved for specific indications such as differentiating those conditions with increased uptake on bone scan that may mimic stress fracture. These include osteoid osteoma, osteomyelitis with a Brodie's abscess, and other malignancies.

CT scans are also particularly valuable in imaging fractures when this may be important in treatment. In particular, CT scanning of the navicular bone is extremely helpful. CT scanning may also be valuable in detecting fracture lines as evidence of stress fracture in long bones (e.g. metatarsal and tibia) where plain radiography is normal and an isotope bone scan shows increased uptake. CT scanning will enable the clinician to differentiate between a stress fracture, which will be visible on CT scan, and a stress reaction. Particularly in the elite athlete, this may considerably affect rehabilitation and forthcoming competition programmes.

As stated, CT scanning is a valuable tool in the assessment of navicular stress fracture. Precise radiological technique is required to demonstrate the tiny navicular stress fractures. A bone algorithm must be used and the gantry angled to the place of the talonavicular joint to take contiguous 1.5 mm slices (Kiss et al. 1993). Cuts should be taken directly parallel to the talonavicular joint. On CT scan, the proximal articular rim of the normal navicular bone appears extremely dense, almost sclerotic, and is ring-like on true axial images. This apparent bone sclerosis may reflect the mechanical load normally borne by the relatively small concave articular surface of the navicular bone during weightbearing. Most stress fractures are linear defects, some have associated bone fragments, and others appear as rim defects without a linear component (Kiss et al. 1993). Saxena and colleagues (2000) proposed a classification system of

navicular stress fractures based on frontal plane CT scan findings: type 1 – dorsal cortical break, type II – fracture propagation into the navicular body, and type III – fracture propagation into another cortex. In their series, type I fractures were more likely to receive conservative treatment and type III fractures took significantly longer to heal than types I and II. The typical CT appearance of a navicular stress fracture is shown in Figure 7-5.

Magnetic Resonance Imaging

MRI has certain advantages in the imaging of stress fractures and is now considered the gold standard for the diagnosis of these injuries. Specific MRI characteristics of stress fracture include new bone formation and fracture lines appearing as very-low-signal medullary bands that are contiguous with the cortex; surrounding marrow haemorrhage and oedema seen as low signal intensity on T1-weighted images and as high signal intensity on T2-weighted and short T1 inversion recovery (STIR) images; and periosteal oedema and haemorrhage appearing as high signal intensity on T2-weighted and STIR images (Figure 7-6). These changes are best seen if the MRI is performed within 3 weeks of symptoms. MRI can also detect stress fracture injuries before symptoms or a fracture become evident (Fredericson et al. 1995; Major 2006).

MRI visualizes marrow haemorrhage and oedema well, a characteristically difficult finding with CT. Although CT scan visualizes bone detail, another advantage of MRI is in distinguishing stress fractures from a suspected bone tumour or infectious process. Furthermore, MRI does not involve the use of ionizing radiation. It is also thought that, compared with bone scans, MRI more precisely defines the anatomical location and extent of injury (Fredericson et al. 1995). In a study of early tibial stress fractures, the sensitivity of MRI was 88% compared with 74% for bone scans and 42% for CT (Gaeta et al. 2005). The specificity, accuracy, and positive and negative predictive values were 100%, 90%, 100%, and 62% respectively for MRI. In particular, it has been reported that axial images of the tibial shaft shows higher rates of diagnostic accuracy in detecting bone stress injuries than coronal images (Ahovuo et al. 2002), as these can detect relative involvement in the periosteum, bone marrow, and

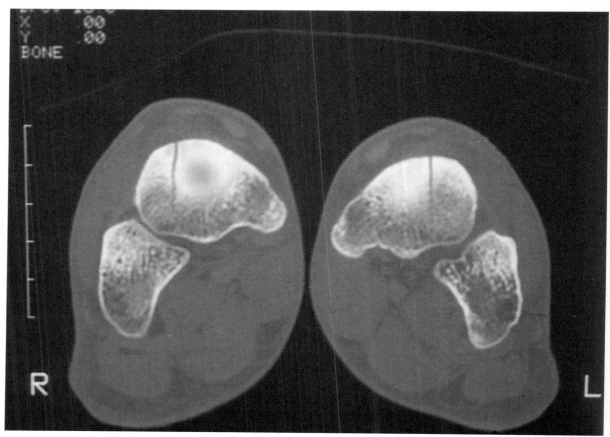

FIGURE 7-5 CT appearance of navicular stress fracture. (Reprinted with permission from Bruckner P and Bennell KL, in O'Connor, F, Wilder R, and Nirschel R (eds) (2001) Textbook of Running Medicine, New York: McGraw-Hill Publishing, p. 249.)

cortical bone (Mammoto et al. 2012). High-resolution MRI of the tibia may be especially useful in the early discrimination of tibial stress injuries with bone marrow abnormalities predictive of later periosteal reactions, suggesting shin splints or stress fractures (Mammoto et al. 2012).

There are limited reports of the use of MRI in diagnosing navicular stress fractures (Burne et al. 2005; Sanders et al. 2004). One study compared CT and MRI scans in their series of 20 navicular stress injuries (Burne et al. 2005). Results showed that CT was more accurate in detecting stress fractures, whereas MRI was able to detect early stress reactions where there was no evidence of abnormality on CT scan. Some authors have recommended that CT scans are ordered first

and, if negative and a high index of clinical suspicion still persists, then an MRI can be obtained to exclude a stress reaction (Mann and Pedowitz 2009).

Ultrasonography

Ultrasonography has the advantages of being easy, fast, non-invasive, and relatively inexpensive and is being increasingly used in sports medicine to assess the musculoskeletal system (Moran et al. 2008). Reports have demonstrated the potential of ultrasound to provide a limited evaluation of superficial bony structures (Banal et al. 2009; Bodner et al. 2005; Howard et al. 1992). A recent pilot study evaluated the sensitivity and specificity of ultrasonography in early diagnosis (average time between onset of symptoms and

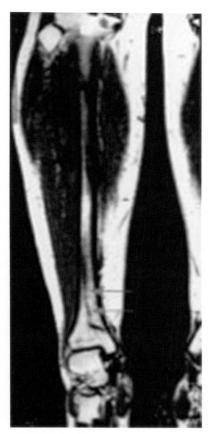

FIGURE 7-6 MRI appearance of a stress fracture of the tibia showing fracture line (arrows). (Reprinted with permission from Brukner P, and Khan K (eds) (2012) Clinical Sports Medicine (4th Ed.) North Ryde, NSW, Australia: McGraw-Hill Publishing, p 744.)

imaging of 3.4 weeks) of 41 metatarsal stress fractures, comparing it with the gold standard of MRI (Banal et al. 2009). The results showed that ultrasound had a sensitivity of 83%, specificity 76%, positive predictive value 59%, and negative predictive value 92%. The authors of this study recommended that this procedure could be performed before MRI or bone scan in metatarsal stress fractures. However, it must be remembered that the sonographer requires considerable experience to ensure adequate skill and competence. Ultrasound may be generally viewed as an imaging alternative in superficial bones where other modalities such as MRI and bone scan cannot be performed (Sofka 2006).

IMPAIRMENTS

Pain is the primary symptom associated with the clinical presentation of stress fractures. The precise nature of the pain experienced is known to vary according to the site of fracture and severity of the underlying bony injury. Indeed, a number of lower limb stress fractures are subclinical (Major 2006; Niva et al. 2009); that is, the affected individual has not sought treatment for their injury, either because the symptoms are not severe enough to impair activity or because no symptoms are experienced.

Typically, the pain associated with stress fracture injury is described as of insidious onset and dull or mild in nature. In the majority of symptomatic cases, pain presents during one-leg hopping (Beck et al. 2008; Swenson et al. 1997) or running (Brukner 2000), most probably due to the relatively high-impact loads this places upon the bones of the lower leg. Early in the pathology continuum – mild to moderate stress reactions – pain may occur only during activity. With a more severe stress reaction or full stress fracture, however, pain often persists following the completion of activity (Brukner 2000; Verma and Sherman 2001). In addition to activity-related pain, palpation of the affected site will illicit localized pain (Brukner 2000; Sterling et al. 1992; Verma and Sherman 2001). In a small number of more severe cases, night pain may be experienced (Brukner 2000).

With relative rest, pain can be expected to dissipate within 4 weeks for mild to moderate stress reactions (Edwards et al. 2005),whereas for those that are more severe 8 to 16 weeks of relative rest is a more realistic expectation (Arendt and Griffiths 1997). When employing a functional progression/relative rest approach, Swenson and colleagues (1997) report that it took up to 92 days to achieve pain-free hopping in athletes presenting with tibial stress fractures, although over half of their cohort achieved this goal within 60 days. Unfortunately, similar data are not currently available for stress fracture injuries of the fibula or foot.

It is generally considered that the pain associated with stress fractures is more severe with injuries involving greater structural damage – that is, those injuries with the presentation of a clear fracture line (or lines) on MRI, X-ray, or CT and well-defined localized uptake on bone scan. With continued bone loading through activity, structural progression of the injury and elevated pain is expected, whereas with rest structural repair of the bony damage will ensue alongside a reduction in the severity of pain. Exceptions to this general pattern exist. It is known that with some mild stress reactions or stress fractures, pain and injury can resolve without the need for relative rest (Burr et al. 1990; Chisin et al. 1987), and in some cases fractures may not resolve despite extended rest or other conservative treatment approaches (Batt et al. 2001; Brukner et al. 2000; Khan et al. 1992). Unfortunately, formal reports of the natural history of pain changes through the course of the disease are not available, as research efforts have primarily focused upon the identification of predisposing factors, and interventions to expedite healing and rehabilitation. This is likely related to the relatively short period it generally takes stress fracture injuries to resolve.

As the majority of stress fracture injuries are associated with a swift and successful recovery, beyond the symptoms of pain, there are only limited accounts of the nature of impairments associated with the injury. In some individuals, particularly those with more-severe stress fractures, an inability to ambulate exists as a result of the pain. Cross-sectional data indicate that tibial stress fractures are not associated with loss of strength, muscular endurance, or range of motion, although these measurements were taken following the cessation of symptoms (Ekenman et al. 1996).

FUNCTION AND QUALITY OF LIFE

To the authors' knowledge, published data regarding function and quality of life in individuals with current stress fractures are not available. Given that symptoms of a typical stress fracture last 8 to 16 weeks (Arendt and Griffiths 1997), it would be reasonable to consider the impact upon quality of life also to be transient in nature. That said, the pain and enforced restriction in weightbearing physical activity associated with the condition may impact upon quality of life for the patient. Moreover, for the patient with an atypical 'high-risk' stress fracture that may not resolve for several months, or years, the impact of the condition upon quality of life is likely to be more persistent and clinically significant. This is of particular concern

for elite athletes and military recruits, as high-risk stress fractures have the potential to jeopardize their chosen career. Work to quantify the implications upon functional and quality of life in this particular subgroup is therefore merited.

MANAGEMENT STRATEGIES

Management strategies vary depending upon the location and severity of the fracture. Stress fractures at the posteromedial tibia, fibula, and first to fourth metatarsals are often termed 'low-risk' fractures as they have a favourable natural history. These stress fractures tend to be on the compressive side of the bone and generally heal without complications. However, there is a group of stress fractures that are prone to recur, become a non-union, or have significant complications should they progress to complete fracture (Diehl et al. 2006). These 'high-risk' stress fractures include those located at the anterior tibial cortex, medial malleolus, navicular, talus, proximal fifth metatarsal, and the sesamoids.

In addition to classifying the fracture as 'low' or 'high risk' based on its anatomical location, the severity of bone damage has prognostic implications regarding healing time and will assist the practitioner in return to play/activity decisions. As previously mentioned, bone stress injuries occur along a continuum from mild microdamage to cortical disruption to complete fractures. Imaging modalities provide information as to the injury severity and existing grading systems can be used to classify the stress fracture as being low or high grade.

The basis of treatment for 'low-risk' stress fractures involves rest from the aggravating activity, a concept known as *relative rest*. This may involve discontinuation of the aggravating activity alone, discontinuation of all training activities, or non-weightbearing using crutches. The extent of relative rest will depend upon the severity of injury and the patient's individual circumstances – such as their level of sporting participation and where they are in the competitive season or their military training. Most 'low-risk' stress fractures with a relatively brief history of symptoms will heal in a straightforward manner, and return to sport or activity should occur within 6 to 8 weeks. Nevertheless, patients with 'low-risk' stress fractures of higher grade (more severe bone injury) have been shown to take significantly longer to return to sport or activity than those with a lower grade (Dobrindt et al. 2012). This may be particularly seen for those who have had confirmed diagnosis by MR imaging (Beck et al. 2012). Conversely, 'high-risk' stress fractures often require more prolonged rest from activity as well as other management strategies such as cast immobilization or surgery, regardless of their severity.

PHARMACOLOGICAL STRATEGIES

Drug therapies do not play a major role in the management of stress fractures. Where drugs are used it is mainly for pain management in the initial stages of recovery. There has also been interest in the use of bisphosphonate drugs to treat and prevent stress fractures, particularly in the elite athlete or military setting.

Pain Management

Pain with stress fractures is seldom severe but can be a problem even with normal walking. Practitioners often suggest non-steroidal anti-inflammatory drugs (NSAIDs) to assist with initial pain reduction and healing of stress fractures. As they inhibit cyclo-oxygenases, NSAIDs will help control inflammatory processes that may accompany injury or overload. However, prostaglandins are essential for normal bone turnover and fracture healing and thus NSAIDs could slow or prevent repair of the stress fracture (Wheeler and Batt 2005). Indeed, a recent animal study showed that both selective COX-2 inhibitors and non-selective NSAIDs adversely influenced bone healing following experimentally induced stress fractures (Kidd et al. 2013). As there is no conclusive evidence in humans to date, the use of NSAIDs in patients with stress fractures is not recommended (Wheeler and Batt 2005; Ziltener et al. 2010). Mild analgesics should be used instead if pain relief is needed.

Bisphosphonates

Bisphosphonates are commonly used in the treatment of postmenopausal osteoporosis. These drugs suppress bone resorption by osteoclasts and thus prevent bone loss during the initial remodelling in response to high bone strains. This may potentially allow increased osteoblastic healing and speed recovery. Intravenous pamidronate has been used successfully on five collegiate athletes who had symptomatic tibial stress fractures. Four of the five athletes were able to continue training without symptoms within 72 hours, suggesting a therapeutic effect (Stewart et al. 2005). However, bisphosphonates are expensive and can have adverse effects such as oesophageal inflammation or severe muscle, bone, and joint pain. Given these contraindications as well as the lack of conclusive evidence, it is prudent to restrict the use of bisphosphonates for the treatment of stress fractures (Shima et al. 2009).

It has also been postulated that bisphosphonates may have a prophylactic effect by preventing stress fractures during intense training, although this is yet to be proven (Ekenman 2009). When military recruits were given a loading dose of 30 mg of risedronate daily for 10 doses during the first 2 weeks of basic training followed by once-a-week maintenance dose for 12 weeks, no reduction in the incidence of stress fractures was seen (Milgrom et al. 2004). Thus bisphosphonates cannot be recommended for preventing stress fractures.

PHYSICAL STRATEGIES

In some cases where activities of daily living are painful it may be necessary for the patient with a stress fracture to be non-weightbearing or partially weightbearing on crutches for a period of up to 7 to 10 days. In the majority of cases this is not necessary and merely avoiding the aggravating activity will be sufficient.

However, there are several 'high-risk' stress fractures where prolonged non-weightbearing with or without cast immobilization may be an option. These include stress fractures of the sesamoid bones (Davis and Alexander 1990) and fractures of the proximal fifth diaphysis (Vu et al. 2006). Although there is some disagreement in the literature as to the best treatment for a navicular stress fracture, a recent systematic review of 23 studies comparing the outcome of conservative versus surgical treatment for navicular stress fractures provides strong evidence to guide management (Torg et al. 2010). The results of the meta-analysis showed that conservative management with weightbearing permitted was significantly less effective in terms of radiographic and/or clinical healing and time to return to activity than either conservative non-weightbearing treatment or surgical treatment. There was no significant difference between conservative non-weightbearing treatment and surgical treatment regardless of the type of fracture, age, sex, or onset of treatment. In fact, there was a statistical trend favouring non-weightbearing management (96% successful outcome) over surgery (82% successful outcome). Thus it is recommended that navicular stress fractures be treated with strict non-weightbearing cast immobilization for at least 6 weeks.

Electrotherapy Modalities

There are several electrotherapy modalities that have been reported in the literature for use in the management of stress fractures. These are generally used for 'high-risk' stress fractures or for 'low-risk' stress fractures involving elite athletes where a speedy return to sport is desirable. However, high-quality evidence to support their efficacy in stress fracture management is generally lacking.

Low-intensity Pulsed Ultrasound. The application of ultrasound therapy is increasingly used to improve the healing of fractures. The sound waves produced are thought to place the bone and surrounding tissue under microstresses and strains, promoting healing. Most reported studies utilize the Sonic Accelerated Fracture Healing System (Exogen®, Piscataway, NJ) with treatment consisting of 20-minute daily sessions of varying duration. A meta-analysis of the effect of low-intensity pulsed ultrasound on the healing of all types of fractures found conflicting results from 13 randomized controlled trials, with evidence that was moderate to very low in quality (Busse et al. 2009). Currently there is only one clinical trial in those with stress fractures. This moderate quality randomized, double-blind placebo-controlled trial failed to find an effect of ultrasound on healing time in 46 tibial stress fractures treated for 20 minutes daily with a commercially available ultrasound system (Rue et al. 2004). This lack of effect may be due to the relatively small sample size. At this stage, ultrasound would not be recommended for routine treatment of stress fractures but might be an option for stress fractures at sites prone to delayed union or non-union, or in elite athletes. Research is needed to assess further the effects of pulsed ultrasound on stress fracture healing, including different dosages and different sites.

Low-power Laser. There has only been one small, short-term study investigating the application of low-power laser treatment of stress fractures/shin splints, with no effect noted upon pain or fracture healing time (Nissen et al. 1994). Although further evidence is required to establish the efficacy of laser therapy for stress-fracture-type injuries, pooled data from a range of soft-tissue injuries indicate some promising results with respect to pain and inflammation (Bjordal et al. 2006).

Magnetic Field Application. Electrical stimulation can be applied to a fracture by direct current stimulation requiring operative placement of an electrode against the fracture site, capacitive-coupled electrical field devices, or pulsed electromagnetic field stimulation of bone. Electric fields are well known to promote bone healing in vitro based upon cellular stimulation (Hartig et al. 2000). In a clinical setting, the use of electricity and electricity-generated magnetic fields has generally been shown to aid the healing of troublesome fractures (Aaron et al. 2004).

There is limited research in stress fractures. In a non-blinded, uncontrolled study, Benazzo et al. (1995) reported on the use of capacitive coupling in stress fractures predominantly of the navicular and fifth metatarsal, which are prone to delayed union or non-union. They claimed that 22 of 25 stress fractures were healed and two more showed improvement. However, a recent randomized controlled trial was unable to detect an effect of capacitively coupled electric field stimulation applied for 15 hours per day on the healing of 44 postero-medial tibial stress fractures (Beck et al. 2008). Nevertheless, the authors commented that greater device use and less weightbearing loading did enhance the effectiveness of the active device. In addition, stress fractures healed more quickly with the electric field stimulation. The authors concluded that, although the use of capacitively coupled electric field stimulation for tibial stress fracture healing may not be efficacious for all, it may be indicated for the more severely injured or elite athlete or military recruit whose incentive to return to activity may motivate superior compliance. Clearly the scientific evidence of the use of electromagnetic fields for the healing of stress fractures is still at an early stage and thus firm conclusions cannot currently be made.

Extracorporeal Shock Wave Therapy. Extracorporeal shock wave therapy (ESWT) involves inducing microtrauma to the affected area by repeated shock waves thereby stimulating neovascularization into the area, which promotes tissue healing. Low-level evidence suggests that ESWT may be beneficial in treating fracture complications such as delayed union and non-union (Zelle et al. 2010). There are limited reports of ESWT used in the management of stress fractures (Albisetti et al. 2010; Moretti et al. 2009; Taki et al. 2007). A relatively recent case series of 10 athletes with chronic stress fractures of the fifth metatarsal and tibia receiving 3–4 sessions of low–middle energy ESWT reported excellent results after 8 weeks (Moretti et al. 2009). However, further research is needed to clarify the role of ESWT, particularly for resistant stress fractures.

Bracing

The use of a pneumatic air brace may assist with stress fracture healing in the leg and reduce the time taken to return to sport. Swenson and colleagues (1997) proposed that the pneumatic leg brace shifts a portion of the weightbearing load from the tibia to the soft tissue, which results in less impact loading with walking, hopping, and running. They also suggested that the brace facilitates healing at the fracture site by acting to compress the soft tissue, thereby increasing the intravascular hydrostatic pressure and resulting in a shifting of the fluid and electrolytes from the capillary space to the interstitial space. This theoretically enhances the piezoelectric effect and enhances osteoblastic bone formation.

Pooled data from three small but very different clinical trials, two in military recruits (Allen et al. 2004; Slayter 1995) and one in athletes (Swenson et al. 1997), showed a significant reduction in the time to recommencing full activity after diagnosis of stress fracture with the use of a pneumatic leg brace (weighted mean difference: −33.4 days; 95% CI: −44.2, −22.6 days) (Rome et al. 2000). However, the results were highly heterogeneous, most probably due to

differences in the trial designs, including study population, control group interventions, and definitions of outcomes. Indeed, the most recent study found no effect of a brace on the time to pain-free hop and time to pain-free 1-mile run in 31 military recruits with tibial stress fracture (Allen et al. 2004). Overall there is some evidence to suggest that a pneumatic brace accelerates return to activity in fibular or tibial stress fractures, but this requires confirmation (Rome et al. 2000). In addition to these 'low-risk' fractures, undisplaced or minimally displaced stress fractures of the medial malleolus can be treated conservatively in a pneumatic leg brace for 6 weeks with unrestricted ambulation (Shelbourne et al. 1988; Schils et al. 1992).

Fitness Maintenance

It is important that the athlete with a stress fracture be able to maintain strength and cardiovascular fitness while undergoing the appropriate rehabilitation programme. It should be emphasized to the athlete that the rehabilitation programme is not designed to maintain or improve fitness, but rather to allow the damaged bone time to heal and gradually develop or regain full strength.

One of the primary considerations in the selection of activities to maintain fitness is the minimization of impact loads upon the affected bone, and thus no weightbearing or low-weightbearing activities are generally preferred. The most common means of maintaining fitness are cycling, swimming, water running, and upper body weight training. These workouts should mimic the athlete's normal training programme as much as possible in both duration and intensity. Water running is particularly attractive to runners for this reason. Water running involves the use of a vest for a flotation device. Stretching should be performed to maintain flexibility during the rehabilitation process. Muscle strengthening is also an important component of the rehabilitation phase. In some elite training facilities, anti-gravity treadmills can also be used to allow runners to continue training but with reduced impact forces. For example, Hoffman and Donaghe (2011) demonstrated that with 50% body-weight support provided by an anti-gravity treadmill, a significant reduction in the loading rate of impact forces was achieved. However, no measurable reduction in the loading rate occurred with 20% body-weight support.

Caution should be exercised in the use of these devices, particularly early in the rehabilitation process, as the impact forces associated with footstrike are reduced and not removed with body-weight support.

As well as maintenance of these parameters of physiological fitness, it is possible in most cases for the athlete to maintain specific sports skills. In ball sports these can involve activities either seated or standing still. This active-rest approach also greatly assists the athlete psychologically.

Muscle Strengthening

Although there are no studies that have evaluated the role of muscle strengthening in the treatment of stress fractures, it is logical to include a specific strengthening programme because of the important role of muscles in shock absorption and to help counteract the effects of detraining. This is obviously vital in those patients in whom the stress fracture has been treated by prolonged non-weightbearing and/or cast immobilization.

A specific programme of muscular-strengthening exercises in muscle groups surrounding the joints above and below the fracture line should be given. Attention should also be paid to developing muscle endurance as muscle fatigue leads to an increase in bone strain (Milgrom et al. 2007). These programmes are usually prescribed for a period of 6–12 weeks and can begin immediately after diagnosis of the stress fracture, provided that the exercises do not involve impact loading. It is also important that the exercises do not cause pain at the stress fracture site.

Manual Therapy

For stress fractures managed by cast immobilization, there will usually be associated stiffness of the talocrural, subtalar, and midtarsal joints following removal of the cast. These can be treated during the rehabilitation period by passive joint mobilization. There will also frequently be soft-tissue tightness, especially in the tibialis posterior and soleus muscles, which can be treated by active stretching and soft-tissue massage techniques including myofascial release.

Modification of Risk Factors

As with any overuse injury, it is not sufficient merely to treat the stress fracture. An essential component of the management of an individual with an overuse injury involves identification of the factors that have potentially contributed to the injury and, when possible, correction or modification of some of these factors to reduce the risk of injury recurrence. The fact that stress fractures have a high rate of recurrence (Korpelainen et al. 2001) is an indication that this part of the management programme is often neglected.

The risk factors for the development of stress fractures have been discussed at length under Predisposing factors. Although not yet supported by rigorous scientific evidence, one possible precipitating factor is training errors or changes in training. Therefore it is important to identify these and to discuss them with both the athlete and the coach when appropriate. Another important contributing factor may be inadequate equipment, especially running shoes. The shoes may be inappropriate for the particular foot type of the athlete, may have general inadequate support, or may be worn out. There is increasing attention to barefoot/minimalist footwear and considerable debate about the relative merits or hazards of minimalist running. Although minimalist footwear has been associated with lower impact loading (Lohman et al. 2011), there is little scientific evidence relating it to injury. A recent case series of 10 experienced runners interviewed about their injuries within 1 year of transitions from traditional to minimalist running footwear highlighted the appearance of 10 new injuries, of which eight were metatarsal stress fractures and one was a calcaneal stress fracture (Salzler et al. 2012).

Biomechanical abnormalities are also thought to be important contributing factors to the development of overuse injuries in general and stress fractures in particular. A heel raise may be needed in those with a leg-length discrepancy. Excessively supinated feet generally give poor shock absorption and require footwear that gives good absorption. Athletes with excessively pronated feet will require appropriate footwear for their foot type and possibly custom-made orthotics.

Gait Retraining

Given the central role that high-impact loading during running-type activities is believed to play in the development and recurrence of lower leg stress fractures, recent work has focused on alterations in running technique to reduce the magnitude of impact loads. In a recent study, 10 runners with high-impact loading underwent a 2-week gait-retraining programme incorporating eight 15–30-minute sessions with real-time feedback of their impact loads (Crowell and Davis 2011). During the retraining sessions, participants ran on a treadmill and received real-time feedback of their tibial acceleration displayed on a screen placed directly in front of them. High tibial accelerations have been associated with tibial stress fractures (Davis et al. 2004; Milner et al. 2006b). Thus, the observed 48% reduction in tibial acceleration from pre- to post-training may assist in reducing the likelihood of tibial stress fracture recurrence (Crowell and Davis 2011). Whereas highly sensitive and accurate accelerometers, such as the one used in the study by Crowell and Davis 2011, are not generally accessible in the clinical setting, new technologies are opening avenues for the use of real-time quantitative feedback devices in the clinical setting. Using an instrumented shoe that provided real-time feedback of the magnitude of impact loading, Cheung and Davis (2011) observed a reduction in impact loading in three runners, and this was maintained at 3 months' post-training.

Interestingly, much of the work focused on the retraining of running gait has not incorporated detailed direction with respect to the suggested kinematic changes required to achieve reductions in impact loads. Conceivably, individuals may adopt varying approaches to achieve reductions in impact loads, yet it is not known whether one approach is more successful than the other. Using a mathematical approach to model tibial load, damage, and repair, Edwards and colleagues (2009, 2010) argued that a lower weekly mileage, slower running speed, and a shorter stride length would reduce the probability of tibial stress fracture. Although mileage and speed reductions are likely to be useful principles in the early stages of rehabilitation, alterations to stride length may be a feasible longer-term adaptation to protect against recurrent fractures. Edwards and colleagues (2009) suggest a reduction in stride length of 10% translates to a 3 to 6% reduction in the probability of tibial stress fracture development. Importantly, before such gait-retraining strategies can be recommended for clinical practice, further research is needed to investigate their clinical efficacy and implications upon running economy.

SURGICAL STRATEGIES

Surgical strategies may be required in the management of 'high-risk' stress fractures depending upon the extent of bone injury, site of the fracture, and previous management.

A variety of surgical techniques have been described in the literature to treat non-union of stress fractures of the anterior tibial cortex. Intramedullary nailing of the tibia has been reported as having a high union rate and a low complication rate, and provides an early return to competitive sports (average of 4 months) in those who have failed conservative management (Varner et al. 2005). Tibial drilling (Orava and Hulkko 1988), bone grafting and internal fixation (Green et al. 1985) have also been described. One more recent study compared antero-medial and lateral tibial drilling with laminofixation in 45 athletes, mainly runners (Liimatainen et al. 2009). Good results were achieved with drilling in only 50% of the operations, whereas with laminofixation good results were achieved in 93% of operations ($p=0.002$). Healing of the stress fracture after laminofixation occurred in less than 6 months. In general, surgery has often been performed in the presence of delayed union or non-union. However, in high-performance athletes who wish to have an earlier return to sport than can be achieved with either conservative management or intramedullary nailing, anterior tension band plating has been used (Borens et al. 2006). A report of four world-class athletes who underwent this procedure showed that fracture healing occurred in all four cases with return to full activity at a mean of 10 weeks. All patients returned to pre-injury competitive levels and there were no complications of infection, non-union, or malunion (Borens et al. 2006).

Displaced medial malleolar stress fractures or those that progress to non-union should be treated operatively. In general these involve open-reduction internal fixation procedures (Orava et al. 1995; Schils et al. 1992; Shelbourne et al. 1988) with motion beginning shortly after fixation and progressing to running activities within 6 weeks and full sports participation within 8 weeks. Shorter recovery time was seen in a study reporting a percutaneous cannulated screw fixation procedure that allowed an athlete to return to competition 24 days after sustaining a displaced medial malleolar stress fracture (Kor et al. 2003).

Although conservative management is recommended for initial management of navicular stress fractures (Torg et al. 2010), those that have failed conservative management may require surgery involving screw fixation, with possible bone graft inlay (Mann and Pedowitz 2009).

For stress fracture of the proximal fifth metatarsal, surgical management with intramedullary screw or other fixation is often preferred, given lower failure rates and shorter times to both clinical union and return to sports than casting (Portland et al. 2003; Zwitser and Breederveld 2010). In athletes who have marked medullary sclerosis (frequently with a lengthy history of symptoms) and established non-union, open reduction and bone grafting is recommended. If non-union occurs in stress fractures of the sesamoids, bone grafting or partial or complete excision of the sesamoid can be performed.

LIFESTYLE AND EDUCATION STRATEGIES
Resumption of Impact-loading Activities

Resumption of the impact-loading activities can begin when normal day-to-day ambulation is pain-free. The rate of resumption of activity is individual and should be modified according to symptoms and physical findings. There are no studies that have compared different return-to-sport programmes. However, since healing bone is weaker, a progressive increase in load is needed so that the bone will adapt with increases in strength. Some studies have evaluated the degree of tibial bone loading during various activities using strain gauges cemented on to the tibia of a small number of healthy volunteers (Milgrom et al. 2000a, 2000b, 2003). The results provide some insight into a possible progression of activities during rehabilitation of tibial stress fractures (Figure 7-7).

For lower limb stress fractures where running is the aggravating activity, a programme that involves initial brisk walking increased by 5–10 minutes per day up

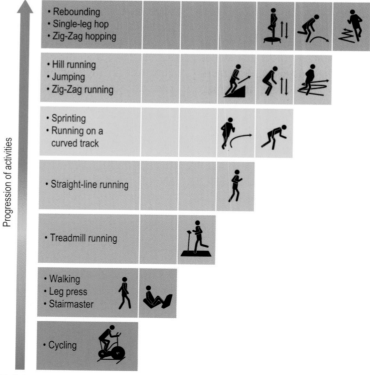

FIGURE 7-7 Schematic for the progression of activities during rehabilitation from tibial stress fracture.

to a length of 45 minutes is recommended. Once 45 minutes of continuous brisk walking is achieved without pain, slow jogging can begin for a period of 5 minutes within the 45-minute walk. Treadmill running provides less tibial strain than running outdoors (Milgrom et al. 2003). The amount of jogging can be increased by 5 minutes per session on a daily or every-other-day basis to a total of 45 minutes at slow jogging pace. The pace can then be increased, initially half pace then gradually increasing to full pace striding. Once full sprinting is achieved pain-free, functional activities such as hopping, skipping, jumping, twisting, and turning can be introduced gradually. It is important that this process is a graduated one and it is important to err on the side of caution rather than try to return too quickly. During this time, attention should be paid to strategies that may enhance faster muscle recovery between training bouts, such as massage and icing. For an uncomplicated lower limb stress fracture, a typical programme for resuming activity after a period of initial rest and activities of daily living is shown in Figure 7-7.

Periodization of running training is also important to reduce the risk of recurrence. This generally follows a 3–4-week cycle with 3 weeks of a progressive increase in intensity, duration or distance followed by an off week of less intense training to allow for rest and subsequent training adaptations to occur before embarking on the next build-up period (Harrast and Colonno 2010).

Resumption of activity should not be accompanied by pain but it is not uncommon to have some discomfort at the site of the stress fracture. If bony pain occurs then activity should be ceased for 1 to 2 days. If pain-free with normal ambulation, the activity is resumed at the volume and pace below the level at which the pain occurred. The patient should be clinically reassessed at 2-weekly intervals, to assess the progress of the training programme and any symptoms related to the stress fracture. It is not necessary to monitor progress by radiography, scintigraphy, CT, or MRI since healing observed by such scanning often lags behind clinical signs and symptoms.

Dietary Factors

Attention to dietary factors is important with an emphasis on calcium intake, vitamin D levels, and energy availability. The latter is particularly relevant in female athletes with hypothalamic amenorrhoea. The most successful strategy for improving bone density and hence bone health in these athletes is to increase energy availability such that body mass is increased and menses resume (Vescovi et al. 2008). An intervention plan that improves energy intake, reduces exercise energy expenditure or both, without dramatic changes in weight, is most desirable (Manore et al. 2007). Consultation with a dietician may assist this process. Hormone replacement therapy offers no benefit and oral contraceptives delay and reduce the likelihood of restoring menstrual patterns (Manore et al. 2007). Bone density evaluation using dual-energy X-ray absorptiometry may be warranted in female athletes with menstrual disturbances or in those with stress fractures at cancellous sites such as the femoral neck, pubic rami, sacrum, and calcaneus. This relates to a study showing that the prevalence of osteopenia was 13% in female athletes whose stress fractures occurred in cortical sites, compared with 89% if the stress fractures occurred in cancellous sites (Marx et al. 2001).

Adequate levels of calcium and vitamin D are needed for bone health. A recent systematic review recommended that female athletes and military recruits ensure their daily calcium intake is upwards of 1500 mg (Tenforde et al. 2010). Although recommended levels for males could not be given based on limited data, it would also be prudent to ensure adequate calcium intake in male patients. Measurement of serum 25(OH)D level is the appropriate screening test in patients in whom vitamin D deficiency is a concern, therapeutic goals for bone health being at least 50 nmol/L (20 ng/mL) and possibly as high as 90 to 100 nmol/L (36 to 40 ng/mL) (McCabe et al. 2012). The amount of vitamin D intake required is highly variable depending on many factors including sun exposure. Although recommended intake levels differ, a recent review on vitamin D and stress fractures recommends that most patients receive 800 to 1000 IU and perhaps as high as 2000 IU of vitamin D_3 since vitamin D is a safe treatment with a high therapeutic index (McCabe et al. 2012).

FUTURE DIRECTIONS

As repeated impact loading to the lower leg bones is an unavoidable consequence of participation in weightbearing activity such as running and marching, stress fractures will always occur in a small number of individuals that frequently participate in these activities. With an improved understanding of the factors that predispose an individual to these injuries however, we will be able to reduce the prevalence of the injury. One promising line of enquiry is the role of genetic factors. In a recent exploratory study of 268 genetic polymorphisms, 25 were found to be significantly different between Israeli military recruits with and without a history of stress fracture (Yanovich et al. 2012). Much work is still required to validate their role, including in other 'at-risk' groups such as runners. Moreover, clinically accessible methods will be required to test for the particular genetic polymorphisms associated with fracture. The benefits of this development will be in the ability to identify individuals at increased risk, modify their exposure to risk factors, and treat mild stress-fracture-like symptoms with a high degree of clinical suspicion.

New commercially available technologies for monitoring training load are also likely to assist in minimizing the incidence of lower leg stress fractures. Wearable technologies such as pedometers, global positioning systems (GPS), and accelerometers allow individuals to record training data, including frequency, duration, altitude ascended/descended, velocities and accelerations. These data can easily be uploaded to online training diaries to monitor training patterns. Given the role that training load is believed to have in stress fracture risk (see Predisposing factors), this improved ability to monitor training load quantitatively may assist in correcting training overload before the development of injury.

As discussed in the Diagnosis section of this chapter, imaging techniques are a useful adjunct to the clinical diagnosis of stress fractures on the basis of symptoms and physical examination. Imaging can be particularly valuable in the differential diagnosis of non-specific leg pain (Edwards et al. 2005); however, the costs associated with imaging often limit its availability to the recreational athlete. With recent developments in MRI technology (including the more cost-effective small gantry machines for extremity imaging), the availability of MRI to the recreational athlete is likely to become more widespread. Given the favourable balance between sensitivity and specificity that MRI offers, it is conceivable that this will become the imaging technology of choice for all clinicians. This will probably assist in more accurate and earlier diagnosis, with subsequent benefits upon patient morbidity.

The fundamentals of stress fracture rehabilitation are unlikely to change in the foreseeable future; however, with research and development work aligned to stress fracture rehabilitation we are likely to see improvements in the efficacy of various adjunct treatments. For example, wearable technologies will facilitate accurate measurement of the progression within a rehabilitation programme, and may also be used to encourage more appropriate running technique to minimize bone load. Improved design of pneumatic braces for tibial fractures may accelerate healing, as may an improved understanding of the effects of various pharmacological aids such as bisphosphonates.

INVITED COMMENTARY

This chapter reviews the key features relating to stress fractures of the lower limb. It is probably the most comprehensive chapter on the subject of stress fractures to date. It goes way beyond the classic elements one would anticipate in a chapter on stress fractures. It has an extensive reference list that is current and contemporary, and also includes some of the classical texts/papers on this often-ignored subject area.

In my opinion, the chapter offers a comprehensive contextual framework of stress fractures of the lower limb and offers readers, no matter their current knowledge of this condition, something new to digest/reflect upon. It would be an excellent adjunct to undergraduate students, clinicians, and academics who may wish to go further in their understanding and knowledge of such a condition. In summary, it does what it sets out to achieve: it gently introduces readers into the somewhat mundane condition of stress fractures and then scholarly exposes them to the complexity of diagnosing and managing this condition.

The introduction is perfectly balanced and scopes out to the reader what to expect in the forthcoming narrative; this includes an outline of the condition's pathology through to treatment. A welcomed additional inclusion is the authors' worthy attempt to comment on patient outcomes, in particular offering commentary on the evidence to treat and

INVITED COMMENTARY (Continued)

prevent. One further additional feature is the emphasis they place on the concept of the spectrum of stress fractures. This is highlighted in the introduction and is lightly touched on occasionally in the preceding text. The chapter is broken down into various headings with additional subheadings throughout. It is logically presented and chronologically follows a traditional medical text format in terms of starting with the known aetiology of the condition. The epidemiology is well covered and easy to follow. The next section explores the predisposing factors associated with stress fractures. This is particularly well covered highlighting the various intrinsic and extrinsic factors associated with this condition. It is round about this point that the chapter begins to excel in its content and presentation: not only are all of the factors explained and described but they are presented in an analytical fashion, readers are offered a contemporary critique of current studies in the area with their relevance to particular theories as well as their various limitations. It is refreshing and indeed comprehensive to see mention of genetic factors, particularly vitamin D and the receptor gene VITD. Given the complexity of this, it would have been nice to have had this concept/theory explained in more detail. In addition to the genetic factors the authors also touch on gender factors associated with the condition: not easy to include and somewhat controversial, and still not entirely clear in terms of some of the issues around gender differences, but certainly worth making reference to (again demonstrating the comprehensiveness of the chapter). In summary, this is an excellent overview of the intrinsic factors. The extrinsic factors are also covered with the same amount of scholarly detail. The authors offer up-to-date literature, they critically assess each of the studies cited and draw out the limitations associated with each.

The diagnosis is also well covered including the information regarding the importance of collecting a thorough history, the differential diagnosis, and the physical examination. All of the main diagnostic tests and imaging techniques are described.

The management strategies described include the full range of modalities for treating and managing this condition. A full range of strategies are given, but I suppose the most important message that this section must highlight, and it does to some extent, is, yes, there are a lot of different treatment regimens available but, to be fully effective in terms of a clinician, patients must be assessed individually and an individual management strategy devised for each. I particularly like the section on surgical strategies; it is quite rare to see this explained in a pragmatic way. One area that the authors could have given some mileage, given the spectrum alluded to in the introduction and the fact that this condition might not be all that disabling, is comment or inclusion on the psychology of managing this patient group.

The future direction heading could have made a reference to the possibility of smart materials for insoles either as a preventative measure or as a rehabilitation treatment regimen. In conclusion this chapter embraces the whole spectrum of stress fractures of the lower limb. It helps explain the complexity of a condition that is sometimes dismissed in the literature as a minor complaint, easily treatable and resolvable in a short period. The chapter stresses this is not always the case and individual cases/patients should be assessed. It gives an insight into the complexity of the condition and draws on literature way beyond basic clinical publications. I would highly recommend this chapter to musculoskeletal students (health care as well as sports science students), clinical practitioners and academics: it is one of the most comprehensive chapters I have read on stress fractures. Other books/chapters are very limited in content and analysis/critique.

Robert L. Ashford DPodM, BA, BEd, MA, MMedSci, PhD, MChS, FCpodMed, FFPM, RCPS
Director of Postgraduate Research Degrees,
Faculty of Health, Birmingham City University,
City South Campus, Birmingham, UK

REFERENCES

Aaron, R.K., Ciombor, D.M., Simon, B.J., 2004. Treatment of nonunions with electric and electromagnetic fields. Clinical Orthopaedics 419, 21–29.

Achermann, J.C., Jameson, J.L., 2003. Human disorders caused by nuclear receptor gene mutations. Pure and Applied Chemistry 75 (11–12), 1785–1796.

Ahovuo, J.A., Kiuru, M.J., Kinnunen, J.J., et al., 2002. MR imaging of fatigue stress injuries to bones: intra- and interobserver agreement. Magnetic Resonance Imaging 20 (5), 401–406.

Albisetti, W., Perugia, D., De Bartolomeo, O., et al., 2010. Stress fractures of the base of the metatarsal bones in young trainee ballet dancers. International Orthopaedics 34 (1), 51–55.

Allen, C.S., Flynn, T.W., Kardouni, J.R., et al., 2004. The use of a pneumatic leg brace in soldiers with tibial stress fractures – a randomized clinical trial. Military Medicine 169 (11), 880–884.

Andrish, J.T., Bergfeld, J.A., Walheim, J., 1974. A prospective study on the management of shin splints. Journal of Bone and Joint Surgery, American Volume 56 (8), 1697–1700.

Arendt, E.A., Griffiths, H.J., 1997. The use of MR imaging in the assessment and clinical management of stress reactions of bone in high-performance athletes. Clinical Sports Medicine 16 (2), 291–306.

Armstrong, D.W., Rue, J.-P.H., Wilckens, J.H., et al., 2004. Stress fracture injury in young military men and women. Bone 35 (3), 806–816.

Banal, F., Gandjbakhch, F., Foltz, V., et al., 2009. Sensitivity and specificity of ultrasonography in early diagnosis of metatarsal bone stress fractures: a pilot study of 37 patients. Journal of Rheumatology 36 (8), 1715–1719.

Barnes, A., Wheat, J., Milner, C., 2008. Association between foot type and tibial stress injuries: a systematic review. British Journal of Sports Medicine 42 (2), 93–98.

Barrow, G.W., Saha, S., 1988. Menstrual irregularity and stress fractures in collegiate female distance runners. American Journal of Sports Medicine 16 (3), 209–216.

Batt, M.E., Kemp, S., Kerslake, R., 2001. Delayed union stress fractures of the anterior tibia: conservative management. British Journal of Sports Medicine 35 (1), 74–77.

Beck, T.J., Ruff, C.B., Mourtada, F.A., et al., 1996. Dual-energy X-ray absorptiometry derived structural geometry for stress fracture prediction in male U.S. Marine Corps recruits. Journal of Bone and Mineral Research 11 (5), 645–653.

Beck, T.J., Ruff, C.B., Shaffer, R.A., et al., 2000. Stress fracture in military recruits: gender differences in muscle and bone susceptibility factors. Bone 27 (3), 437–444.

Beck, B.R., Matheson, G.O., Bergman, G., et al., 2008. Do capacitively coupled electric fields accelerate tibial stress fracture healing? A randomized controlled trial. American Journal of Sports Medicine 36 (3), 545–553.

Beck, B.R., Bergman, A.G., Miner, M., et al., 2012. Tibial stress injury: relationship of radiographic, nuclear medicine bone scanning, MR imaging, and CT Severity grades to clinical severity and time to healing. Radiology 263 (3), 811–818.

Benazzo, F., Mosconi, M., Beccarisi, G., et al., 1995. Use of capacitive coupled electric fields in stress fractures in athletes. Clinical Orthopaedics 310, 145–149.

Bennell, K.L., Malcolm, S.A., Thomas, S.A., et al., 1996a. The incidence and distribution of stress fractures in competitive track and field athletes. American Journal of Sports Medicine 24, 211–217.

Bennell, K.L., Malcolm, S.A., Thomas, S.A., et al., 1996b. Risk factors for stress fractures in track and field athletes. A twelve-month prospective study. American Journal of Sports Medicine 24 (6), 810–818.

Bensel, C., Kaplan, D.B., 1986. Wear test of boot inserts. Report No. STRNC-ICH. US Army Natrick Research and Development Laboratories, Natrick (MA).

Bijur, P.E., Horodyski, M., Egerton, W., et al., 1997. Comparison of injury during cadet basic training by gender. Archives of Pediatric and Adolescent Medicine 151, 456–461.

Bjordal, J.M., Johnson, M.I., Iversen, V., et al., 2006. Photoradiation in acute pain: A systematic review of possible mechanisms of action and clinical effects in randomized placebo-controlled trials. Photomedicine and Laser Surgery 24 (2), 158–168.

Bodner, G., Stockl, B., Fierlinger, A., et al., 2005. Sonographic findings in stress fractures of the lower limb: preliminary findings. European Radiology 15 (2), 356–359.

Borens, O., Sen, M.K., Huang, R.C., et al., 2006. Anterior tension band plating for anterior tibial stress fractures in high-performance female athletes: a report of 4 cases. Journal of Orthopaedic Trauma 20 (6), 425–430.

Brudvig, T.J., Gudger, T.D., Obermeyer, L., 1983. Stress fractures in 295 trainees: a one-year study of incidence as related to age, sex, and race. Military Medicine 148 (8), 666–667.

Brukner, P., 2000. Exercise-related lower leg pain: bone. Medicine and Science in Sports and Exercise 32 (S2), S15–S26.

Brukner, P., Bennell, K.L., 2001. Textbook of running medicine. McGraw-Hill, New York, pp. 239, 241, 249.

Brukner, P., Fanton, G., Bergman, A.G., et al., 2000. Bilateral stress fractures of the anterior part of the tibial cortex. Journal of Bone and Joint Surgery 82 (2), 213–218.

Brunet, M.E., Cook, S.D., Brinker, M.R., et al., 1990. A survey of running injuries in 1505 competitive and recreational runners. Journal of Sports Medicine and Physical Fitness 30 (3), 307–315.

Burne, S.G., Mahoney, C.M., Forster, B.B., et al., 2005. Tarsal navicular stress injury: long-term outcome and clinicoradiological correlation using both computed tomography and magnetic resonance imaging. American Journal of Sports Medicine 33 (12), 1875–1881.

Burr, D.B., Milgrom, C., Boyd, R.D., et al., 1990. Experimental stress fractures of the tibia. Journal of Bone and Joint Surgery 72, 370–375.

Burr, D.B., Milgrom, C., Fyhrie, D., et al., 1996. In vivo measurement of human tibial strains during vigorous activity. Bone 18 (5), 405–410.

Busse, J.W., Kaur, J., Mollon, B., et al., 2009. Low intensity pulsed ultrasonography for fractures: systematic review of randomised controlled trials. British Medical Journal 338, b351.

Carbon, R., Sambrook, P.N., Deakin, V., et al., 1990. Bone density of elite female athletes with stress fractures. Medical Journal of Australia 153, 373–376.

Chatzipapas, C., Boikos, S., Drosos, G.I., et al., 2009. Polymorphisms of the Vitamin D Receptor Gene and Stress Fractures. Hormone Metabolism Research 41 (8), 635–640.

Cheung, R.T., Davis, I.S., 2011. Landing pattern modification to improve patellofemoral pain in runners: a case series. Journal of Orthopaedic and Sports Physical Therapy [Case Reports] 41 (12), 914–919.

Chisin, R., Milgrom, C., Giladi, M., et al., 1987. Clinical significance of nonfocal scintigraphic findings in suspected tibial stress fractures. Clinical Orthopaedics 220, 200–205.

Cobb, K., Bachrach, L., Sowers, M., et al., 2007. The effect of oral contraceptives on bone mass and stress fractures in female runners. Medicine and Science in Sports and Exercise 39 (9), 1464–1473.

Courtney, A.C., Davis, B.L., Manning, T., et al., 1997. Effects of age, density, and geometry on the bending strength of human metatarsals. Foot and Ankle International 18 (4), 216–221.

Cranney, A., Weiler, H.A., O'Donnell, S., et al., 2008. Summary of evidence-based review on vitamin D efficacy and safety in relation to bone health. American Journal of Clinical Nutrition 88 (Suppl.), S513–S519.

Crossley, K., Bennell, K.L., Wrigley, T., et al., 1999. Ground reaction forces, bone characteristics, and tibial stress fracture in male runners. Medicine and Science in Sports and Exercise 31 (8), 1088–1093.

Crowell, H.P., Davis, I.S., 2011. Gait retraining to reduce lower extremity loading in runners. Clinical Biomechanics [Research Support, N.I.H., Extramural Research Support, Non-U.S. Gov't Research Support, U.S. Gov't, Non-P.H.S.] 26 (1), 78–83.

Davis, A.W., Alexander, I.J., 1990. Problematic fractures and dislocations in the foot and ankle of athletes. Clinics in Sports Medicine 9 (1), 163–181.

Davis, I., Milner, C.E., Hamill, J., 2004. Does increased loading during running lead to tibial stress fractures? A prospective study. Medicine and Science in Sports and Exercise 36 (Suppl.), S58.

Diehl, J.J., Best, T.M., Kaeding, C.C., 2006. Classification and return-to-play considerations for stress fractures. Clinics in Sports Medicine 25 (1), 17–28, vii.

Dixon, S.J., Collop, A.C., Batt, M.E., 2000. Surface effects on ground reaction forces and lower extremity kinematics in running. Medicine and Science in Sports and Exercise 32 (11), 1919–1926.

Dixon, S.J., Waterworth, C., Smith, C.V., et al., 2003. Biomechanical analysis of running in military boots with new and degraded insoles. Medicine and Science in Sports and Exercise 35 (3), 472–479.

Dobrindt, O., Hoffmeyer, B., Ruf, J., et al., 2012. Estimation of return-to-sports-time for athletes with stress fracture – an approach combining risk level of fracture site with severity based on imaging. BMC Musculoskeletal Disorders 13 (1), 139.

Drinkwater, B.L., Nilson, K., Chesnut lll, C.H., et al., 1984. Bone mineral content of amenorrheic and eumenorrheic athletes. New England Journal of Medicine 311 (5), 277–281.

Edwards, P.H., Wright, M.L., Hartman, J.F., 2005. A practical approach for the differential diagnosis of chronic leg pain in the athlete. American Journal of Sports Medicine 33 (8), 1241–1249.

Edwards, W.B., Taylor, D., Rudolphi, T.J., et al., 2009. Effects of stride length and running mileage on a probabilistic stress fracture model. Medicine and Science in Sports and Exercise 41 (12), 2177–2184.

Edwards, W.B., Taylor, D., Rudolphi, T.J., et al., 2010. Effects of running speed on a probabilistic stress fracture model. Clinical Biomechanics (Bristol, Avon) 25 (4), 372–377.

Ekenman, I., 2009. Do not use bisphosphonates without scientific evidence, neither in treatment nor prophylactic, in the treatment of stress fractures. Knee Surgery, Sports Traumatology, Arthroscopy 17 (5), 433–434.

Ekenman, I., Tsai-Fellander, L., Westblad, P., et al., 1996. A study of intrinsic factors in patients with stress fractures of the tibia. Foot and Ankle International 17 (8), 477–482.

Ekenman, I., Milgrom, C., Finestone, A., et al., 2002. The role of biomechanical shoe orthoses in tibial stress fracture prevention. American Journal of Sports Medicine 30 (6), 866–870.

Finestone, A., Milgrom, C., 2008. How stress fracture incidence was lowered in the Israeli army: a 25-yr struggle. Medicine and Science in Sports and Exercise 40 (S11), S623–S629.

Finestone, A., Giladi, M., Elad, H., et al., 1999. Prevention of stress fractures using custom biomechanical shoe orthoses. Clinical Orthopaedics 360, 182–190.

Franklyn, M., Oakes, B., Field, B., et al., 2008. Section modulus is the optimum geometric predictor for stress fractures and medial tibial stress syndrome in both male and female athletes. American Journal of Sports Medicine 36 (6), 1179–1189.

Fredericson, M., Bergman, A.G., Hoffman, K.L., et al., 1995. Tibial stress reaction in runners. Correlation of clinical symptoms and scintigraphy with a new magnetic resonance imaging grading system. American Journal of Sports Medicine 23 (4), 472–481.

Friedl, K.E., Nuovo, J.A., Patience, T.H., et al., 1992. Factors associated with stress fracture in young army women: indications for further research. Military Medicine 157 (7), 334–338.

Fyhrie, D.P., Milgrom, C., Hoshaw, S.J., et al., 1998. Effect of fatiguing exercise on longitudinal bone strain as related to stress fracture in humans. Annals of Biomedical Engineering 26 (4), 660–665.

Gaeta, M., Minutoli, F., Scribano, E., et al., 2005. CT and MR imaging findings in athletes with early tibial stress injuries: comparison with bone scintigraphy findings and emphasis on cortical abnormalities. Radiology 235 (2), 553–561.

Gam, A., Goldstein, L., Karmon, Y., et al., 2005. Comparison of stress fractures of male and female recruits during basic training in the Israeli anti-aircraft forces. Military Medicine 170 (8), 710–712.

Giladi, M., Milgrom, C., Simkin, A., et al., 1987. Stress fractures and tibial bone width. A risk factor. Journal of Bone and Joint Surgery, British Volume 69 (2), 326–329.

Giza, E., Mithöfer, K., Farrell, L., et al., 2005. Injuries in women's professional soccer. British Journal of Sports Medicine 39 (4), 212–216.

Goldberg, B., Pecora, C., 1994. Stress fractures. A risk of increased training in freshman. The Physician and Sportsmedicine 22, 68–78.

Green, N.E., Rogers, R.A., Lipscomb, B., 1985. Nonunions of stress fractures of the tibia. American Journal of Sports Medicine 13, 171–176.

Groves, A.M., Cheow, H.K., Balan, K.K., et al., 2005. 16-Detector multislice CT in the detection of stress fractures: a comparison with skeletal scintigraphy. Clinical Radiology 60 (10), 1100–1105.

Haris Phuah, A., Schache, A.G., Crossley, K.M., et al., 2010. Sagittal plane bending moments acting on the lower leg during running. Gait and Posture 31 (2), 218–222.

Harrast, M.A., Colonno, D., 2010. Stress fractures in runners. Clinics in Sports Medicine 29 (3), 399–416.

Hartig, M., Joos, U., Wiesmann, H.P., 2000. Capacitively coupled electric fields accelerate proliferation of osteoblast-like primary cells and increase bone extracellular matrix formation in vitro. European Biophysics Journal 29 (7), 499–506.

Hetsroni, I., Finestone, A., Milgrom, C., et al., 2008. The role of foot pronation in the development of femoral and tibial stress fractures: a prospective biomechanical study. Clinical Journal of Sport Medicine 18 (1), 18–23.

Hoffman, J.R., Chapnik, L., Shamis, A., et al., 1999. The effect of leg strength on the incidence of lower extremity overuse injuries during military training. Military Medicine 164, 153–156.

Hoffman, M.D., Donaghe, H.E., 2011. Physiological responses to body weight-supported treadmill exercise in healthy adults. Archives of Physical Medicine and Rehabilitation 92 (6), 960–966.

Howard, C.B., Lieberman, N., Mozes, G., et al., 1992. Stress fracture detected sonographically. American Journal of Roentgenology 159 (6), 1350–1351.

Hughes, L.Y., 1985. Biomechanical analysis of the foot and ankle predisposition to developing stress fractures. Journal of Orthopaedic Research and Sports Physical Therapy 7, 96–101.

Jones, B.H., Bovee, M., Harris, J., et al., 1993. Intrinsic risk factors for exercise-related injuries among male and female army trainees. American Journal of Sports Medicine 21 (5), 705–710.

Karamanidis, K., Arampatzis, A., Bruggemann, G.P., 2006. Adaptational phenomena and mechanical responses during running: effect of surface, aging and task experience. European Journal of Applied Physiology 98, 284–298.

Kawamoto, R., Ishige, Y., Watarai, K., et al., 2002. Influence of curve sharpness on torsional loading of the tibia in running. Journal of Applied Biomechanics 18 (3), 218–230.

Kelsey, J.L., Bachrach, L.K., Procter-Gray, E., et al., 2007. Risk factors for stress fracture among young female cross-country runners. Medicine and Science in Sports and Exercise 29 (9), 1457–1463.

Khan, K.M., Fuller, P.J., Brukner, P.D., et al., 1992. Outcome of conservative and surgical management of navicular stress fracture in athletes. American Journal of Sports Medicine 20 (6), 657–666.

Khan, K.M., Brukner, P.D., Kearney, C., et al., 1994. Tarsal navicular stress fracture in athletes. Sports Medicine 17, 65–76.

Kidd, L.J., Cowling, N.R., Wu, A.C., et al., 2013. Selective and non-selective cyclooxygenase inhibitors delay stress fracture healing in the rat ulna. Journal of Orthopaedic Research 31 (2), 235–242. Epub 2012 Jul 30.

Kiss, Z.A., Khan, K.M., Fuller, P.J., 1993. Stress fractures of the tarsal navicular bone: CT findings in 55 cases. American Journal of Roentgenology 160, 111–115.

Kiuru, M.J., Pihlajamaki, H.K., Hietanen, H.J., et al., 2002. MR imaging, bone scintigraphy, and radiography in bone stress injuries of the pelvis and the lower extremity. Acta Radiologica 43 (2), 207–212.

Kor, A., Saltzman, A.T., Wempe, P.D., 2003. Medial malleolar stress fractures. Literature review, diagnosis, and treatment. Journal of the American Podiatric Medical Association 93 (4), 292–297.

Korpelainen, R., Orava, S., Karpakka, J., et al., 2001. Risk factors for recurrent stress fractures in athletes. American Journal of Sports Medicine 29 (3), 304–310.

Langdahl, B.L., Løkke, E., Carstens, M., et al., 2000. A TA repeat polymorphism in the estrogen receptor gene is associated with osteoporotic fractures but polymorphisms in the first exon and intron are not. Journal of Bone and Mineral Research 15 (11), 2222–2230.

Lappe, J., Davies, K., Recker, R., et al., 2005. Quantitative ultrasound: use in screening for susceptibility to stress fractures in female army recruits. Journal of Bone and Mineral Research 20 (4), 571–578.

Lappe, J., Cullen, D., Haynatzki, G., et al., 2008. Calcium and vitamin D supplementation decreases the incidence of stress fractures in female Navy recruits. Journal of Bone and Mineral Research 23, 741–749.

Leffers, D., Collins, L., 2009. An overview of the use of bone scintigraphy in sports medicine. Sports Medicine and Arthroscopy Review 17 (1), 21–24.

Liimatainen, E., Sarimo, J., Hulkko, A., et al., 2009. Anterior midtibial stress fractures. Results of surgical treatment. Scandinavian Journal of Surgery 98 (4), 244–249.

Liu, S.L., Lebrun, C.M., 2006. Effect of oral contraceptives and hormone replacement therapy on bone mineral density in premenopausal and perimenopausal women: a systematic review. British Journal of Sports Medicine 40 (1), 11–24.

Lloyd, T., Triantafyllou, S.J., Baker, E.R., et al., 1986. Women athletes with menstrual irregularity have increased musculoskeletal injuries. Medicine and Science in Sports and Exercise 18, 374–379.

Lohman, E.B., 3rd, Balan Sackiriyas, K.S., Swen, R.W., et al., 2011. A comparison of the spatiotemporal parameters, kinematics, and biomechanics between shod, unshod, and minimally supported running as compared to walking. Physical Therapy in Sport 12 (4), 151–163.

Loucks, A.B., 2007. Low energy availability in the marathon and other endurance sports. Sports Medicine 37 (4–5), 348–352.

Loud, K.J., Micheli, L.J., Bristol, S., et al., 2007. Family history predicts stress fracture in active female adolescents. Pediatrics 120 (2), e364–e372.

Major, N.M., 2006. Role of MRI in prevention of metatarsal stress fractures in collegiate basketball players. American Journal of Roentgenology 186 (1), 255–258.

Mammoto, T., Hirano, A., Tomaru, Y., et al., 2012. High-resolution axial MR imaging of tibial stress injuries. Sports Medicine, Arthroscopy, Rehabilitation, Therapy and Technology 4 (1), 16.

Mann, J.A., Pedowitz, D.I., 2009. Evaluation and treatment of navicular stress fractures, including nonunions, revision surgery, and persistent pain after treatment. Foot and Ankle Clinics 14 (2), 187–204.

Manore, M.M., Kam, L.C., Loucks, A.B., 2007. The female athlete triad: components, nutrition issues, and health consequences. Journal of Sports Science 25 (Suppl. 1), S61–S71.

Maquirriain, J., Ghisi, J.P., 2006. The incidence and distribution of stress fractures in elite tennis players. British Journal of Sports Medicine 40 (5), 454–459.

Marti, B., Vader, J.P., Minder, C.E., et al., 1988. On the epidemiology of running injuries. The 1984 Bern Grand-Prix study. American Journal of Sports Medicine 16, 285–294.

Marx, R.G., Saint-Phard, D., Callahan, L.R., et al., 2001. Stress fracture sites related to underlying bone health in athletic females. Clinical Journal of Sport Medicine 11 (2), 73–76.

Matheson, G.O., Clement, D.B., Kenzie, D.C., et al., 1987a. Stress fractures in athletes. A study of 320 cases. American Journal of Sports Medicine 15 (1), 46–58.

Matheson, G.O., Clement, D.B., McKenzie, D.C., et al., 1987b. Scintigraphic uptake of 99m Tc at non-painful sites in athletes with stress fractures. Sports Medicine 4, 65–75.

Mattila, V.M., Niva, M., Kiuru, M., et al., 2007. Risk factors for bone stress injuries: a follow-up study of 102,515 person-years. Medicine and Science in Sports and Exercise 39 (7), 1061–1066.

McCabe, M.P., Smyth, M.P., Richardson, D.R., 2012. Current concept review: vitamin D and stress fractures. Foot and Ankle International 33, 526–533.

Milgrom, C., Giladi, M., Kashtan, H., et al., 1985. A prospective study of the effect of a shock-absorbing orthotic device on the incidence of stress fractures in military recruits. Foot and Ankle 6 (2), 101–104.

Milgrom, C., Giladi, M., Stein, M., et al., 1985. Stress fractures in military recruits. A prospective study showing an unusually high incidence. Journal of Bone and Joint Surgery, British Volume 67 (5), 732–735.

Milgrom, C., Giladi, M., Simkin, A., et al., 1988. An analysis of the biomechanical mechanism of tibial stress fractures among Israeli infantry recruits. A prospective study. Clinical Orthopaedics 231, 216–221.

Milgrom, C., Giladi, M., Simkin, A., et al., 1989. The area moment of inertia of the tibia: a risk factor for stress fractures. Journal of Biomechanics 22 (11–12), 1243–1248.

Milgrom, C., Finestone, A., Shlamkovitch, N., et al., 1992. Prevention of overuse injuries of the foot by improved shoe shock attenuation. Clinical Orthopaedics 281, 189–192.

Milgrom, C., Finestone, A., Levi, Y., et al., 2000a. Do high impact exercises produce higher tibial strains than running? British Journal of Sports Medicine 34 (3), 195–199.

Milgrom, C., Finestone, A., Simkin, A., et al., 2000b. In vivo strain measurements to evaluate the strengthening potential of exercises on the tibial bone. Journal of Bone and Joint Surgery, British Volume 82, 591–594.

Milgrom, C., Finestone, A., Segev, S., et al., 2003. Are overground or treadmill runners more likely to sustain tibial stress fracture? British Journal of Sports Medicine 37 (2), 160–163.

Milgrom, C., Finestone, A., Novack, V., et al., 2004. The effect of prophylactic treatment with risedronate on stress fracture incidence among infantry recruits. Bone 35 (2), 418–424.

Milgrom, C., Radeva-Petrova, D.R., Finestone, A., et al., 2007. The effect of muscle fatigue on in vivo tibial strains. Journal of Biomechanics 40, 845–850.

Milner, C.E., Davis, I.S., Hamill, J., 2006a. Free moment as a predictor of tibial stress fracture in distance runners. Journal of Biomechanics 39 (15), 2819–2825.

Milner, C.E., Ferber, R., Pollard, C.D., 2006b. Biomechanical factors associated with tibial stress fracture in female runners. Medicine and Science in Sports and Exercise 38 (2), 323–328.

Milner, C.E., Hamill, J., Davis, I.S., 2007. Are knee mechanics during early stance related to tibial stress fracture in runners? Clinical Biomechanics 22, 697–703.

Milner, C.E., Hamill, J., Davis, I.S., 2010. Distinct hip and rearfoot kinematics in female runners with a history of tibial stress fracture. Journal of Orthopaedic and Sports Physical Therapy 40 (2), 59–66.

Moran, D.S., Evans, R.K., Hadad, E., 2008. Imaging of lower extremity stress fracture injuries. Sports Medicine 38 (4), 345–356.

Moran, D.S., Finestone, A.S., Arbel, Y., et al., 2012. A simplified model to predict stress fracture in young elite combat recruits. Journal of Strength and Conditioning Research 26 (9), 2585–2592.

Moretti, B., Notarnicola, A., Garofalo, R., et al., 2009. Shock waves in the treatment of stress fractures. Ultrasound in Medicine and Biology 35 (6), 1042–1049.

Morrison, N.A., Qi, J.C., Tokita, A., et al., 1994. Prediction of bone density from vitamin D receptor alleles. Nature 367 (284–287).

Muehleman, C., Lidtke, R., Berzins, A., et al., 2000. Contributions of bone density and geometry to the strength of the human second metatarsal. Bone 27 (5), 709–714.

Mündermann, A., Nigg, B.M., Humble, R.N., et al., 2003. Foot orthotics affect lower extremity kinematics and kinetics during running. Clinical Biomechanics 18 (3), 254–262.

Myburgh, K.H., Hutchins, J., Fataar, A.B., et al., 1990. Low bone density is an etiologic factor for stress fractures in athletes. Annals of Internal Medicine 113 (10), 754–759.

Nattiv, A., Puffer, J.C., Casper, J., et al., 2000. Stress fracture risk factors, incidence and distribution: a 3-year prospective study in collegiate runners. Medicine and Science in Sports and Exercise 32 (Suppl. 5), S347.

Nguyen, T.V., Eisman, J.A., 2000. Genetics of fracture: challenges and opportunities. Journal of Bone and Mineral Research 15 (7), 1253–1256.

Nielsen, M.B., Hansen, K., Holmer, P., et al., 1991. Tibial periosteal reactions in soldiers. A scintigraphic study of 29 cases of lower leg pain. Acta Orthopaedica Scandinavica 62 (6), 531–534.

Nieves, J.W., Melsop, K., Curtis, M., et al., 2010. Nutritional factors that influence change in bone density and stress fracture risk among young female cross-country runners. Physical Medicine and Rehabilitation 2 (8), 740–750.

Nigg, B.M., Herzog, W., Read, L.J., 1988. Effect of viscoelastic shoe insoles on vertical impact forces in heel-toe running. American Journal of Sports Medicine 16 (1), 70–76.

Nigg, B.M., Stergiou, P., Cole, G., et al., 2003. Effect of shoe inserts on kinematics, center of pressure, and leg joint moments during running. Medicine and Science in Sports and Exercise 35 (2), 314–319.

Nilsson, J., Thorstensson, A., 1989. Ground reaction forces at different speeds of human walking and running. Acta Physiologica Scandinavica 136 (2), 217–227.

Nissen, L.R., Astvad, K., Madsen, L., 1994. Lavenergi-laserbehandling af medialt tibialt stress-syndrom [Low energy laser treatment of shin splints]. Ugeskrift for Laeger 156, 7329–7331.

Niva, M.H., Mattila, V.M., Kiuru, M.J., et al., 2009. Bone stress injuries are common in female military trainees: a preliminary study. Clinical Orthopaedics 467 (11), 2962–2969.

Norman, A.W., 1990. Intestinal calcium absorption: a vitamin-D-hormone-mediated adaptive response. American Journal of Clinical Nutrition 51, 290–300.

Orava, S., Hulkko, A., 1988. Delayed unions and nonunions of stress fractures in athletes. American Journal of Sports Medicine 16 (4), 378–382.

Orava, S., Karpakka, J., Taimela, S., et al., 1995. Stress fracture of the medial malleolus. Journal of Bone and Joint Surgery, American Volume 77 (3), 362–365.

Pavlov, H., Torg, J.S., Freiberger, R.H., 1983. Tarsal navicular stress fractures: radiographic evaluation. Radiology 148 (3), 641–645.

Pester, S., Smith, P.C., 1992. Stress fractures in the lower extremities of soldiers in basic training. Orthopaedic Review 21 (3), 297–303.

Pohl, M.B., Mullineaux, D.R., Milner, C.E., 2008. Biomechanical predictors of retrospective tibial stress fractures in runners. Journal of Biomechanics 41 (6), 1160.

Popp, K.L., Hughes, J.M., Smock, A.J., et al., 2009. Bone geometry, strength, and muscle size in runners with a history of stress fracture. Medicine and Science in Sports and Exercise 41 (12), 2145–2150.

Portland, G., Kelikian, A., Kodros, S., 2003. Acute surgical management of Jones' fractures. Foot and Ankle International 24 (11), 829–833.

Prather, J.L., Nusynowitz, M.L., Snowdy, H.A., et al., 1977. Scintigraphic findings in stress fractures. Journal of Bone and Joint Surgery 59-A, 869–874.

Protzman, R.R., Griffis, C.G., 1977. Stress fractures in men and women undergoing military training. Journal of Bone and Joint Surgery 59-A (825).

Radin, E.L., 1986. Role of muscles in protecting athletes from injury. Acta Medica Scandinavica. Supplementum 711, 143–147.

Rome, K., Handoll, H.H., Ashford, R., 2005. Interventions for preventing and treating stress fractures and stress reactions of bone of the lower limbs in young adults [update of Cochrane Database Systemic Reviews 2000;2:CD000450; PMID: 10796367]. Cochrane Database of Systematic Reviews (2), CD000450.

Ross, R.A., Allsopp, A., 2002. Stress fractures in Royal Marines recruits. Military Medicine 167 (7), 560–565.

Rue, J.P., Armstrong, D.W., Frassica, F.J., et al., 2004. The effect of pulsed ultrasound in the treatment of tibial stress fractures. Orthopedics 27, 1192–1195.

Salzler, M.J., Bluman, E.M., Noonan, S., et al., 2012. Injuries observed in minimalist runners. Foot and Ankle International 33 (4), 262–266.

Sanders, T.G., Williams, P.M., Vawter, K.W., 2004. Stress fracture of the tarsal navicular. Foot and Ankle International 169 (7), viii–xiii.

Sasimontonkul, S., Bay, B.K., Pavol, M.J., 2007. Bone contact forces on the distal tibia during the stance phase of running. Journal of Biomechanics 40 (15), 3503–3509.

Saxena, A., Fullem, B., Hannaford, D., 2000. Results of treatment of 22 navicular stress fractures and a new proposed radiographic classification system. Journal of Foot and Ankle Surgery 39 (2), 96–103.

Schils, J.P., Andrish, J.T., Piraino, D.W., et al., 1992. Medial malleolar stress fractures in seven patients: review of the clinical and imaging features. Radiology 185 (1), 219–221.

Schnackenburg, K.E., MacDonald, H.M., Ferber, R., et al., 2011. Bone quality and muscle strength in female athletes with lower limb stress fractures. Medicine and Science in Sports and Exercise 43 (11), 2110–2119.

Schneiders, A.G., Sullivan, S.J., Hendrick, P.A., et al., 2012. The ability of clinical tests to diagnose stress fractures: a systematic review and meta-analysis. Journal of Orthopaedic and Sports Physical Therapy 42 (9), 760–771. Epub 19 Jul 2012.

Schwellnus, M.P., Jordaan, G., Noakes, T.D., 1990. Prevention of common overuse injuries by the use of shock absorbing insoles. A prospective study. American Journal of Sports Medicine 18 (6), 636–641.

Scott, S.H., Winter, D.A., 1990. Internal forces of chronic running injury sites. Medicine and Science in Sports and Exercise 22 (3), 357–369.

Shaffer, R.A., Rauh, M.J., Brodine, S.K., et al., 2006. Predictors of stress fracture susceptibility in young female recruits. American Journal of Sports Medicine 34 (1), 108–115.

Shelbourne, K.D., Fisher, D.A., Rettig, A.C., et al., 1988. Stress fractures of the medial malleolus. American Journal of Sports Medicine 16 (1), 60–63.

Shima, Y., Engebretsen, L., Iwasa, J., et al., 2009. Use of bisphosphonates for the treatment of stress fractures in athletes. Knee Surgery, Sports Traumatology, Arthroscopy 17 (5), 542–550.

Simkin, A., Leichter, I., Giladi, M., et al., 1989. Combined effect of foot arch structure and an orthotic device on stress fractures. Foot and Ankle 10 (1), 25–29.

Slayter, M., 1995. Lower limb training injuries in an army recruit population [PhD thesis]. University of Newcastle, Newcastle, UK.

Snyder, R.A., DeAngelis, J.P., Koester, M.C., et al., 2009. Does shoe insole modification prevent stress fractures? A systematic review. Hospital for Special Surgery Journal 5, 92–98.

Sofka, C.M., 2006. Imaging of stress fractures. Clinics in Sports Medicine 25 (1), 53–62, viii.

Sterling, J.C., Edelstein, D.W., Calvo, R.D., et al., 1992. Stress fractures in the athlete. Diagnosis and management. Sports Medicine 14, 336–346.

Stewart, G.W., Brunet, M.E., Manning, M.R., et al., 2005. Treatment of stress fractures in athletes with intravenous pamidronate. Clinical Journal of Sport Medicine 15 (2), 92–94.

Sullivan, D., Warren, R.F., Pavlov, H., et al., 1984. Stress fractures in 51 runners. Clinical Orthopaedics 187, 188–192.

Swenson, E.J., DeHaven, K.E., Sebastianelli, W.J., et al., 1997. The effect of a pneumatic leg brace on return to play in athletes with tibial stress fractures. American Journal of Sports Medicine 25, 322–328.

Taki, M., Iwata, O., Shiono, M., et al., 2007. Extracorporeal shock wave therapy for resistant stress fracture in athletes: a report of 5 cases. American Journal of Sports Medicine 35 (7), 1188–1192.

Tenforde, A.S., Sayres, L.C., Sainani, K.L., et al., 2010. Evaluating the relationship of calcium and vitamin d in the prevention of stress fracture injuries in the young athlete: a review of the literature. American Academy of Physical Medicine and Rehabilitation 2 (10), 945–949.

Torg, J.S., Moyer, J., Gaughan, J.P., et al., 2010. Management of tarsal navicular stress fractures: conservative versus surgical treatment: a meta-analysis. American Journal of Sports Medicine 38 (5), 1048–1053.

Uitterlinden, A.G., Burger, H., Huang, Q., et al., 1998. Relation of alleles of the collagen type Ialpha1 gene to bone density and the risk of osteoporotic fractures in postmenopausal women. New England Journal of Medicine 338 (15), 1016–1021.

Välimäki, V.-V., Alfthan, H., Lehmuskallio, E., et al., 2005. Risk factors for clinical stress fractures in male military recruits: A prospective cohort study. Bone 37 (2), 267–273.

Varner, K.E., Younas, S.A., Lintner, D.M., et al., 2005. Chronic anterior midtibial stress fractures in athletes treated with reamed intramedullary nailing. American Journal of Sports Medicine 33 (7), 1071–1076.

Verma, R.B., Sherman, O., 2001. Athletic stress fractures, part I: history, epidemiology, physiology, risk factors, radiography, diagnosis, and treatment. American Journal of Orthopedics 30, 798–806.

Vescovi, J.D., Jamal, S.A., De Souza, M.J., 2008. Strategies to reverse bone loss in women with functional hypothalamic amenorrhea: a systematic review of the literature. Osteoporosis International 19 (4), 465–478.

Vu, D., McDiarmid, T., Brown, M., et al., 2006. Clinical inquiries. What is the most effective management of acute fractures of the base of the fifth metatarsal? Journal of Family Practice 55 (8), 713–717.

Walter, S.D., Hart, L.E., McIntosh, J.M., et al., 1989. The Ontario cohort study of running-related injuries. Archives of Internal Medicine 149, 2561–2564.

Warden, S.J., Burr, D.B., Brukner, P.D., 2006. Stress fractures: pathophysiology, epidemiology, and risk factors. Current Osteoporosis Reports 4, 103–109.

Warden, S.J., Burr, D.B., Brukner, P.D., 2009. Repetitive stress pathology – bone. In: Magee, D.J., Zachazewski, J.E., Quillen, W.S. (Eds.), Pathology and intervention in musculoskeletal rehabilitation. Saunders Elsevier, St Louis, pp. 686.

Weaver, C., Teegarden, D., Lyle, R., et al., 2001. Impact of exercise on bone health and contraindication of oval contraceptive use in young women. Medicine and Science in Sports and Exercise 33, 873–880.

Wentz, L., Liu, P.Y., Haymes, E., et al., 2011. Females have a greater incidence of stress fractures than males in both military and athletic populations: a systemic review. Military Medicine 176 (4), 420–430.

Wentz, L., Liu, P.Y., Ilich, J.Z., et al., 2012. Dietary and training predictors of stress fractures in female runners. International Journal of Sport Nutrition and Exercise Metabolism 22 (5), 374–382.

Wheat, J.S., Bartlett, R.M., Milner, C.E., et al., 2003. The effect of different surfaces on ground reaction forces during running: a single-individual design approach. Journal of Human Movement Studies 44 (5), 353–364.

Wheeler, P., Batt, M.E., 2005. Do non-steroidal anti-inflammatory drugs adversely affect stress fracture healing? A short review. British Journal of Sports Medicine 39, 65–69.

Wiegerinck, J.I., Boyd, J., Yoder, J.C., et al., 2009. Differences in plantar loading between training shoes and racing flats at a self-selected running speed. Gait and Posture 29 (3), 514–519.

Williams, D.S., 3rd, McClay Davis, I., Baitch, S.P., 2003. Effect of inverted orthoses on lower-extremity mechanics in runners. Medicine and Science in Sports and Exercise 35 (12), 2060–2068.

Windle, C.M., Gregory, S.M., Dixon, S.J., 1999. The shock attenuation characteristics of four different insoles when worn in a military boot during running and marching. Gait and Posture 9 (1), 31–37.

Withnall, R., Eastaugh, J., Freemantle, N., 2006. Do shock absorbing insoles in recruits undertaking high levels of physical activity reduce lower limb injury? A randomized controlled trial. Journal of the Royal Society of Medicine 99 (1), 32–37.

Yanovich, R., Friedman, E., Milgrom, R., et al., 2012. Candidate gene analysis in Israeli soldiers with stress fractures. Journal of Sports Science and Medicine 11 (1), 147–155.

Zadpoor, A.A., Nikooyan, A.A., 2011. The relationship between lower-extremity stress fractures and the ground reaction force: a systematic review. Clinical Biomechanics 26 (1), 23–28.

Zanker, C.L., Swaine, I.L., 1998a. Relation between bone turnover, oestradiol, and energy balance in women distance runners. British Journal of Sports Medicine 32, 167–171.

Zanker, C.L., Swaine, I.L., 1998b. Bone turnover in amenorrheic and eumenorrheic women distance runners. Scandinavian Journal of Medicine and Science in Sport 8, 20–26.

Zelle, B.A., Gollwitzer, H., Zlowodzki, M., et al., 2010. Extracorporeal shock wave therapy: current evidence. Journal of Orthopaedic Trauma 24 (Suppl. 1), S66–S70.

Ziltener, J.L., Leal, S., Fournier, P.E., 2010. Non-steroidal anti-inflammatory drugs for athletes: an update. Annals of Physical and Rehabilitation Medicine 53 (4), 278–282, 82–88.

Zwitser, E.W., Breederveld, R.S., 2010. Fractures of the fifth metatarsal; diagnosis and treatment. Injury 41 (6), 555–562.

Chapter 8

Cerebral Palsy

N. Susan Stott

Chapter Outline

INTRODUCTION

DEFINITION AND INCIDENCE

Sir William Little was the first to recognize the condition of 'cerebral paresis' in a paper presented to the Obstetrical Society of London in 1861, entitled 'On the influence of abnormal parturition, difficult labours, premature birth, and asphyxia neonatorum, on the mental and physical condition of the child, especially in relation to deformities' (Little 1861). This paper contained the classic description of spastic cerebral palsy (CP), which became eponymously known as Little's disease for many years.

Although improved definitions of cerebral palsy were provided by McKeith and Polani (1959) and then Bax (1964), the definition of cerebral palsy has continued to challenge clinicians, as it is not an aetiological diagnosis but rather a term that represents a constellation of clinical signs and symptoms. In 2004, an International Workshop on Definition and Classification of Cerebral Palsy was held in Bethseda, Maryland, with the task of revisiting and updating the definition/classification of cerebral palsy to reflect the increased knowledge in the field and changing perceptions of impairment, function, and participation (Bax et al. 2005). The working group chaired by Bax reported a revised definition of cerebral palsy as 'a group of permanent disorders of the development of movement and posture, causing activity limitation, that are attributed to non-progressive disturbances that occurred in the developing fetal or infant brain. The motor disorders of cerebral palsy are often accompanied by disturbances of sensation, cognition, communication, perception, and/or behavior, and/or by a seizure' (Bax et al. 2005). Following clinician and researcher feedback, this definition was further revised to acknowledge the substantive secondary musculoskeletal pathologies that occur as a result of the disorders in movement and posture seen in cerebral palsy (Rosenbaum et al. 2007). The updated 2007 definition now reads: 'a group of permanent disorders of the development of movement and posture, causing activity limitation, that are attributed to non-progressive disturbances that occurred in the developing fetal or infant brain. The motor disorders of cerebral palsy are often accompanied by disturbances of sensation, perception, cognition, communication and behavior; by epilepsy and by secondary musculoskeletal problems'.

Thus, cerebral palsy is an umbrella term that covers a heterogeneous group of non-progressive neurological disorders, the hallmark of which is that they are acquired within the first few years of life (Gibson et al. 2007). These neurological disorders lead to characteristic effects on motor function and posture, which adversely influence the development of the growing musculoskeletal system. This, in turn, leads to secondary musculoskeletal impairments, which then impact on the individual's activity and participation throughout life and, potentially, quality of life.

Despite improvements in neonatal care, the incidence of cerebral palsy has not decreased and may even have risen over the last few decades. In the 1960s, the incidence was reported at less than 1.6 cases per 1000 live births, but by the 1990s the measured incidence had increased to 2.5 cases per 1000 live births (Odding et al. 2006). Some cerebral palsy registers now report an incidence as high as 3.5 per 1000 live births, making cerebral palsy the most common cause of physical disability in children (Blair 2010; Paneth et al. 2006). Ninety-six percent of all children with cerebral palsy now survive into adulthood, with an estimated direct and indirect cost to the economy of Aus$43 431 per person with cerebral palsy per year (Access Economics 2008). If the value of lost wellbeing is included, the cost to the economy is over Aus$115 000 per person with cerebral palsy per annum, with 76% of the costs borne by the individual with cerebral palsy.

PREDISPOSING FACTORS

Predisposing factors to cerebral palsy are many and include premature birth, multiple gestations, perinatal adverse events, and maternal infection/inflammation during pregnancy (Himmelmann et al. 2011). A comprehensive study by Thorngren-Jerneck and Herbst (2006), using data from the Swedish Medical Birth Register, calculated the odds ratios together with 95% confidence intervals for a large number of risk factors for cerebral palsy. The study reported that infants born pre-term had a highly increased risk of cerebral palsy, making up 35% of all children with cerebral palsy, even though pre-term births represent only 2 per 1000 births. The odds ratio for cerebral palsy was 34 (95% CI 29–39) for infants born at weeks 23–27 of gestation, 37 for infants born at weeks 28–29 of gestation, and 3.9 for infants born at weeks 32–36 of gestation (Thorngren-Jerneck and Herbst 2006). For those infants born at term, low Apgar scores were strongly associated with a higher risk of cerebral palsy (Table 8-1).

Socioeconomic gradient has also been linked to the incidence of cerebral palsy, with children born in households with a low socioeconomic status being reported to have a higher risk of cerebral palsy (OR

TABLE 8-1 Perinatal Factors Associated with Cerebral Palsy

Infants Born Pre-term (Before 37 Weeks)	Odds Ratio (95% Confidence Interval)
23–27 weeks	34 (29–39)
28–29 weeks	37 (32–42)
30–31 weeks	26 (23–30)
32–36 weeks	3.9 (3.4–4.4)
Infants Born at Term	**Odds Ratio (95% Confidence Interval)**
Low Apgar scores	
Apgar score 6 at 5 minutes	62 (52–74)
Apgar score 3 at 5 minutes	498 (458–542)
Breech presentation at vaginal birth	3.0 (2.4–3.7)
Instrumental delivery	1.9 (1.6–2.3)
Emergency caesarean section	1.8 (1.6–2.0)

Reprinted from Thorngren-Jerneck K and Herbst A (2006) Perinatal factors associated with cerebral palsy in children born in Sweden, Obstetrics and Gynaecology, 108(6):1499-1505, with permission from Wolters Kluwer Health.

1.49) compared with higher socioeconomic status after adjustment for demographic confounders (Hjern and Thorngren-Jerneck 2008). Although in vitro fertilization has been linked to a higher risk of cerebral palsy, this result appears largely due to the high proportions of pre-term deliveries following in vitro fertilization, primarily for twins but also for singletons (Hvidtjorn et al. 2006). A recent systematic review by McIntyre et al. (2013) identified 10 factors common to all reviewed studies that were statistically associated with increased risk of cerebral palsy following term birth; these included low birth weight, meconium aspiration, presence of major and minor birth defects, neonatal seizures or hypoglycaemia, and presence of infection.

Thus, in summary pre-term birth remains a major risk factor for the subsequent diagnosis of cerebral palsy. However, across all series, at least half of the children with cerebral palsy will have been born at term, with only 35 to 45% being delivered pre-term (i.e. at less than 37 weeks) (Krageloh-Mann and Cans 2009). Cerebral palsy can also be acquired postnatally owing to events such as acquired or traumatic brain injury, encephalitis, neonatal stroke, etc. occurring in the first 2 years of life. However, about 10% of cerebral palsy is attributable to disorders of neuronal migration that occur early in fetal life as the neuronal precursor cells leave their site of origin and migrate towards their final location within the brain (Spalice et al. 2009). Failure of normal migration leads to structural brain malformations that range from a few heterotopic neurons to complete cortical disorganization (Couillard-Despres et al. 2001; Liu 2011). An increasing number of genetic mutations have been linked with neuronal migration disorders, many of which involve genes involved in cytoskeletal reorganization (Liu 2011).

Over the years there has been considerable interest in understanding the association between normal genetic polymorphisms in the infant and the relative risks of subsequent cerebral palsy, after a predisposing event such as pre-term birth or maternal infection. Despite many studies, to date the published literature has not been able to identify significant associations between genetic variance and susceptibility to cerebral palsy. Wu et al. (2011) recently reported on a study of a population derived from total births at >36 weeks

at Kaiser Permanente Medical Care Program and the association between certain genetic polymorphisms and subsequent diagnosis of cerebral palsy. Although they found that the apoE ε4 allele and the iNOS-231 T allele were more common in patients diagnosed with cerebral palsy than in controls, they could not demonstrate a significant association once statistical corrections was made for multiple comparisons. A similar study from Australia looked at 35 candidate single-gene polymorphisms. They found that the only genetic association marginally associated with risk of hemiplegia in term infants born to mothers with a reported infection during pregnancy was fetal carriage of a prothrombin gene mutation (O'Callaghan et al. 2012).

DIAGNOSIS AND CLASSIFICATION

As noted above, cerebral palsy represents a heterogeneous group of conditions resulting from injury or insult to the developing brain before birth or in early childhood; therefore there is no one unifying investigation that can confirm the diagnosis. Given the lack of a single diagnostic test for all cases of cerebral palsy, the clinician still must use clinical signs and symptoms as the key components of their diagnostic pathway for cerebral palsy. Several possible algorithms for clinical screening for cerebral palsy have been published, but have not yet been sufficiently tested to determine validity and generalizability across different practices and countries. These are recommended to the reader only for interest to highlight the clinical thinking applied by paediatric neurologists and developmental paediatricians to the challenge of diagnosing cerebral palsy in the young child (Cottalorda et al. 2012).

In practice, the first clinical signs of cerebral palsy are usually evident before the age of 2 to 3 years, although the occasional child with very mild clinical signs (e.g. impacting only the foot and ankle) may present later to the clinician. Difficulty with swallowing, poor motor skills, and poor quality of general movement are among the first identifiable symptoms in the newborn period, but are not specific for cerebral palsy and not always apparent to new parents. These signs often precede the more obvious features of motor impairments such as delays in developmental milestones (e.g. sitting, rolling over, crawling, and walking). Children who have very mild cerebral palsy may have developmental milestones that fit within the continuum of normal but can present with specific alterations in gait patterns, such as toe walking (unilateral or bilateral) and hypertonia on clinical examination (see below).

By the time of the appearance of delays in motor milestones, considerable time may have passed since the original insult to the brain in utero or at delivery. Professor Heinz Prechtl has published extensively on the assessment of general movements (GM) in the new-born 'infant at risk' as a guide to subsequent development of cerebral palsy (Ferrari et al. 2002; Prechtl 2001). For the first 2 months post-term, GMs are generally referred to as writhing movements. At about 9 weeks corrected age, the 'writhing movements' change to what is termed 'fidgety movements'. In turn these are replaced by movements that reflect voluntary motor activity and anti-gravity movements around 15–20 weeks. Abnormalities in early movement patterns, such as cramped synchronized general movements and the absence of fidgety or spontaneous movement at 2–4 months corrected age, can be used to identify infants with neurodevelopmental disabilities, with reported sensitivity of >92% and specificity of >83% (Burger and Louw 2009). Such abnormal patterns of movement are thought more predictive of cerebral palsy than oromotor difficulties in the young infant.

GMs appear highly sensitive for neurodevelopmental disabilities. Early cranial ultrasounds have been used with some success to predict later development of cerebral palsy, as has neonatal MRI (Hnatyszyn et al. 2010; Mathur and Inder 2009). However, GMs appear to be more sensitive to the subsequent development of cerebral palsy than are cranial ultrasounds in a neonate (although less specific). GMs are quick to perform and non-invasive, and can be assessed from appropriate video of the infant's movements (Bosanquet et al. 2013). At the moment, the General Movements Trust requires that clinicians complete a 4-day training course in general movements before they can apply these to their practice. Information on the available courses is accessible through the General Movements Trust website http://www.general-movements-trust.info/5/HOME.html.

In 2004, the American Academy of Neurology published a practice guideline that advocated routine neuroimaging for all children who are suspected of having cerebral palsy (Russman and Ashwal 2004). This recommendation has proved controversial in practice, as routine imagining of the brain in children diagnosed with cerebral palsy is unlikely to lead to findings that alter clinical management. However, neuroimaging has contributed significantly to our understanding of the neuroanatomical pathology seen in children with cerebral palsy, with abnormal findings present in 80% to 90% of children (Korzeniewski et al. 2008). A systematic review of neuroimaging studies found that about 30% of cerebral palsy resulted from prenatal insults, 40% from insults around the time of birth and the rest from post-natal events (Korzeniewski et al. 2008). However, the review also highlighted four pervasive problems in the current literature: (i) inconsistent language used to describe radiological findings, (ii) study designs that were not generalizable owing to non-population-based samples, (iii) aetiological assumptions about the cause of the neuroanatomical findings that may not be accurate, and (iv) assumptions about timing of neurological events from neuroimaging findings with bias towards the early end of the age spectrum. The authors concluded that the 'primary contribution of neuroimaging to cerebral palsy diagnosis is to rule out progressive or genetic disorder'. However, they also noted that neuroimaging can be beneficial to clinicians, providing reassurance and greater clinical certainty about the diagnosis for both the clinician and parents.

Different patterns of damage to the developing brain have been identified within the umbrella of cerebral palsy. These depend on the presumed timing of the neurological insult, due to different neuronal susceptibilities as brain development proceeds (Ferriero 2004; Stolp et al. 2012). For example, injury to the developing brain in the late third trimester leads to grey matter loss as well as damage to the hippocampus and cerebellum (Gunn and Bennet 2008; Volpe 2009), and is more probably associated with hemiplegia (unilateral involvement). Pre-term injury is associated with white matter and subcortical grey matter damage and often manifests as spastic diplegia (bilateral involvement) and is more likely to occur in the early third trimester (Krageloh-Mann and Horber 2007).

Animal models of maternal inflammation at a time point equivalent to the latter part of the second trimester lead to diffuse demyelination and cystic lesions in the fetal brain that look similar to the periventricular leukomalacia seen commonly on MRI scans of pre-term infants who develop cerebral palsy (Rezaie and Dean 2002). This appearance is thought due to the susceptibility of oligodendrocytes at that time point in brain development. As neuroimaging modalities advance, it is likely that neuroimaging will further improve our understanding of the aetiologies and timing of insults that cause cerebral palsy and ultimately will contribute to the clinical algorithm of management (Arnfield et al. 2013).

Of note, up to 17–29% of children who have clinical features consistent with cerebral palsy will have normal or non-specific findings on MRI scans (Benini et al. 2012). Children with specific subtypes of cerebral palsy such as ataxic or dyskinetic cerebral palsy seem especially likely to have normal or non-specific findings on structural MRI (Ashwal et al. 2004). For these children, further testing for metabolic and genetic conditions such as Rett's syndrome, Angelman syndrome, hereditary spastic paraplegia, and neurometabolic disorders such as congenital lactic acidaemia and urea cycle defects has been recommended (Ashwal et al. 2004). Such testing is best carried out by paediatric neurologists, rehabilitation specialists, or developmental pediatricians, as the number of tests available is increasing year by year and the indications for use of such tests is outside the scope of the general clinician. However, despite advances in diagnostic testing, comprehensive metabolic and genetic testing still fails to clarify the aetiology of cerebral palsy for many children. It is possible that, with better and more advanced imaging techniques such as diffusion imaging, MRI may detect abnormalities that have previously been below the limits of detection (Scheck et al. 2012). Such abnormalities may fall into the category of alterations in functional pathways in the brain rather than structural abnormalities. In this regard, new imaging techniques such as high-angular diffusion imaging (HARDI), functional MRI (fMRI), and trans-magnetic stimulation (TMS) hold promise for the detection of causes that currently cannot be defined (Ment et al. 2009). Also possible, however, is that, with more developments in this area, a larger proportion of children with 'cerebral palsy' and normal MRI scans will be shown to have alternative aetiologies such as metabolic abnormalities or previously unrecognized inherited neurological conditions or movement disorders.

Several classification systems exist for cerebral palsy. Traditionally, it has been classified by both motor type and distribution. The topographic distributions include monoplegia (one limb), hemiplegia (i.e. unilateral involvement of one arm and leg), diplegia (lower limbs more involved than upper limbs), triplegia (involvement of three limbs), and quadriplegia (total body involvement with involvement of all four limbs). Phrases such as double hemiplegia are also present in the older published literature, reflecting the child with bilateral but very asymmetric involvement. An early study in the 1980s showed that there was only poor to moderate agreement on topographical pattern between experienced neurodevelopmental paediatricians, with the terms diplegia and quadriplegia creating most confusion (Blair and Stanley 1985). Previous studies (Reid et al. 2011; Rosenbaum et al. 2007) suggest the use of the terms 'unilateral' and 'bilateral' rather than categories 'diplegia' and 'quadriplegia', although there is recognition that even the distinction between unilateral and bilateral can be blurred, as many children with primarily unilateral cerebral palsy have some degree of involvement of the contralateral limb and some children with bilateral cerebral palsy can be very asymmetric (Reid et al. 2011; Rosenbaum et al. 2007).

Classification of cerebral palsy by alterations in motor type and distribution including hypertonia (spasticity, dystonia, or rigidity) and movement disorders [e.g. dyskinetic cerebral palsy (dystonia, chorea, athetosis)] is also problematic as many children have a combination of hypertonia and movement disorders. However, improved accuracy of classification of an individual patient by tone and motor involvement can be achieved with careful standardization of definitions and appropriate training, as demonstrated by the SCPE (Surveillance of Cerebral Palsy in Europe) Collaboration (Sellier et al. 2012), which is considered to be the gold standard internationally. Nevertheless, although classification by topography and motor type provides some useful guide for the clinician, it may not predict the underlying brain pathology and timing of the brain insult (Grant and Barkovich 1998) and as yet may not provide a definite guide to clinical management (Holmefur et al. 2013; Rose et al. 2011).

One of the key advances in cerebral palsy management in the last 15 years has been the development of reliable and valid methods of classification based not on impairment but rather on functional ability. In the lower limb, this work has underpinned the ability to predict risk of secondary musculoskeletal consequences such as hip subluxation and scoliosis (Persson-Bunke et al. 2012) and to accurately judge outcomes of various treatments of cerebral palsy (Shore et al. 2012). In turn, this has allowed the development of treatment algorithms that are based on gross motor functional ability in the lower limbs. The key functional classification for the lower limb is the Gross Motor Function Classification System (GMFCS), which is a five-level ordinal scale developed by Rosenbaum et al. (2008). Table 8-2 outlines the descriptors of the GMFCS classification across three different age bands. The GMFCS classifies children with cerebral palsy according to 'usual' (not best) motor ability in the lower limbs and was first reported in 1997 (Palisano et al. 1997). An expanded and revised version was reported in 2008, allowing development of a 12–18-year-old age band (Palisano et al. 2008). The originators of the scale reported moderate intra-rater reliability in children less than 2 years of age (weighted $\kappa=0.55$) and excellent reliability in children from age 2 to 12 years (weighted $\kappa=0.75$) (Palisano et al. 1997). High levels of reliability for proxy-reporting by parents and by video or medical chart review have also been reported (Bodkin et al. 2003; Morris and Bartlett 2004). Jewell et al. (2011) reported precise agreement of 77% and a chance-corrected agreement of $\kappa=0.7$ between therapists and parents using the GMFCS descriptors for children with cerebral palsy. Although not developed for adults with cerebral palsy, the GMFCS levels have also been reported to have high inter-rater reliability in adults with cerebral palsy when self-reports are compared with professional ratings, with ICCs of 0.93–0.95 (Jahnsen et al. 2006).

The validity of the GMFCS is also high. The GMFCS level observed at the age of 12 years is highly predictive of ambulatory function as an adult (McCormick et al. 2007). The positive predictive value of the GMFCS at 12 years of age to predict walking without mobility aides by adulthood is 0.88. Conversely, if a child is using a wheelchair at the age of 12 years as the usual mode of mobility then the positive predictive value is 0.96 that he/she will still use a wheelchair as an adult. The motor patterns/topography overlap the GMFCS definitions with the majority of children with spastic hemiplegia fitting into GMFCS levels I and III and the majority of children with spastic quadriplegia fitting into GMFCS levels IV and V. Although the GMFCS has been widely adopted, it has been suggested that children may need to be re-classified at the ages of 2 and 5 years as the distinction between different levels, particularly levels II and III, may be more difficult when classifying children below the age of 4 years (Palisano et al. 2006).

IMPAIRMENTS

Cerebral palsy is an upper motor lesion, and is characterized by features of the upper motor neuron syndrome, which is divided into positive and negative signs. Negative signs include muscle weakness, loss of selective motor control, sensory deficits, poor co-ordination, bradykinesia, and poor balance. The common positive signs include hypertonia, which is subdivided into spasticity, dystonia, and rigidity and hyperkinetic features, such as chorea, dystonia, and athetosis.

CHANGES IN MUSCLE TONE AND MOVEMENT PATTERNS

Abnormal muscle tone is a common diagnostic feature of cerebral palsy. Older textbooks identified that a small percentage of children with cerebral palsy had low tone or hypotonia (termed hypotonic cerebral palsy) but suggest that the majority will have increased tone or hypertonia. Current literature suggests that children with hypotonia often have movement disorders by the age of 5 years or do not have cerebral palsy (Nelson and Ellenberg 1982), or, in those children who acquire cerebral palsy antenatally or at birth, a change in tone becomes evident somewhere from the first 6 to 24 months of life. The most severe cases are often diagnosed as early as around the age of 6 months and children with milder clinical phenotypes are often not diagnosed until the age of 18 months to 2 years or beyond. The general term 'hypertonia' (increased

TABLE 8-2	Gross Motor Function Classification System (GMFCS) Levels for Children				
	Age 4–6*	Age 6–12*	Age 12–18*	Risk of Hip Subluxation** (%)	Risk of Scoliosis*** (%); Cobb Angle >40°
GMFCS level 1.	Independent, without support Balance, speed and co-ordination are limited; Emerging ability to run and jump	Independent, without support Runs/jumps but speed, balance, and co-ordination limited May participate in physical activities/sport	Independent, without support Runs/jumps but speed, balance and coordination limited May participate in physical activities/sport	0–5	—
GMFCS level II	Independent on short distances/level surfaces Unable to run or jump Stairs with handrail	Difficulty with long distances, on uneven terrain, inclines, crowded areas, confined spaces or when carrying objects Hand-held mobility device or physical assistance or wheeled mobility for long distances Stairs with handrail or physical assistance	Environmental factors and personal choice influence mobility choices Hand-held mobility device Wheeled mobility for long distances Stairs with handrail or physical assistance	8–17	—
GMFCS level III	Hand-held mobility device on level surfaces Transported for long distances or uneven terrain	Hand-held mobility device in most indoor settings Wheeled mobility for long distances Stairs with rails and supervision or assistance	Environmental factors and personal choice influence mobility choices Self-mobility using manual or powered wheelchair Transported on manual wheelchair	39–50	—
GMFCS level IV	Indoor mobility at best with walker and adult supervision Transported in the community Powered wheelchair	At home: floor mobility, or walk short distance with assistance Powered wheelchair – or transported on manual wheelchair	Powered wheelchair or transported on manual wheelchair	45–69	20
GMFCS level V	Adaptive seating Transported in manual wheelchair – for some: powered wheelchair with extensive adaptations	At home: floor mobility or carried by adult Transported in manual wheelchair For some: powered wheelchair with extensive adaptations	Transported in manual wheelchair For some: powered wheelchair with extensive adaptations	68–90	40

*Palisano et al. (2007); **Terjesen (2012); ***Persson-Bunke et al. (2012).

muscle tone) includes spasticity, dystonia, and rigidity with more than one type of movement disorder existing within the same patient. Overall, at least 20% of children with cerebral palsy will have an element of secondary dystonia as well as spasticity (Rice et al. 2009), with this figure increasing as knowledge of the features of dystonia broadens. Rigidity appears to be relatively uncommon in individuals with cerebral palsy.

The Hypertonia Assessment Tool (HAT) is a seven-item clinical assessment tool developed to differentiate the subtypes of paediatric hypertonia in children between the ages of 4 and 19 (Jethwa et al. 2010). Each limb is evaluated separately in the Hypertonia Assessment Tool and is scored according to seven items. Two spasticity items, two rigidity items, and three dystonia items are present within the tool. If one sub-item is scored as present, then the child has some form of hypertonia. If another item is scored as present, then the child has mixed hypertonia. The internal consistency of the tool is high for dystonia ($\alpha = 0.79$) and moderate for spasticity ($\alpha = 0.58$). The developers of the tool have reported the test–retest reliability, the inter-rater reliability, and the validity when compared with the judgement of an expert neurologist (Jethwa et al. 2010). For spasticity, the test–retest reliability is high [prevalence-adjusted bias adjusted kappa (PABAK) of 1.0], the inter-rater reliability substantial (PABAK 0.65), and validity moderate to good (PABAK 0.57–0.74). For dystonia, the test–retest reliability is moderate (PABAK 0.43), the inter-rater reliability fair (PABAK 0.3), and validity of mixed outcomes with agreement ranging from fair to substantial (PABAK 0.3–0.65). For the absence of rigidity the tool has excellent test–retest and inter-rater reliability and validity (PABAK 0.91–1.0). Although further work is required, the HAT is a useful screening tool in the clinic for different types of hypertonia in the four limbs and has highlighted that dystonia may be present in conjunction with spasticity, but not necessarily in the same distribution in the four limbs. The HAT has not been extensively tested in adults.

Spasticity has been characterized as 'a velocity-dependent increase in the tonic stretch reflexes (muscle tone) with exaggerated tendon jerks, resulting from the hyperexcitability of the stretch reflex' (Lance 1980). Spasticity commonly leads to secondary effects on the growing musculoskeletal system, with evolving muscle and joint contractures due to the restriction in muscle excursion with active use of the limb. Clinicians evaluate the presence of spasticity by testing the degree of resistance to passive movement of the limb when performed at different speeds. Typically, when spasticity is present, 'resistance to externally imposed movement increases with increasing speed of stretch and varies with the direction of joint movement; secondly, resistance to externally imposed movement rises rapidly above a threshold speed or joint angle' (Gibson et al. 2007). At the ankle, spasticity in the calf muscle is manifested by increased ankle reflex and resistance to rapid passive dorsiflexion, seen sometimes as beats of clonus. Spasticity in other muscle groups in the foot and ankle, such as tibialis posterior, can also be detected by rapid movement but is difficult to quantify more accurately owing to the small size of the muscles.

The resistance to movement felt by the examiner when testing for spasticity reflects both the neural component of spasticity and the degree of soft-tissue compliance (i.e. degree of secondary muscle contracture). Differentiating between the two is important to establish the type of treatment that might most benefit the patient and ways to quantify spasticity are therefore important. The Ashworth and Modified Ashworth scales are the most widely used scales to rank spasticity (Biering-Sorensen et al. 2006). The original five-item Ashworth scale was expanded by Bohannon and Smith (1987) into a six-item modified Ashworth scale that grades spasticity from 0 (no increase in muscle tone) through to 4 (impaired parts/s rigid in flexion or extension). Spasticity is tested with the patient in a supine position and starts with the joint either maximally flexed (if the muscle is a primary joint flexor) or maximally extended (if the muscle is a primary joint extensor). The joint is then moved to the opposite maximal position (either extension or flexion) over the period of 1 second (Box 8-1). Although widely used to assess muscle tone, the inter-rater agreement for the modified Ashworth scale varies between muscle groups, with ICCs that range from >0.75 for the hamstrings and <0.5 for other limb muscles (Clopton et al. 2005).

When used to assess spasticity in the ankle plantarflexors in children with cerebral palsy, the inter-rater

BOX 8-1 DESCRIPTION OF ASHWORTH, MODIFIED ASHWORTH, AND TARDIEU SCALES

ASHWORTH SCALE (ASHWORTH 1964)

0   No increase in tone
1   Slight increase in tone giving catch when the limb is moved in flexion and extension
2   More marked increase in tone, but limb is easily fixed
3   Considerable increase in tone; passive movement difficult
4   Limb rigid in flexion or extension

MODIFIED ASHWORTH SCALE (BOHANNON AND SMITH 1987)

0   No increase in muscle tone
1   Slight increase in muscle tone, manifested by a catch, followed by minimal resistance at the end of range of motion when the part is moved in flexion or extension/abduction or adduction, etc.
1+   Slight increase in muscle tone, manifested by a catch, followed by minimal resistance throughout the remainder (less than half) of the range of motion
2   More marked increase in muscle tone through most of the range of motion, but the affected part is easily moved
3   Considerable increase in muscle tone; passive movement is difficult
4   Affected part is rigid in flexion or extension (e.g. abduction or adduction)

MODIFIED TARDIEU SCALE (FOSANG ET AL. 2003)

For each muscle group, reaction to stretch is rated at a specific stretch velocity with two parameters (X and Y)

Quality of Muscle Reaction (X)

0   No resistance throughout the course of the passive movement
1   Slight resistance through the course of the passive movement; no clear catch at a precise angle
2   Clear catch at a precise angle, interrupting the passive movement, followed by release
3   Fatigable clonus (<10 s when maintaining the pressure) appearing at a precise angle
4   Unfatigable clonus (>10 s when maintaining the pressure) at a precise angle
5   Joint immovable

Angle of Muscle Reaction (Y)

Measure relative to the position of minimal stretch of the muscle (corresponding to angle zero) for all joints except the hip and ankle, where it is relative to the resting anatomical position (e.g. angle zero corresponds to the ankle at 90°)

R1 Angle of muscle reaction
R2 Angle of full range of motion (passive range of motion)

Definition of Velocities Used

V1 As slow as possible (slower than the natural drop of the limb segment under gravity)
V2 Speed of the limb segment falling under gravity
V3 As fast as possible (faster than the rate of the natural drop of the limb segment under gravity)

---

reliability of the modified Ashworth scale has been reported to be at best only moderate, with ICCs of 0.56 with the knee extended and 0.46 with the knee flexed (Yam and Leung 2006). Similar findings were reported by Mutlu et al. (2008) and by Clopton et al. (2005) who identified that the gastrocnemius and soleus had the lowest reliability of all the muscle groups tested in their study. The validity of the modified Ashworth and the Ashworth scales has also been questioned as they do not address the velocity-dependent nature of the stretch reflex and are unable to 'differentiate' between the 'neural and peripheral contributions' to passive resistance to stretch (Vattanasilp et al. 2000). Until recently, there have been few other options to grade spasticity and the Ashworth and the modified Ashworth scales therefore remain in current use despite concerns about reliability. Recently, the Australian Spasticity Assessment has been reported to be a more reliable measure of spasticity than the

Ashworth scale (Williams et al. 2008), with clearer definitions of the different grades within the scale. However this measurement tool has been published only in abstract form and has yet to be tested by other groups for reliability and validity.

More recently, clinicians have utilized the Tardieu scale as a way to qualify the effect of spasticity on joint arc of motion (Fosang et al. 2003). The Tardieu scale involves assessment of resistance to passive movement at both slow and fast speeds, thus adhering more closely to Lance's (1980) definition of spasticity. This scale has been taken up into everyday clinical practice, with use of the scale to discriminate between the joint angle achieved with a slow stretch (R2) and the joint angle achieved with a fast stretch (R1). R2 is the angle of full-range of motion (passive range of motion) and R1 is the angle of muscle reaction or 'catch' following a fast stretch. The difference between the two is thought to represent the degree of spasticity that can be addressed with focal injections of botulinum toxin A or other systemic treatments for spasticity. However, a systematic review in 2006 on use of the Tardieu scale in adults noted that there has been no rigorous testing of the reliability and validity of the Tardieu scale (Haugh et al. 2006). The authors also noted that there were relatively few publications that had reported use of the Tardieu scale (only 31 by 2006), none of which included adults. The review identified two papers that looked at aspects of the scale, noting considerable variation in the measured angles achieved due to variations in the speed of applied stretch (Fosang et al. 2003; Mackey et al. 2004). Since that review there have been a number of papers that have further investigated the reliability of the Tardieu scale in cerebral palsy (Gracies et al. 2010; Numanoglu and Gunel 2012; Yam and Leung 2006). Yam and Leung found that the inter-rater reliability of the Modified Tardieu scale was low, with ICCs of 0.22 for ankle plantarflexion with the knee extended and 0.44 for ankle plantarflexion with the knee flexed. Conversely, Gracies et al. (2010) have argued that the reliability of the Tardieu scale in adult stroke can be improved by training but did not report ICCs for their study. Despite these issues, the Tardieu scale is increasingly being used in preference to the Ashworth in the literature owing to its ability to quantify a dynamic catch.

Individuals with cerebral palsy commonly have a secondary dystonia associated with their spasticity. Dystonia is a movement disorder in which there is 'involuntary sustained or intermittent muscle contractions (causing) twisting and repetitive movements, abnormal postures or both' (Gibson et al. 2007). Dystonic movements and postures are often superimposed on, or substituted for, voluntary movements and postures and may be related to specific tasks or movements. Dystonic movements and postures are not random; rather they are characteristic for that individual and are repetitive, with overflow of activity into extraneous muscles leading to abnormal patterns of muscle activation during a voluntary movement or posture. Dystonia is not present during sleep and is associated with less development of muscle and joint contracture than spasticity.

Injury to the basal ganglia is most commonly associated with dystonia but other areas of the brain have been implicated including the cerebellum (Sadnicka

et al. 2012), brainstem (Blood et al. 2012), and sensorimotor cortex (Tamura et al. 2008). In children with cerebral palsy, the onset of secondary dystonia is typically later than spasticity and may present first between the ages of 3 and 5 years, with progression into late childhood or adolescence (Burke et al. 1980). A common dystonic posture in cerebral palsy is an equino-varus foot deformity; this often appears in children with hemiplegia around the age of 5–8 years.

Dystonia can be quantified by the Barry–Albright Dystonia Scale (BADS). This scale was developed to define the severity of involuntary movements and postures that are a consequence of dystonia. It is a five-point ordinal scale that assesses secondary dystonia in eight regions of the body: eyes, mouth, neck, trunk, and the four extremities (Barry et al. 1999). In each region, dystonia is rated on a scale from 0 (no dystonia) through to a score of 4 (severe dystonia); with a maximum score of 24, which is a sum of all regions measured. The reliability of this scale has been assessed by the developers in a small group of patients with generalized secondary dystonia. The intra-rater reliability was reported as excellent with mean ICCs for total BAD scores of 0.967 and 0.978 for the two raters studied, although reliability across the individual items was more variable (Barry et al. 1999). Inter-rater reliability is less satisfactory but can be improved with training (Sellier et al. 2012).

JOINT RANGE OF MOTION

Children with cerebral palsy are not born with restrictions in range of motion and will have a full range of motion in all their joints at birth unless they have other medical conditions or associated syndromes. However, there is strong evidence for increasing abnormality in lower limb muscles in cerebral palsy over time, secondary to the altered neurological environment within which the muscles function (Barrett and Lichtwark 2010). Lower limb muscles in children with cerebral palsy show both impaired longitudinal muscle growth and reduced physiological cross-sectional area, leading to muscles that are significantly smaller and shorter than those seen in typically developing children (Oberhofer et al. 2010; Smith et al. 2013). At the foot and ankle, calf muscle shortening leads to reduction in measured ankle dorsiflexion over time. A recent population-based study from Sweden has reported that the passive range of ankle dorsiflex-ion decreases by an average of 19° in the first 18 years of life in children with cerebral palsy, with a significant association between higher Ashworth scores (indicat-ing increased spasticity) and greater reduction in ankle dorsiflexion (Hagglund and Wagner 2011). Much of this decrease in ankle dorsiflexion occurs in the first 5 years of life, a finding that the authors postulate is due to higher rate of growth of the bony skeleton during that time and the higher levels of spasticity recorded at younger ages (Hagglund and Wagner 2008). The figures from this study probably under-represent the true natural history of development of calf muscle contracture in cerebral palsy, given that all of the children in the study group were receiving on-going monitoring and treatment from health pro-fessionals, including physiotherapists.

Calf muscle hypertonia, coupled with loss of passive ankle dorsiflexion, leads to abnormal foot postures in standing and gait, such as either equinus (increased plantarflexion) or hindfoot varus or valgus to accommodate the decreased functional range of the gastrocnemius–soleus muscle complex. Ini-tially these postures are dynamic and correctable to neutral with passive manipulation when the child is non-weightbearing. However, over time fixed muscle contracture develops, with shortening of the gastrocnemius–soleus muscle complex, manifested by fixed plantarflexion, or equinus, at the ankle on passive range of motion testing. Ultrasound studies have suggested that this shortening may differentially impact on the muscle belly, with a longer-than-nor-mal Achilles tendon and shorter-than-normal medial gastrocnemius muscle belly in children with spastic diplegia cerebral palsy (Wren et al. 2010).

If untreated, equinus contracture at the ankle can finally lead to true joint capsular contracture, although this is very rare at the ankle in children and adoles-cents with cerebral palsy. Secondary compensations elsewhere in the foot are more common, particularly at the level of the midfoot, as a consequence of the development of valgus or varus positioning of the hindfoot (Davids 2010). Valgus positioning of the hindfoot coupled with equinus at the ankle can be associated with a deformity known as midfoot break. Midfoot break is characterized by a forefoot position that is dorsiflexed, abducted, and supinated relative to

the hind foot. As part of the deformity, the navicular bone is subluxated dorsally and laterally on the talus (Maurer et al. 2013). Conversely hindfoot varus sec-ondary to ankle equinus can lead to pronation of the forefoot and a higher arch, a deformity known as cavus (i.e. an equino-cavovarus foot).

Passive range of motion at the ankle is most typi-cally measured with a goniometer at the ankle, with the hindfoot held in subtalar joint neutral. Subtalar joint neutral has been defined as the position of the subtalar joint in which the talocalcaneal joint, the talonavicular joint, and the calcaneocuboid are all congruously aligned (Elveru et al. 1988). Clinically, this represents the position in which the navicular is centred on the talus. If the hindfoot cannot be aligned to neutral, measures of range of motion at the ankle will be inaccurate (Tiberio 1987). Ankle range of motion is documented both with the knee flexed to 90° and with the knee extended. The maximum ankle dorsiflexion with the knee flexed represents the length of the soleus muscle. The maximum ankle dorsiflexion with the knee extended reflects the length of both the soleus muscle and the gastrocnemius muscle. The dif-ference between these two measures has been termed the Silfverskiold test (Silfverskiold 1924). Although these measures are commonly performed by clini-cians, the intra-rater reliability between sessions is variable, with ICCs of 0.63–0.69 for ankle dorsiflexion with the knee extended and 0.75–0.90 for ankle dor-siflexion with the knee flexed (Kilgour et al. 2003). Mean absolute differences in measures between ses-sions (by the same rater) were reported by the same authors as 6±5.8° for ankle dorsiflexion with the knee extended and 5.9±5.6° for ankle dorsiflexion with the knee flexed. These ranges lead to a wide 95% CI of almost 20°. The normative ranges of ankle dorsiflexion are 40–50° in infants and only 25° in children aged 2–17 years (Kilgour et al. 2002) making these errors in measurement more significant than other joints with greater ranges of motion. Another potential cause of error is secondary deformity in the subtalar or mid-tarsal joints, which can make it difficult to assess accu-rately the range of motion at the ankle. It is important therefore to stabilize the hindfoot in the correct posi-tion before measurement.

Measurement of subtalar joint range of motion is more difficult and can have a high level of inaccuracy

(Elveru et al. 1988). Elveru et al. (1988) reported ICCs for inter-rater reliability of 0.25 for measurement of subtalar joint neutral position, 0.32 for subtalar joint inversion and 0.17 for subtalar joint eversion. These ICCs are considerably lower than ICCs reported by the same authors for measures of passive ankle range of motion and were equally low regardless of whether the subject had a neurological diagnosis or not. Overall the authors recommended that one therapist should take all repeated measures and that clinical decisions based on these measures should be carefully considered.

MUSCLE STRENGTH

Reduced muscle strength is present in many adults with cerebral palsy, with a recent systematic review showing that young adults with cerebral palsy have 34–60% lower muscle strength, 21–52% lower muscle endurance, and 14% lower cardiorespiratory endurance compared with their peers (Hombergen et al. 2012). The authors of this systematic review postulate several reasons for the lower muscle strength and endurance in individuals with cerebral palsy. First, the normal reciprocal synchronization that occurs between agonist and antagonist muscle groups in voluntary movement may be compromised; secondly, the presence of a hypersensitive tonic stretch reflex may limit normal muscle excursion during use; thirdly, there may be atrophy of type II muscle fibres, leading to greater proportion of type I fibres; and fourthly, muscle growth is impaired during childhood, leading to muscle volumes in adulthood that are reduced by as much as 50% compared with age-matched peers (Brooke and Engel 1969; Shortland 2009).

Historically, it was believed that manual muscle strength testing could not be performed in individuals with cerebral palsy because of inability to isolate movements, lack of full joint range of motion, and accompanying changes in tone. Eek and Beckung (2008) have shown that children who function at GMFCS levels I to III can initiate muscle contraction in isolation, although children who function at GMFCS level III find the task more challenging. Thus, individual muscle strength can be graded in ambulatory individuals with cerebral palsy using the Medical Research Council (MRC) scale for muscle strength. This scale rates patients' effort to contract a muscle on a scale of 0 to 5. [Grade 5: muscle contracts normally against full resistance; grade 4: muscle strength is reduced but can move the joint against gravity and resistance; grade 3: muscle strength is such that the joint can be moved against gravity but not if there is any further resistance from the examiner; grade 2: muscle can move the joint only if gravity is eliminated; grade 1: only a trace or flicker of movement is seen; grade 0: no movement is observed (Medical Research Council 1943).] However, the MRC scale does have limitations in this patient population as muscle strength is often graded within a limited arc of motion, rather than the full range, owing to coexistent contracture and spasticity. Although used in this patient population, there are no reported studies of the reliability of manual muscle charting and no studies linking the measured grade of muscle strength to other measures of muscle strength in this group of patients.

Another way to assess muscle function in individuals with cerebral palsy is the use of measurements by a hand-held dynamometer. This is a device that can be held between the hand of the examiner and the patient's body part, similar to the positioning for manual muscle testing. Unlike manual muscle charting, the hand-held dynamometer provides a quantified measure of muscle force generation, which has been shown to have good validity when compared with the gold standard isokinetic dynamometry (Stark et al. 2011). In recent years, several authors have shown that a hand-held dynamometer can be used to assess muscle strength in children with cerebral palsy with good reliability and ICCs consistently above 0.8 for intra- and inter-sessional testing (Berry et al. 2004). Normative values are also now available for children of different ages, allowing comparisons of different patient groups (Eek et al. 2006). Testing of independently ambulatory children with cerebral palsy with hand-held dynamometry has shown that they have significantly reduced lower limb muscle strength, ranging from 46% to 84% of predicted normal depending on the muscle group tested (Eek et al. 2008). The same authors found that muscle weakness appears most pronounced at the ankle, with substantive weakness in both ankle dorsiflexion and ankle plantarflexors. Overall muscle strength in the lower limbs is associated with the GMFCS level, being 75–100% of predicted normal values in children who function at

GMFCS level 1, 50–75% of predicted normal values in children who function at GMFCS level II, and below 50% of predicted normal values for children who function at GMFCS level III (Eek and Beckung 2008).

Typical values for hand-held dynamometry in adults with cerebral palsy have not been established. However, normative values for able-bodied adults are available for a clinician to compare individual patient data together with estimates of inter-sessional variability, which varies between muscle groups (van der Ploeg et al. 1991).

PAIN

Both adolescents and adults with cerebral palsy report significant prevalence of pain. The foot and ankle appears to be one of the most common sites to experience pain, along with back and hip (Opheim et al. 2011). A systematic appraisal of the literature found that three in four children with cerebral palsy report pain, which was present at all levels of physical disability (Novak et al. 2012). The pain experienced by children with cerebral palsy has qualities suggesting a nociceptive origin and is activity-related (Russo et al. 2008). Reported pain is associated with lower reported quality of life and self-perception in children with congenital hemiplegia cerebral palsy (Russo et al. 2008) and is linked to behavioural problems and reduced participation (Novak et al. 2012). The presence and severity of pain would most commonly be assessed with the visual analogue scale, which is utilized in many patient groups. However, the evaluation of pain in the more severely disabled child or adult with cerebral palsy, who are often non-verbal, can be more challenging. Clinicians commonly use observer-reported changes in behaviour, such as vocalizations, facial expression, and irritability as indicators of pain, or sometimes other cues such as decreased attention, withdrawal, and changes in sleeping or eating (Swiggum et al. 2010). Although proxy reporting is utilized for non-verbal individuals it is thought that proxies significantly under-report pain in disabled adults with cerebral palsy (Parkinson et al. 2010).

GROSS MOTOR FUNCTION AND GAIT

Gross motor function improves in all children with cerebral palsy in the first few years of life, but plateaus somewhere between ages 3 and 7 years depending on the GMFCS level. In 1989, the 88-item Gross Motor Function Measure (GMFM-88) was developed to specifically assess the acquisition of motor function skills in children with cerebral palsy (Russell et al. 1989). It is a criterion-referenced observational measure that has five dimensions: A – lying and rolling, B – sitting, C – kneeling and crawling, D – standing, and E – walking, running, and jumping. From these five dimensions, a total score can be obtained to score the child's motor ability. Although widely used, this measure has several limitations, including variable clinician interpretation of the total score and reduced reliability and validity when dimension scores are reported separately. In 2000, the GMFM-88 was Rasch analysed and converted to a 66-item one-dimensional hierarchical scale, creating the GMFM-66 (Russell et al. 2000). The test–retest reliability of this scale is higher than the GMFM-88, with reported ICCs ranging from 0.96 to 0.99 (Russell et al. 2000; Wei et al. 2006). High-longitudinal construct validity has also been reported in the context of a long-term follow-up study (Lundkvist Josenby et al. 2009).

Ross and Engsberg (2007) have looked at the relationship between the total GMFM-66 score in children with spastic diplegia cerebral palsy and ankle plantarflexor spasticity and strength, finding only a 'weak relationship' ($r=0.23$) between ankle plantarflexor spasticity and scores on the GMFM-66 when data were analysed by individual muscle group. Overall, strength rather than spasticity accounted for most of the variance in gross motor function, with isolated ankle plantarflexor strength explaining 11% of the variance in the GMFM-66 total scores. These data are similar to other studies in the literature, which place greater emphasis on muscle strength than spasticity as a contributor to gross motor functional ability (Damiano et al. 2001).

Gross motor curves with reference percentiles are now available online and map the rate of acquisition of gross motor milestones by children with cerebral palsy, based on changes in the GMFM-66 score with age (Hanna et al. 2008). These curves demonstrate that there is a wide range of gross motor function possible within the broader GMFCS levels, with some overlap between the different GMFCS levels. When assessed on the GMFM-66, children who function at

GMFCS level V may show a plateau in functioning after the age of 3 years; conversely, children with cerebral palsy who are independently ambulatory may continue to gain gross motor skills until the age of 5–7 years (similar to typically developing peers). The gross motor function of children who function at GMFCS level I and II appears to remain stable through adolescence and into the early adult years. However, children who function at GMFCS levels III, IV, and V are at risk of loss of function (as measured by the GMFM-66) as they move into their adult years (Hanna et al. 2008). This loss of function may be due to the adverse effects of increasing height and weight in the pubertal growth spurt, without the accompanying increase in muscle strength. As well, many children have by then developed contractures in the lower limbs that also increase the energy demands of motor tasks.

Both children and adults with cerebral palsy have gait impairments that reduce efficiency of community ambulation. In the clinic, the 6-minute walk test (6MWT) is an easy tool to assess overall walking endurance in both children and adults with cerebral palsy and has high levels of reliability and validity (Andersson et al. 2006; Maher et al. 2008; Maltais et al. 2012; Nsenga Leunkeu et al. 2012). Children with cerebral palsy have reduced walk distances compared with age-matched peers, with mean distances walked in 6 minutes ranging from a mean of 541 m for children who function at GMFCS level I to 248 m in children who function at GMFCS level III (i.e. using a walking aid) (Chong et al. 2011). Adults with cerebral palsy have similarly reduced 6-minute walk distances, ranging from a median of 611 m in adults who function at GMFCS level I to 376 m in adults who function at GMFCS level III (Maanum et al. 2010). There are also a number of patient questionnaires specific to cerebral palsy that focus on locomotor skill such as the ABILOCO-Kids, the Functional Mobility Scale (FMS) and the Gillette Functional Assessment Questionnaire (FAQ) (Caty et al. 2008; Chong et al. 2011; Gorton et al. 2011; Harvey 2010; Harvey et al. 2010). These latter questionnaires have been developed for children with cerebral palsy and have not been validated for use in adults with cerebral palsy, although they have been used in studies with adult participants (Maanum et al. 2010). The reader is referred to an extensive review by Harvey et al. (2008) for more details of the reliability and validity of these questionnaires in children with cerebral palsy (Harvey et al. 2008). Targeted questionnaires to measure ankle and foot function in children or adults with cerebral palsy are not available, but one study has used scales developed by the American Orthopedic Foot Ankle Society (AOFAS) to score the results of surgical intervention for hallux valgus in children with cerebral palsy (Davids et al. 2001). The reliability and validity of the use of such questionnaires in the population with cerebral palsy are not known.

Deficits in individual joint movements during gait can be quantified through observational gait analysis using two-dimensional (2D) gait videos or through three-dimensional (3D) gait analysis. Several observational video rating scales are available to quantify the findings on 2D videos with reported moderate reliability between raters (Brunnekreef et al. 2005; Mackey et al. 2003). Commercial software is also available to calculate joint angles from 2D gait video, with reported high test–retest reliability (ICC>0.89) for dynamic joint motion (Cronin et al. 2006). However, 2D video can give misleading information, as gait deviations in the frontal or transverse planes affect the visual assessment of sagittal plane motion. Three-dimensional (3D) gait analysis provides the most comprehensive assessment of joint angles, moments and powers, but the clinical interpretation is challenging, given the large data set generated by one analysis (Sagawa et al. 2013). Various algorithms have been developed to collapse the data collected during gait analysis into a single variable, such as the Gait Deviation Index (GDI) or the Gait Performance Score (GPS) (Schwartz and Rozumalski 2008). These single measures quantify the degree of variation from normal gait but have only low correlations with clinical measures such as the 6-minute walk test (6MWT), suggesting that gait deviations and walking endurance are different constructs in this patient group (Maanum et al. 2012). However, recent work has suggested some link between clinical measures and the GDI, with greater spasticity and weakness in the calf muscle acting as one predictor of a lower GDI – that is, more severe deviation of gait pattern from normal (Sagawa et al. 2013).

The repeatability of 3D gait analysis is high in the sagittal and frontal planes and slightly lower in the transverse planes owing to errors in defining the hip joint centres (Mackey et al. 2005; Steinwender et al. 2000). At the ankle, measures of dynamic ankle dorsiflexion have a test–retest repeatability of ±2° over a period of 1–2 weeks, with adjusted coefficients of multiple correlations (CMCs) of 0.87 for within-day repeatability and 0.83 for between-day repeatability (Mackey et al. 2005; Steinwender et al. 2000). The pattern of ankle motion is also repeatable from week to week. However, valid measurement of dynamic ankle motion is compromised in gait analysis by the underlying kinematic foot models, which fail to take into account the alterations in position of the hindfoot and midfoot that are commonly present in individuals with cerebral palsy. Commercially available clinical gait analysis software models the foot as a single segment in gait analysis, based on the assumption that the foot is rigid (Kadaba et al. 1990). This assumption is simply not true for individuals with foot deformities, with over 90% of children with cerebral palsy developing some form of foot deformity due to the abnormal forces that are applied to the immature skeleton by increased muscle tone (O'Connell et al. 1998).

For this reason, the correlation between passive range of motion measures and dynamic range of motion measures at the ankle in individuals with cerebral palsy is poor. For example, children with cerebral palsy may have a fixed equinus at the ankle when tested by goniometric measurement of passive range of motion but a gait analysis result that shows excessive ankle dorsiflexion in gait. This is because tightness in the gastrocnemius–soleus complex pulls the talus into significant equinus, while the forefoot collapses into supination, abduction, and dorsiflexion on weightbearing (Maurer et al. 2013). The measured 'ankle dorsiflexion' on 3D gait analysis thus reflects motion through the midfoot, not the ankle. Conversely, if there is a fixed hindfoot varus then there may be an exaggeration of the equinus appearance of the ankle on 3D analysis, which reflects the compensatory plantarflexion and pronation of the forefoot, particularly the first ray, rather than the ankle position. Multiple solutions to model the foot in three dimensions have been reported in the literature, all of which aim to address these issues and improve assessment of ankle and foot kinematics in individuals with foot deformities including those with cerebral palsy (Maurer et al. 2013; Stebbins et al. 2006). With this

work, it is hoped that improvement in this aspect of modelling should overcome this significant limitation of 3D gait analysis.

Foot plantar pressure distribution can provide further information about dynamic foot function and can be used to determine pre- and post-intervention change in foot functioning. There are many different plantar pressure systems available in the marketplace, with two common configurations: pressure distribution platforms based in research laboratories and portable in-shoe systems, both wired and wireless (Razak et al. 2012). These devices provide information on the dynamic loading of the whole foot, as well as information specific to different areas of the foot. Multiple variables can be derived from plantar pressure analysis to assess the loading characteristics of the foot, including measures of foot contact pattern (e.g. total contact area, contact length, and contact width), measures of plantar pressure distributions across different foot segments, and centre of pressure (COP) trajectories in the medio-lateral and antero-posterior plane as the body weight moves over the foot (Chiu et al. 2013; Han et al. 1999). Specific measures of plantar pressure distribution include peak pressure and force, which can be reported both for the total foot and selected foot regions (e.g. lateral heel, medial heel, midfoot, first metatarsophalangeal joint, second to fifth metatarsophalangeal joints, hallux, and lesser toes). These values can be further integrated with time to provide the pressure–time and force–time integrals, which give an indication of the duration of the peak loading values (Cousins et al. 2012).

Moderate to good within-session reliability has been reported for measures of peak pressure and force across all segments of the foot in children (ICCs of 0.69–0.93), except for the lesser toes (Cousins et al. 2012). The same study reported high between-session reliability yielding ICC values greater than 0.79, again except for the lesser toes. Similar levels of between-day reliability of plantar pressure distribution measurements have also been reported for normal adults, with ICCs >0.9 for areas with high loading characteristics [e.g. central forefoot (Gurney et al. 2008)]. Although small children have quite variable plantar pressures, children over the age of 6–7 years have more consistent patterns with loading characteristics that are similar to an adult foot and therefore can be assessed with plantar pressure measurements (Alvarez et al. 2008; Hennig et al. 1994).

Park et al. (2006) reported on the results of 67 lower limb surgeries for foot deformities in children with cerebral palsy using a computerized in-sole system. They found that those parameters reflecting asymmetry in the medial and lateral columns of the foot, such as the COPI (centre of pressure index) and coronal index, best differentiated changes in the frontal plane such as changes in heel varus or valgus. Conversely, total contact area, contact length, and contact width of the hindfoot and antero-posterior displacement of the centre of pressure appeared to be the most sensitive measures to assess improvements in the sagittal plane after corrective surgery. For example, improved weightbearing on the heel after surgery for equinus contracture led in their study to a 22% increase in mean total contact area and a 20% increase in contact length, but no change in the medio-lateral displacement of the centre of pressure. Further work by the same authors has also found that dynamic foot pressures are sensitive enough to detect differences in outcome between two different surgical procedures for a valgus hindfoot (Park et al. 2008). More work is still needed though, to test the association between improvements in foot pressure distribution and clinically important changes in the functioning of the foot.

QUALITY OF LIFE

The measurement of quality of life (QOL) is a controversial one in individuals with cerebral palsy. There are a number of generic and condition-specific questionnaires for children and adolescents with cerebral palsy. However, many of these instruments have been developed with minimal involvement of families with children with cerebral palsy, were developed to assess function rather than wellbeing, and have negatively worded items that can cause distress (Waters et al. 2009). Different reports of the quality of life of a child with cerebral palsy can be obtained depending upon the measure used and the perspective of the person reporting it. Measures that emphasize objectively observed aspects of health-related quality of life (HRQOL) consistently score children with cerebral palsy lower on QOL than their typically developing

peers. For example, Varni et al. (2005) used the paediatric quality of life inventory (PedsQL) to report on the HRQOL of children and adolescents with cerebral palsy and showed that the HRQOL of children with cerebral palsy is lower than typically developing children and similar to that of children diagnosed with cancer who are undergoing treatment (Varni et al. 2005). However, when assessed using the Kidscreen Quality of Life measure, 8- to 12-year-olds with cerebral palsy report similar levels of QOL to their typically developing peers (Dickinson et al. 2012). Children with cerebral palsy often also report a higher QOL than is obtained from a proxy report (e.g. parents or caregivers). It has been argued that parent proxy reports of QOL are more influenced by the level of parental distress, with parental depression being negatively correlated with parent-proxy-reported QOL (Davis et al. 2012). This may mean that parents who are depressed view their child's life negatively, or conversely that if a child with cerebral palsy has a poor QOL that this then leads to greater depression within the parent. Due to the difficulty in interpretation of proxy report, it is advised that, where possible, children and adolescents should be allowed to self-report QOL rather than report through a proxy (Livingston et al. 2007). Other authors recommend collection of both viewpoints (Davis et al. 2013).

There has been little in the way of research into QOL for adults with cerebral palsy. Roebroeck et al. (2009) reported that young adults with cerebral palsy perceive reductions in both HRQOL and global QOL with restricted participation in activities of daily life, particularly paid work, intimate relationships, and independent housing. They noted that young adults with cerebral palsy can have difficulty with the transition process from childhood to adulthood, which may impact on their reported QOL. Studies in older adults with cerebral palsy are even more limited. A recent mapping review of studies of long-term outcomes has noted that most research studies include very wide age ranges and have a cross-sectional design, with very few prospective longitudinal studies (Novak et al. 2012). Gaskin and Morris (2008) reviewed HRQOL in 51 adults with cerebral palsy, aged from 19 to 66 years, and reported lower levels of HRQOL than in the general population. However, there were only weak associations between HRQOL and measures of psychosocial functioning, suggesting a level of psychological adaptation to the diagnosis of cerebral palsy. Because of the wide age band, the authors had difficulty interpreting the results for narrower age bands (Gaskin and Morris 2008). They also found that adults with spastic cerebral palsy perceive a low HRQOL for physical functioning but not for mental health. Overall, greater self-efficacy appears to be associated with greater participation and higher physical and mental HRQOL (van der Slot et al. 2010) suggesting a possible target for clinical intervention.

MANAGEMENT STRATEGIES

Clinical decision making for the management of foot deformities in children and adults with cerebral palsy requires assessment and integration of data from a number of sources. The management algorithm is based on the integration of information from clinical history, physical examination, plain radiographs (weightbearing), and observed gait patterns [(+/−2D video) and on occasion, 3D gait analysis]. Features of the clinical history specific to the foot and ankle include whether pain is present either with or without weightbearing, any difficulty with shoe or orthotic fitting, and problems in gait (e.g. instability in stance with tripping and falling). Physical examination on the examination couch will involve assessment of passive range of motion, determination of the range of motion of the joints of the foot and ankle, and the presence of muscle contracture or increased tone. As always, the vascular status of the foot should be checked.

The position of the foot and ankle with weightbearing in gait should be noted as these can vary from the position when non-weightbearing. Weightbearing antero-posterior (AP) and lateral radiographs of the foot and ankle can help determine the alignment of the foot in standing. Specific angles to measure on the weightbearing film include Meary's angle, or talo first metatarsal angle (normal values 0±4°), on the lateral weightbearing film and the talocalcaneal (Kite's) angle on the AP view (normal values 15–30°). A Meary's angle of >4° convex downwards is indicative of planus, with an angle of 15–30° considered moderate planus and >30° severe planus (Pedowitz and Kovatis 1995). An angle of >4° convex upwards is indicative of cavus. The talocalcaneal angle should be in the

range of 15–30° on a weightbearing AP radiograph. An angle <15° indicates hindfoot varus and an angle greater than 30° hindfoot valgus.

2D gait video can be useful to determine ankle and knee and hip position in the sagittal plane during walking and is easily applied to the clinic setting. However, 3D gait analysis remains the preferred analysis to delineate complex malalignments of the limb in both stance and swing phase, but needs to be interpreted by experts with the knowledge of the limitations of underlying software models.

PHARMACOLOGICAL STRATEGIES

Early spasticity management is an integral part of management of foot and ankle deformities in younger children with cerebral palsy and can also be helpful in adults with focal spasticity. Focal botulinum toxin A injections into the calf muscle are widely used to control spasticity, either in isolation or with other muscle groups (e.g. toe flexors, tibialis posterior), and often in conjunction with the use of orthoses or serial casting (Love et al. 2010). Botulinum toxin A is taken up at the cholinergic nerve terminal when injected intramuscularly and blocks the release of acetyl choline, temporarily causing selective focal muscle denervation. This leads to a temporary reduction in muscle tone that provides a window of opportunity to strengthen opposing muscles, apply further stretch to the calf muscle through orthotics or serial casting, and perhaps allow children with cerebral palsy time to learn new patterns of movement (Desloovere et al. 2012). Factors thought to predict a more favourable response to focal botulinum toxin A injections for spastic equinus gait include children with less severe functional deficits, fair to good selective motor control of dorsiflexion at the ankle, and 'mild' equinus gait (Satila and Huhtala 2010). The need for botulinum toxin A injections to manage focal spasticity is best judged by use of the Tardieu scale to record the R2 and R1 for dorsiflexion range of motion at the ankle, using a goniometer to measure the angle of the joint both after a slow stretch (R2=full passive range of motion) and after a fast stretch (R1=angle at first catch). The difference between R2 and R1 is felt to represent the change in dynamic dorsiflexion of the ankle that can be reasonably achieved with spasticity management. The European Journal of Neurology has recently published international consensus statements for the assessment, treatment, and aftercare associated with the use of botulinum toxin A in both children and adults with cerebral palsy (Love et al. 2010; Olver et al. 2010). These provide useful guidelines for the clinician considering botulinum toxin A injections for their client.

Despite widespread use, the evidence for botulinum toxin A injections at the foot and ankle in both children and adults is still somewhat restricted. The number of studies in adults is limited and there is no information on effect sizes in this group of patients. However, there are a greater number of published studies in children, which allows calculation of effect sizes for botulinum toxin A injections into the calf muscle for children with cerebral palsy (Koog and Min 2010). Koog and Min (2010) reported that the current data indicate that botulinum toxin A is more effective than non-sham control in reducing calf muscle tone, increasing passive ankle range of motion, gait speed, and activity for approximately 2 to 4 months following injection. The effect sizes for muscle tone at 1 month were −2.3 and at 3 months −1.72. For passive ankle range of motion, the effect size at 1 month was 3.29 and at 3 months 1.0. The effect on gait speed was 0.91 at 1 month and at 3 months 0.61. The effect on gross motor function at 2 months was 2.02.

However, when compared with a sham injection many of the significant effects of botulinum toxin A injection were not found apart from an effect on gross motor function at 4 months, effect size 0.98. Koog and Min (2010) noted that this finding suggested that 'the efficacy of botulinum toxin A may be lower than is commonly believed'. However, the authors noted that there were only a small number of studies that were sham controlled (seven) and a smaller number (two) that satisfied the sample calculations. Also, the authors had to estimate the necessary values on four of the five non-sham controlled studies and three of the seven sham-controlled studies. The authors of this review caution that, due to the small number of studies and small sample sizes, their results could be affected by a type II error, and noted that further studies with sufficient statistical power, optimal age range and dose, and appropriate outcome measures are needed.

One study has looked at the effect on calf muscle passive stiffness after botulinum toxin A injection, finding a small but significant decrease in the torque required to achieve either plantar grade position or 5° of dorsiflexion of the ankle but no significant difference in myo-tendinous stiffness or hysteresis (Alhusaini et al. 2011). The authors concluded from these findings that, despite any effect on neurally mediated responses, the compliance of the calf muscle is not changed by botulinum toxin A injections. This supports the clinical experience that children with cerebral palsy often present with a combination of hypertonia plus evolving contracture of the calf muscle. Thus, additional treatment approaches such as serial casting followed by orthoses are needed to supplement the effects of botulinum toxin A injections when managing children with calf muscle spasticity. Figure 8-1 presents an algorithm for clinical decision making for therapies post botulinum toxin A injections.

PHYSICAL STRATEGIES
Physiotherapy

Physiotherapy is one of the key services for children with cerebral palsy and is an important part of management by a multidisciplinary team. The general aims of physiotherapy for children with cerebral palsy are to maintain or improve motor skills and motor functional level, minimize development of muscle contractures and deformities, and provide education to families on the condition, including early management, through a family-centred approach. Physiotherapists may not be routinely involved in the care of adults with cerebral palsy but on occasion will be asked to review and assess adults with cerebral palsy. Varying techniques are used in physiotherapy including conventional techniques such as muscle stretching and strengthening, gait retraining, and functional activities to promote motor learning, coupled with adjuncts such as hydrotherapy (aquatic therapy), therapeutic horse riding (hippotherapy), and electrical stimulation. As well, there are several older conceptual approaches derived from early theories of motor learning such as neurodevelopmental treatment (NDT), Vojta therapy, and conductive education. A full description of these alternative approaches is outside the remit of this chapter, but the interested reader is referred to the review article by Franki et al. (2012) for further information.

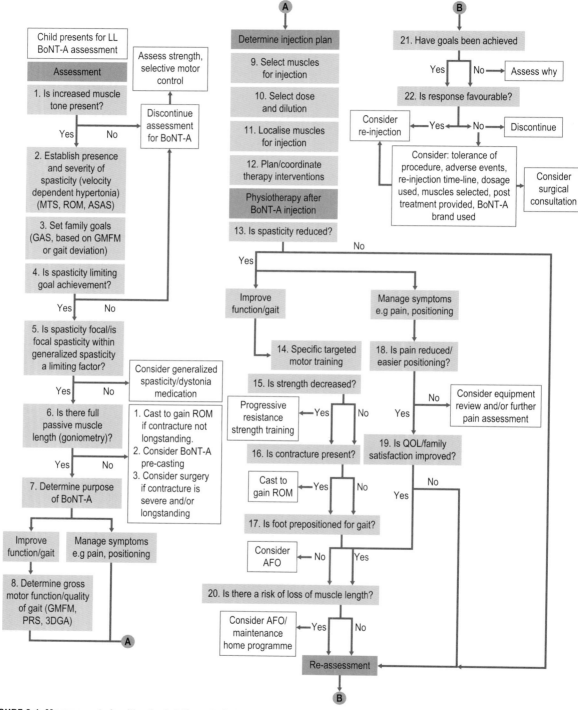

FIGURE 8-1 Management algorithm for botulinum toxin A injections in the lower limb. (Reprinted from Love SC, Novak I, Kentish M, et al. (2010) Botulinum toxin assessment, intervention and after care for lower-limb spasticity in children with cerebral palsy: international consensus statement. European Journal of Neurology, 17 suppl 2, 9–37, with permission of John Wiley and Sons ©2010 The Authors. Journal compilation ©2010 EFNS.)

At the foot and ankle, ambulatory children with cerebral palsy require sufficient passive ankle dorsiflexion to allow for foot clearance in swing and a stable foot position in early- to mid-stance. Calf muscle contractures lead to loss of ankle dorsiflexion and on occasion secondary foot deformities, either equino-varus or equino-valgus. Passive stretching of the calf muscle is therefore a common component of therapy programmes and is designed to prevent or reduce the onset of calf muscle contractures. Typical strategies include either intermittent manual passive stretching (i.e. holding the joint at end range manually for a set time, often seconds or minutes, and then releasing the joint), or providing sustained muscle stretch over hours through the use of mechanical means such as standing frames or positioning orthoses (i.e. solid AFOs used for 5–7 hours per day during periods of rest). The timeframe of 5–7 hours is often quoted but is based on only one study, which suggested that the soleus must be stretched for 6 hours a day to avoid progressive contracture (Tardieu et al. 1988).

The long-term effect of passive stretching on changes in range of motion is unclear. Pin et al. (2006) reviewed the effectiveness of passive stretching to reduce contracture and found only small positive effect sizes in some studies, with others showing no difference in joint range pre and post stretching. Although the studies were weak, Pin et al. (2006) felt that the evidence supported sustained stretching over intermittent manual stretching in improving range of motion and reducing spasticity in targeted joints. Given the lack of strong evidence for sustained stretching, Maas et al. (2012) are currently undertaking a randomized controlled trial to look at the effect of use of orthotics at rest on calf muscle length, incorporating measures of muscle length by ultrasound as well as measures of ankle dorsiflexion and gross motor function. The results of this study should better inform the practice of passive stretching as a therapy regimen.

Strengthening has become an increasingly popular intervention for children with cerebral palsy (Damiano and Abel 1998). Early fears that strengthening would increase hypertonicity have not been confirmed and strengthening is now proposed as an important feature of therapy for cerebral palsy. Resistance training is a specific type of strengthening 'which involves the progressive use of a wide range of resistive loads and a variety of training modalities designed to enhance health, fitness and sports performance' (Verschuren et al. 2011). Several earlier reviews supported the concept of progressive muscle resistance training in children with cerebral palsy, reporting positive outcomes (Dodd et al. 2002; Mockford and Caulton 2008; Taylor et al. 2004; Verschuren et al. 2011). However, the most recent review in 2009, a systematic review with meta-analysis, looked critically at the question 'do strengthening interventions increase strength without increasing spasticity and improve activity, and is there any carryover after cessation in children and adolescents with cerebral palsy?' (Scianni et al. 2009). Six studies were identified, of which five could be included in a meta-analysis. The authors concluded that strengthening interventions in the lower limb had no effect on muscle strength (SMD 0.20), no effect on walking speed (MD 0.02 m/s), and had only a small statistically significant, but not clinically significant effect, on Gross Motor Function Measure (MD 2%, 95% CI 0–4). The effect on spasticity could not be ascertained as only one study assessed spasticity in the study group.

Subsequent to that review, a well-executed study of functional progressive resistance training of the knee extensors and hip abductors in children with cerebral palsy was reported (Scholtes et al. 2012). This randomized controlled trial showed that training led to early improvements in isometric muscle strength, but that these gains did not translate over into improvements in functional walking ability when measured by tests such as the timed 10 m walk test and the timed stair test (Boyd 2012; Scholtes et al. 2012). The message from this study is that it is not enough to provide training that lacks context; rather, functional activities must be trained in a context-specific manner that enhances motor learning in combination with the resistance training. Training to improve gait, for example, must incorporate context, such as walking across uneven surfaces and slopes, and consider the intensity and number of repetitions required to achieve the desired response. Progressive resistance training must be tailored to the functional ability of the client and may require greater rest periods and greater emphasis on single joints rather than multi-joint exercises. An up-to-date guide in this area is provided by Verschuren et al. (2011) who discuss how current

National Strength and Conditioning Association (NSCA) strength-training guidelines for typically developing children and adolescents might be adapted for children and adolescents with cerebral palsy (Faigenbaum et al. 2009).

Overall, evaluating the effect of varying physiotherapy approaches on a young child's development and motor function has not been easy for researchers and studies of different physiotherapy programmes have had inconsistent results (Stanger and Oresic 2003). The research in this area is difficult to interpret owing to methodological issues such as heterogeneity in patient samples, lack of non-treatment groups, and lack of satisfactory outcome measures (Anttila et al. 2008). Only three studies in the review by Anttila et al. (2008) had published effect sizes, and of those only one involved the lower limb solely. The American Academy of Cerebral Palsy and Developmental Medicine (AACPDM) has published several reviews of therapy interventions in children with cerebral palsy, including reviews of neurodevelopmental treatment and conductive education (Bagley et al. 2007; Butler et al. 2001; Darrah et al. 2004). The authors of the review of conductive education concluded that 'the present literature base does not provide conclusive evidence either in support of or against conductive education as an intervention strategy'. Similarly, the review of NDT concluded that NDT has failed to produce 'consistent clinically significant effects on activity or demonstrate superiority over alternative approaches'. Given the lack of evidence for one specific approach, clinicians should incorporate a variety of interventions in therapy programmes for both adults and children with cerebral palsy including strengthening, adjunctive sustained stretching through orthotic use, and functional tasks designed to enhance motor learning.

Serial Casting

'Serial casting' or serial application of below-knee walking casts with progressive increases in ankle dorsiflexion has been used for many years in the management of equinus contracture of the ankle in children with cerebral palsy. A prerequisite for successful serial casting is the ability to bring the hindfoot to subtalar neutral and inability to do this means that stretch cannot be effectively applied to the ankle. The technique of serial casting is illustrated in Figure 8-2 with sequential application of the cast to hold the hindfoot in neutral, dorsiflex the ankle to the maximum possible with the knee flexed, and then to level the sole of the cast in the sagittal and frontal planes to allow an efficient gait pattern with the sole set at 10° dorsiflexion relative to the shank. It is the author's experience that serial casting works best in independently ambulatory children. This suggests that ambulation in the cast is an important aspect of the casting protocol to facilitate better knee position in gait and stretching of the gastrocnemius muscle. The author's personal protocol is to change the cast every 2 weeks for a period of 6 weeks, with the commencement thereafter of gait retraining and fabrication of an appropriate orthoses. However, other clinicians have argued for a shorter period of casting and more frequent changing intervals (Pohl et al. 2002).

The underlying scientific rationale of serial casting is that normal muscle grows with stretch and conversely that prolonged positioning of a muscle in the shortened position, either passively or by sustained contracture (as in spasticity), will lead to reduced growth over time and finally fixed contracture. Although there is evidence for muscle length increases with stretching when there is no underlying pathology present, there is less evidence that stretching of a spastic muscle can lead to improved growth (Biering-Sorensen et al. 2006; Gajdosik et al. 2007). Although serial casting is a widely used intervention, there is relatively little reporting in the literature on the outcomes. A systematic review of the effects of casting of equinus in children with cerebral palsy identified 22 articles, including seven randomized control trials (Blackmore et al. 2007). The study found little evidence that casting was superior to no casting, but noted that current protocols of casting had not been compared with 'no treatment' in the randomized clinical trials. There was also no strong existing evidence that combined casting and botulinum toxin A injections was superior to one intervention alone. Finally, the authors could not identify evidence to determine whether the order of the treatment (i.e. serial casting before botulinum toxin A injection or botulinum toxin A injection followed by serial casting) affected the patient outcome. This review noted that the studies included within the review had three major

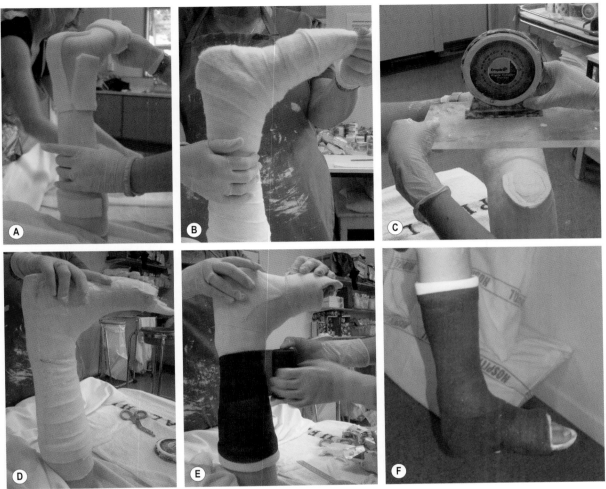

FIGURE 8-2 (A–F) Example of application of a below-knee cast as part of a serial casting programme.

limitations. These were: (i) small sample sizes with lack of power calculations, (ii) lack of blinding, and (iii) inadequate treatment of dropouts. Generalizability outside of the studies was also limited because of considerable variation in casting protocols (i.e. the timing of co-interventions, the angle of dorsiflexion to which the cast was applied, whether the cast was a one-off, serial or progressive, and finally the length of casting). Overall, the evidence was felt insufficient to allow the calculation of effect sizes and the current research was noted to be flawed, with major methodological weaknesses. The study's authors felt that such evidence was 'potentially harmful' for informed clinical decision making and that much better-designed studies are required in this area.

Orthoses

Ankle foot orthoses (AFOs) are routinely used in children with cerebral palsy to minimize development of calf muscle contractures, improve dynamic efficiency of gait, improve stance phase stability, and facilitate swing phase clearance. A systematic review of the effects of AFOs on gait found that studies of orthotic use have predominantly adopted a cross-sectional design, with generally poor-quality studies that lacked randomization procedures, were not blinded, and did not control patient attrition from the group (Figueiredo et al. 2008). The review also noted confusing terminology for ankle–foot orthoses, with up to 12 different terms used. The authors were able to collapse these terms down into a small number of ankle–foot orthoses (hinged AFO, posterior leaf spring AFO, dynamic AFO, ground reaction AFO, and supra-malleolar orthoses). Although there are no reported effect sizes, the review noted that studies have generally agreed that gait velocity, step, and stride length and single-support time show a modest 5–10% increase with the use of AFOs when compared with barefoot walking (White et al. 2002). All AFOs, except supra-malleolar orthoses (SMOs), can improve ankle position during heelstrike either by decreasing ankle plantarflexion or by increasing dorsiflexion. They also reduce excessive equinus during mid-stance and can lead to increased dorsiflexion at terminal stance with better positioning of the ankle in the swing phase of gait. The fine-tuning of AFOs can also improve knee position in gait: AFOs set in ankle dorsiflexion act to reduce knee hyperextension and AFOs set in plantarflexion increase the plantarflexor knee extensor couple and reduce knee flexion (Butler et al. 2007). Radiographic studies have also shown small improvements in static foot alignment with the use of orthoses of children with cerebral palsy in the range of <6° (Westberry et al. 2007).

A useful guide to the clinical decision making on foot orthoses has been published by Davids et al. (2007). Their recommendation is that supra-malleolar orthoses have little to no indications for use in cerebral palsy. A quantitative gait analysis assessment of patients walking with supra-malleolar orthoses show no kinematic or kinetic improvements that could be attributed to the orthoses (Crenshaw et al. 2000). The SMO is designed to treat excessive supination or pronation of the foot in patients without significant spasticity and, for this reason, could be expected to be relatively ineffective in controlling foot position in children with cerebral palsy. Posterior leaf spring orthoses (PLSO) are frequently used in cerebral palsy and are best suited for feet that have mild and passively correctable deformities, and relatively mild spasticity. They are designed to have contact with the plantar aspect of the foot with the posterior line extending to the proximal third of the calf. The posterior shell is narrowed from the distal tibial segment to the hindfoot allowing bending of the orthosis to accommodate ankle dorsiflexion in mid- to late-stance. Quantitative gait analysis studies have shown that posterior leaf spring orthoses reduce excessive ankle plantarflexion in swing phase while allowing ankle dorsiflexion in stance phase (Buckon et al. 2004; Ounpuu et al. 1996; Sienko Thomas et al. 2002).

Hinged ankle–foot orthoses have a similar contour to that of the PLSO, but the posterior shell captures both the hindfoot and the posterior half of the calf. There is separation of the foot portion from the tibial portion and the two portions are connected by hinges, either metal or plastic. These orthoses also prevent excessive ankle plantarflexion in swing phase (foot drop), but allow ankle dorsiflexion in stance. Hinged AFOs can be either free or constructed to allow limited dorsiflexion. The primary contraindication to the hinged AFO is excessive ankle dorsiflexion in mid-stance during second rocker. This pattern of movement is commonly seen in older children with cerebral palsy, making this an unsuitable orthosis for the older child. It should also be noted that the hinged AFO is more labour-intensive and expensive to fabricate than the PLSO and more difficult to tolerate, owing to the thicker plastic and the hinges that necessitate greater modifications in the footwear.

Ground reaction AFOs (also termed floor reaction AFOs) are useful for control of crouch gait pattern but, in practice, are often difficult for children to tolerate unless spasticity in the hamstrings can be reduced either through intramuscular botulinum toxin A injections or through surgical means. These orthoses are, however, useful in the post-surgical phase where more support is required at the ankle and knee.

Orthotic use will probably change as the child grows and is influenced by the GMFCS level of the child. Young children (<3 years) with little fixed contracture, but dynamic tone, often benefit from an off-the-shelf dynamic orthosis that can allow squatting and developmentally appropriate tasks. Several such orthotic designs are available and the reader is directed to company websites for further information (Cascade Orthotics 2013). Older children require more standard AFOs such as the posterior leaf spring; those with greater level of impairments (e.g. children who function at GMFCS level III or IV) often need greater orthotic support (e.g. solid AFOs or two-piece orthoses, incorporating a wrap-around inner shell and a stiff posterior outer frame to resist both dorsiflexion and block plantarflexion).

Neuromuscular Electrical Stimulation

The use of electrical stimulation dates back to the Ancient Greeks, who reportedly used rubbed amber to produce muscular contractions (Wright et al. 2012). There are a number of types of electrical stimulation ranging from subthreshold electrical stimulation, where low levels of stimulation are applied over a prolonged duration, through to neuromuscular electrical stimulation (NMES), which produces muscle contraction. NMES can be used either cyclically as a strengthening exercise (and is then usually high in intensity and short in duration) or for the purpose of producing a contraction and subsequent movement. The latter type of NMES is often combined with performance of a functional task such as walking or cycling and is then known as functional electrical stimulation (FES). In FES, stimulation is applied peripherally to muscles and/or nerves with impaired motor control for the purpose of overcoming an inability to contract the muscle and thus improve timing of muscle activation during tasks (Doucet et al. 2012). In the lower limb, FES has been incorporated into an in-home cycling programme and, in gait, has been used as a peroneal nerve stimulator (Johnston and Wainwright 2011; Leidinger et al. 2011). Most reported electrical stimulation work involves surface electrodes. There have, however, been some studies that used percutaneous implant stimulation systems (Doucet et al. 2012). The majority of the literature on electrical stimulation is targeted towards adults with disability, ranging from conditions such as chronic stroke through to spinal cord injury and multiple sclerosis. However, there is increasing literature on the use of electrical stimulation in children (Wright et al. 2012). Neuromuscular electrical stimulation (NMES) has been applied to patients with cerebral palsy to improve swing-phase ankle dorsiflexion, through targeting either the tibialis anterior muscles during swing or conversely the calf muscle during stance (Chen et al. 2006; Wright et al. 2012). Also, studies are underway to assess the use of NMES as an adjunct to botulinum toxin A injections (Kazon et al. 2012).

A recent systematic review and meta-analysis on the effect of the three types of electrical stimulation protocols on gait impairment in children with cerebral palsy has been reported (Cauraugh et al. 2010); this showed an overall moderate effect size of 0.62, with similar effect sizes for functional electrical stimulation (0.62) and neuromuscular electrical stimulation (0.70). A separate meta-analysis (Cauraugh et al. 2010) focused on 15 studies reporting activity limitations found an overall moderate effect size of 0.64, again with similar effect sizes for functional electrical stimulation (0.72) and neuromuscular electrical stimulation (0.79). The authors concluded that this indicated that electrical stimulation revealed medium effect sizes on gait outcomes for children with cerebral palsy with both functional and neuromuscular electrical stimulation treatments minimizing impairment and activity limitations in walking. Given the small number of studies, the authors cautiously advocated the electrical stimulation be used to minimize impaired activity limitations in gait in individuals with cerebral palsy. However, the study also highlighted the deficits in the literature and suggested further research needs to be done to determine the best practice guidelines with larger scale and wider perspective trials (Cauraugh et al. 2010).

SURGICAL STRATEGIES

Although this section is focused on the foot–ankle, readers should be aware that foot and ankle surgery is often combined with more proximal surgery, often termed single-event multilevel surgery. Interested readers are referred to other review articles and publications for more information in this area (Firth et al. 2013; Gage 2004; Schwartz et al. 2004).

Equinus Deformity

Fixed equinus at the ankle is defined as the inability to dorsiflex the ankle passively to plantargrade with the hindfoot in subtalar neutral and the knee extended. However, the term 'equinus' is also often used to describe equinus posturing in gait (i.e. a plantarflexed position of the ankle in gait), which may or may not reflect a lack of dorsiflexion at the ankle. Equinus posturing in gait, or toe walking, can be due to either 'true equinus' (i.e. the ankle is in plantarflexion) or 'apparent equinus', where the heels are off the ground but the ankle is at neutral position relative to the shank. 'Apparent equinus' is commonly seen in children with more proximal involvement at the hip and knee joints, and management should be directed at the hip and knee position rather than the ankle. 'True equinus' in gait is either dynamic (i.e. due to increased tone in the calf muscle) or fixed (i.e. due to static contracture in the calf muscle).

Equinus overall is a very common and visible problem in children with cerebral palsy. As a result there is a large amount of published literature on the management of equinus, much of which is confusing for the reader. Surgical procedures can be carried out at different levels or zones in the calf muscle: zone 1 is the most proximal zone beginning proximal to the gastrocnemius heads, zone 2 represents the mid-portion between the Tendo Achilles and the gastrocnemius heads, and zone 3 is the Tendo Achilles (Shore et al. 2010). The major complications of surgery for equinus include both recurrence of deformity and overlengthening of the calf muscle. Overlengthening is particularly deleterious, impairing force generation by the calf and contributing to the development of crouch gait, with excessive ankle dorsiflexion and increased hip and knee flexion.

A recent systematic review of the management of equinus found that most surgical studies provided low levels of positive evidence (Shore et al. 2010). The authors did not calculate any effect sizes, but noted that the topographical distribution of cerebral palsy may well be the strongest determinant of outcome of the surgical intervention, with results being worse in children with bilateral involvement (diplegia). The results also appeared better when early surgery was avoided, with the authors commenting that delaying surgical intervention to over the age of 6 years may significantly improve outcomes and reduce the risk of recurrent equinus and overlengthening. Overall, the rate of overcorrection with time averaged only 1% of children with spastic hemiplegia, compared with 15% (range 0% to 41%) in children with spastic diplegia. Procedures that lengthen the Tendo Achilles should be avoided in individuals with spastic diplegia who are less than 8 years, as they seem to have the highest rate of overcorrection with time (Borton et al. 2001).

Overall, several key principles should be applied to the management of equinus: (i) define whether the equinus is fixed or dynamic or a combination of both, (ii) avoid early surgery and continue with conservative management for as long as possible, (iii) remember that surgery for fixed equinus often needs to be combined with multilevel surgery at the hip or knee rather than being performed in isolation, and (iv) lengthening interventions at higher levels in the calf minimize detrimental effects on calf muscle power generation but give less correction of equinus.

Calcaneus Deformity

Although equinus is common in cerebral palsy, calcaneal gait has been reported in a significant proportion in children (i.e. a gait characterized by excessive ankle dorsiflexion with secondary increased hip and knee flexion). Increased body weight and hamstring tightness both contribute to development of a calcaneal gait (Huh et al. 2010). Other risk factors for development of a calcaneal gait following surgery are lengthening of the Tendo Achilles, age at operation of less than 8 years, and a diagnosis of spastic diplegia (Borton et al. 2001). Management of calcaneal gait is challenging but includes therapy to maintain plantarflexor muscle strength, reduction in hamstring tightness through pharmacological or surgical means, and blocking of excessive ankle dorsiflexion with ground reaction AFOs or solid AFOs.

Equino-varus Deformity

Equino-varus foot deformity is more common in children with hemiplegia than in those with diplegia and may relate to the development of dystonic posturing of the foot and ankle in the age range from 5 to 10 years. This deformity is initially dynamic and can respond to spasticity management and orthotics. However, over time the deformity becomes fixed with further imbalance in tendon pull, the development of contracture in the gastrocnemius soleus complex, and secondary deformity of the hindfoot. Overactivity in tibialis posterior was thought to be the most common cause of equino-varus foot deformity. However, recent dynamic EMG studies suggest a higher prevalence of tibialis anterior dysfunction, either isolated or in combination with tibialis posterior dysfunction (Michlitsch et al. 2006). Hoffer et al. (1974) recommended considering split tendon transfers for phasic muscle overactivity but intramuscular lengthening if there was continuous activity on EMG. However, determination of timing of muscle overactivity is not possible without the use of fine-wire EMG. For that reason, some surgeons prefer the combined treatment of the lengthening of the posterior tibial tendon and split transfer of the anterior tibial tendon, such as that reported by Barnes and Herring (1991). In addition to tendon rebalancing, secondary bony deformities often need to be addressed through combinations of bony osteotomies, such as a calcaneal osteotomy to correct fixed hindfoot varus.

Equino-valgus Deformity

Equino-valgus foot deformity is the most common foot deformity observed in children with cerebral palsy (O'Connell et al. 1998) and is characterized by a complex three-dimensional malalignment of the subtalar joint, which has been described as consisting of plantarflexion of the talus and calcaneus along with valgus and external rotation of the calcaneus. Furthermore, abduction of the navicular bone on plantarflexed talus creates a shorter lateral column relative to the medial column of the foot. Other features are supination of the forefoot relative to the hindfoot and a tight gastrocnemius–soleus complex. This deformity leads to reduced power in ankle plantarflexion at the time of push-off and instability of the foot during the stance phase. Early management of the equino-valgus foot includes spasticity management and casting plus orthosis for the mild deformity. For the more significant deformity, surgical procedures are required and include lateral column lengthening or subtalar fusion of the hindfoot. More commonly though in adults, a triple arthrodesis (fusion) will be required owing to accompanying deformity within the midfoot (fusion of the talocalcaneal joint, the talonavicular joint, and the calcaneocubiod joint). Most patients will still require the use of orthotics such as a posterior leaf spring orthosis as a long-term aide to walking after surgery.

The technique of lateral column lengthening has been described by Mosca (1995). During surgery, a calcaneal osteotomy is carried out about 1.5 centimetres proximal to the calcaneocuboid joint through the interval between the anterior and middle facets. A bone graft is obtained from the iliac crest and trimmed into a trapezoidal shape before being hammered into the osteotomy to lengthen the lateral column of the foot. If there is residual supination deformity in the forefoot, medial plication of the talonavicular joint capsule can be performed together with a plantarflexion osteotomy of the medial cuneiform (Figure 8-3). Once the valgus hindfoot has been corrected, the contracture in the gastrocnemius–soleus complex can be appreciated and addressed by surgical lengthening.

Children with more limited ambulatory demands may benefit from a subtalar fusion rather than a lateral column lengthening. In children, subtalar fusions need to preserve the growth potential of the foot. Hence, a modified Grice extra-articular arthrodesis of the subtalar joint is performed (Dennyson and Fulford 1976). In this procedure, the tarsal sinus is exposed and the calcaneus rotated on the talus and held in the corrected neutral position with a screw. Both lateral column lengthening and subtalar fusion lead to improved radiograph indices. However, the supination deformity of the forefoot appears better corrected by lateral column lengthening than by extra-articular subtalar arthrodesis (Park et al. 2008).

Hallux Valgus

Hallux valgus is common in children and adults with cerebral palsy. It is one component of a complex multisegment malalignment of the foot that is acquired during the growing years, as a result of loss of extrinsic muscle balance around the foot coupled with abnormal loading that occurs in individuals with cerebral palsy. Common deformities associated with hallux valgus in individuals with cerebral palsy include external tibial torsion, hindfoot valgus with excessive forefoot supination, and flexed knees in gait. Hallux valgus is not only a cosmetic deformity but can also cause problems with pain, difficulty with footwear, and alterations in gait patterns. There is no one method of managing hallux valgus in children and adults with cerebral palsy that is universally recognized as effective at preventing or reducing the deformity. Surgical procedures dominate in the published literature and have included soft-tissue-balancing procedures, osteotomies of the first metatarsal, and first-MTP arthrodesis. There is little published on the results of these surgeries and the decision-making paradigms are often derived from similar surgeries performed in the typically developing adolescent and able-bodied adults who have hallux valgus.

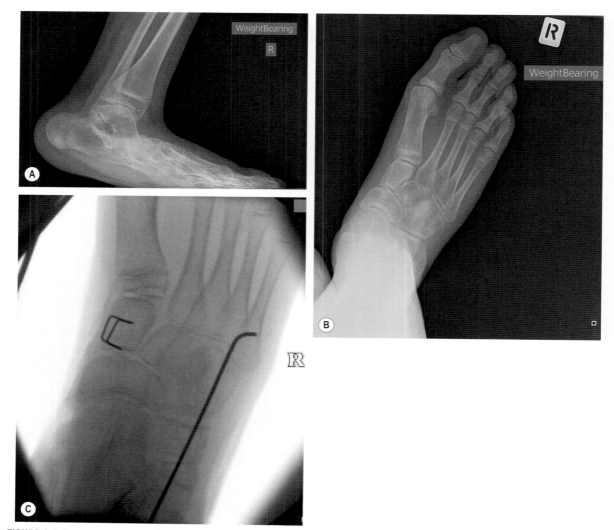

FIGURE 8-3 Radiographs of a 12 year old boy with equino valgus foot. (A, B) Preoperative AP and lateral weight bearing radiographs and (C) postoperative AP radiograph after lateral column lengthening and medial cuneiform plantar closing osteotomy.

Arthrodesis of the first MTP joint appears to have the most reliable outcome for hallux valgus in adolescents and adults with cerebral palsy. Davids et al. (2001) reported on 26 cases of hallux valgus deformities in 16 children with cerebral palsy, managed by first-MTPJ arthrodesis. They reported significant improvement in the mean hallux valgus angle (pre-operative 36°, post-operative 9.6°) and the mean intermetatarsal angle (pre-operative 12°, post-operative 8.4°). They

also documented a significant improvement in the modified American Orthopedic Foot and Ankle Society Hallux Metatarsophalangeal–Interphalangeal Scale with a pre-operative mean score of 46.2 and post-operative means score of 90.9, and patient-, parent-, and caregiver-reported improvements in fitting of footwear, hygiene, activity, and pain, with levels of satisfaction ranging from 81% to 100%. Similar results were reported by Bishay et al. (2009) in 20 ambulatory patients (24 feet) with painful forefeet and restricted footwear secondary to spastic hallux valgus. Using the modified American Orthopedic Foot and Ankle Society Hallux Metatarsophalangeal–Interphalangeal Scale, 18 feet (75%) were classified as excellent and six feet (25%) as good.

Soft-tissue realignment and corrective osteotomies that are popular for able-bodied adolescents and adults with hallux valgus appear to have a lower rate of success in the cerebral palsy population. Jenter et al. (1998) reported on 26 feet treated by four different techniques, finding that a first-MTPJ arthrodesis provided the best results (mean 89% correction). Other combinations of metatarsal osteotomies, soft-tissue releases, and exostectomies had lower rates of correction, ranging from 83% to only 36% correction. Overall, the surgeon needs to consider all aspects of foot alignment when correcting the position of the great toe.

LIFESTYLE AND EDUCATION STRATEGIES

Prevention of further functional decline and disability is an important goal for adults with cerebral palsy, with adults with cerebral palsy wanting greater knowledge and understanding about their condition so that they can make good decisions on ways to enhance or maintain their health (Horsman et al. 2010; Jones 2009). Unfortunately, there is a paucity of information available for adults with cerebral palsy regarding the effects of ageing with cerebral palsy. However, the available data suggest a higher mortality rate from other medical disorders and a high prevalence of secondary musculoskeletal conditions compared with the general population. Peterson et al. (2013) have noted that there are few national surveillance programmes that monitor health in adults with cerebral palsy, but that mortality records show a greater prevalence of coronary artery disease compared with the general population. They postulate this increased prevalence may reflect the impact of lifestyle factors such as habitual sedentary behaviour, obesity, and muscle wasting from disuse. Despite this risk, it appears that fewer adults with cerebral palsy engage in screening for cardiovascular risk factors than do their able-bodied peers (Turk 2009). Similarly there is reduced participation in screening programmes for conditions such as breast and cervical cancer owing to environmental,

attitudinal, and information barriers. These influence both the adults with cerebral palsy and their treating physicians (Nosek and Howland 1997).

Individuals with cerebral palsy also have a higher incidence of secondary musculoskeletal disorders in adulthood such as osteoporosis, early osteoarthritis, and soft-tissue or bony injuries (Sheridan 2009). Contributing factors include decreased bone density due to lower levels of physical activity, abnormal joint stresses with weightbearing, and increased risk of falls. Strategies to increase bone density in childhood and adulthood need to be considered, recognizing that increasing physical activity is often not an option. The presence of musculoskeletal pain needs to be identified and managed effectively, with investigations and treatments as appropriate. This has been poorly recognized in previous years, but it is now known that up to 50% of adults with cerebral palsy will have some pain and discomfort, particularly in the back and foot and ankle (Murphy 2009; Vogtle 2009).

An early deterioration in physical abilities in adulthood is often seen in individuals with cerebral palsy and has been postulated to be due to physiological burn-out caused by ongoing high-energy consumption (Pimm 1992). Fatigue is characteristic of young adults with cerebral palsy. Adults with cerebral palsy report substantially more physical, but not mental, fatigue than the general population (Jahnsen et al. 2003). Of note, the energy required to wheel a wheelchair is similar to the energy required to walk (Zwiren and Bar-Or 1975), whereas the energy required to utilize crutches is considerably higher. Treatment programmes for adults with cerebral palsy should thus address energy conservation on the one hand and increasing physical fitness on the other. Reducing the energy demands for mobilization through mobility aides such as mobility scooters allows emphasis on other aspects of life such as participation in the community.

In children, lifestyle and education strategies should focus on early motor activity to reduce the negative impact of limited mobility on personal and social development. Such motor activity can include the use of power wheelchairs, which allow children the independence to explore their environment and have been shown to enhance 'can do' attitudes (Damiano 2006). Strength training, fun activities that involve weightbearing through the lower limbs, and the maintenance of good nutrition are all important to ameliorate the adverse effects of reduced activity on bone density and muscle growth. Also, there needs to be an early focus on the transition from paediatric to adult care so that adolescents with cerebral palsy can become informed consumers of healthcare and responsible for their own healthcare needs.

FUTURE DIRECTIONS

The understanding of the consequences of cerebral palsy in terms of the impact on activity limitations, participation restrictions, and community function has increased markedly in the last few years. We now have better ways to classify the functional impact of cerebral palsy, a wider range of early interventions, and stronger evidence for our outcomes than ever before. Inroads are also being made into understanding the different patterns of disability in infants and the reasons for differing clinical presentations of the same structural change within the brain on MRI. Advances in brain imaging, including functional MRI, diffusion-tensor-weighted imaging (DTI), and other modalities such as trans-magnetic stimulation (TMS), have made it possible to classify and quantify the nature of the brain lesion but also the brain reorganization that may have occurred due to the early timing of the injury. These technologies are predominantly research tools but will come increasingly available into the clinical setting in the decades to come. They have the potential to unravel further the relationships between the initial neurological event, the neurological damage (brain lesion severity), and the subsequent brain reorganization, which leads to the final clinical phenotype (Johnston 2009).

Developing a robust evidence base for early interventions is also likely to have a greater impact on the prevalence and severity of cerebral palsy in the future. For example, recent research has suggested that infants with unilateral brain lesions may develop progressive loss of surviving corticospinal projections from the injured cortex over the first 2 years of life as ipsilesional pathways, according to early motor experiences. This explains the often 'late' presentation of the signs of mild hemiplegia, with apparent progression over the first few years of life (Eyre et al. 2007). Very early detection of such lesions makes early intervention/s feasible in the clinical setting. However, further research work is needed to understand better how to promote neuroplasticity to improve functional outcomes for these infants who have early brain lesions. As the research work advances over the next 10–20 years, knowledge of how to better target early interventions should lead to a reduction in the secondary neurological and musculoskeletal consequences of cerebral palsy and, ultimately, have positive impacts throughout the adult years.

INVITED COMMENTARY

In the book 'Management of chronic musculoskeletal conditions of the foot and lower leg', the chapter on cerebral palsy provides a comprehensive overview for multidisciplinary allied health and medical clinicians and students. The author provides a detailed review on the most recent definition of cerebral palsy highlighting the importance of the substantive secondary musculoskeletal pathologies that may progress with age, the incidence of cerebral palsy, and its recent decline in infants born pre-term due to improving medical management with reference to recent meta-analyses of aetiology in term-born infants and population-based registers. The section of diagnosis and classification of cerebral palsy as based on early clinical signs and symptoms followed by classification of general movements as the best predictive tool are well presented. The increasing role of both structural MRI and advanced imaging (including diffusion MRI) in understanding the nature, presumed timing, as well as brain lesion severity and subsequent functional correlates, are presented with important reference to recent reviews. The more predictive classification by motor type, distribution, and functional classification with the gross motor function classification are outlined. Next the author provides a comprehensive overview of the clinical measurement of impairments by the positive (hypertonia, dystonia) and negative signs (strength, muscle contracture by joint range of motion) of the upper motor neuron syndrome (UMNS) including reference to systematic reviews in both adults and children with the UMNS. A potential limitation of the chapter is to highlight clearly the differences in psychometric properties of clinical measurement, signs, and symptoms between children and adults with the UMNS. Next the author outlines the importance of measurement of pain, gross motor function (with GMFM), and gait in children with cerebral palsy,

INVITED COMMENTARY (Continued)

emphasizing a clinical approach to gait observation (6-minute walk test, 2D video) with reference to more comprehensive approaches such as three-dimensional gait analysis (3DGA). Quite correctly, the author emphasizes the poor correlation between the measurement of joint range of motion and functional gait in 3DGA, highlighting the need for consideration of the biomechanical lessons that clinicians must learn from 3DGA in order to inform their clinical decision making. Next the author reports current valid measures of quality of life and the limitations of generic rather than condition-specific measures and the potential differences between child self-report and parent report. In such a comprehensive chapter, there is limited room to report measures of participation in relation to foot and lower limb management. The later part of the chapter focuses on management strategies with a general overview on the current evidence for contemporary use of intramuscular botulinum toxin A, physiotherapy motor training, strength training, serial casting, and lower limb orthoses. Preliminary evidence is provided for the use of neuromuscular electrical stimulation (NMES); however, currently this is mostly in a research setting. A broad overview of the context of orthopaedic surgery for specific lower limb deformities is described and quite rightly the author refers to comprehensive texts such as Gage for a more comprehensive overview of surgery and 3DGA in children with cerebral palsy. The section of future directions focuses on potential contribution of early intervention, advanced neuroimaging to

measure brain reorganization, and neuroplasticity, something that is beyond the scope of this text. Overall this chapter provides a comprehensive overview on the state of the clinical science for clinicians in the orthopaedic management of ambulant children with cerebral palsy. Future interventions on the horizon for the management of ambulant children with cerebral palsy may include higher intensities of activity-based training at a younger age (<2 years during periods of early white matter development), judicious use of interventions to reduce the positive features of the UMNS (spasticity), and better interventions to improve the negative features (i.e. strength training in context of motor learning); medical treatments may focus less on reducing spasticity and more on maintaining/increasing muscle mass and 3DGA along with surgical interventions will provide a one-stop comprehensive assessment/management strategy at the right time for correction of residual deformity. In future, a greater emphasis may be placed on multimodal activity-based training for fitness, endurance in the home and community, combined with facilitation of behavioural change to enhance participation and maintain a healthy lifestyle into adulthood.

Roslyn N. Boyd BSc, BAppSc, MSc, PhD, PGRad
Professor of Cerebral Palsy and Rehabilitation Research;
Scientific Director, Queensland Cerebral Palsy and
Rehabilitation Research Centre, School of Medicine,
University of Queensland, Brisbane, Australia

REFERENCES

Access Economics, 2008. The economic impact of cerebral palsy in Australia in 2007. Online. Available: <http://www.cpresearch.org.au/pdfs/access_economics_report.pdf>.

Alhusaini, A.A., Crosbie, J., Shepherd, R.B., et al., 2011. No change in calf muscle passive stiffness after botulinum toxin injection in children with cerebral palsy. Developmental Medicine and Child Neurology 53 (6), 553–558.

Alvarez, C., De Vera, M., Chhina, H., et al., 2008. Normative data for the dynamic pedobarographic profiles of children. Gait and Posture 28 (2), 309–315.

Andersson, C., Asztalos, L., Mattsson, E., 2006. Six-minute walk test in adults with cerebral palsy. A study of reliability. Clinical Rehabilitation 20 (6), 488–495.

Anttila, H., Suoranta, J., Malmivaara, A., et al., 2008. Effectiveness of physiotherapy and conductive education interventions in children with cerebral palsy: a focused review. American Journal of Physical Medicine and Rehabilitation 87 (6), 478–501.

Arnfield, E., Guzzetta, A., Boyd, R., 2013. Relationship between brain structure on magnetic resonance imaging and motor outcomes in children with cerebral palsy: a systematic review. Research in Developmental Disabilities 34 (7), 2234–2250.

Ashwal, S., Russman, B.S., Blasco, P.A., et al., 2004. Practice parameter: diagnostic assessment of the child with cerebral palsy: report of the Quality Standards Subcommittee of the American Academy of Neurology and the Practice Committee of the Child Neurology Society. Neurology 62 (6), 851–863.

Ashworth, B., 1964. Preliminary trial of carisoprodol in multiple sclerosis. The Practitioner 192, 540–542.

Bagley, A.M., Gorton, G., Oeffinger, D., et al., 2007. Outcome assessments in children with cerebral palsy, part II: discriminatory ability of outcome tools. Developmental Medicine and Child Neurology 49 (3), 181–186.

Barnes, M.J., Herring, J.A., 1991. Combined split anterior tibial-tendon transfer and intramuscular lengthening of the posterior tibial tendon. Results in patients who have a varus deformity of the foot due to spastic cerebral palsy. Journal of Bone and Joint Surgery, American Volume 73 (5), 734–738.

Barrett, R.S., Lichtwark, G.A., 2010. Gross muscle morphology and structure in spastic cerebral palsy: a systematic review. Developmental Medicine and Child Neurology 52 (9), 794–804.

Barry, M.J., VanSwearingen, J.M., Albright, A.L., 1999. Reliability and responsiveness of the Barry-Albright Dystonia Scale. Developmental Medicine and Child Neurology 41 (6), 404–411.

Bax, M., 1964. Terminology and classification of cerebral palsy. Developmental Medicine and Child Neurology 6, 295–297.

Bax, M., Goldstein, M., Rosenbaum, P., et al., 2005. Proposed definition and classification of cerebral palsy, April 2005. Developmental Medicine and Child Neurology 47 (8), 571–576.

Benini, R., Dagenais, L., Shevell, M.I., 2012. Normal imaging in patients with cerebral palsy: what does it tell us? Journal of Pediatrics 162 (2), 369–374.e1.

Berry, E.T., Giuliani, C.A., Damiano, D.L., 2004. Intrasession and intersession reliability of handheld dynamometry in children with cerebral palsy. Pediatric Physical Therapy 16 (4), 191–198.

Biering-Sorensen, F., Nielsen, J.B., Klinge, K., 2006. Spasticity-assessment: a review. Spinal Cord 44 (12), 708–722.

Bishay, S.N., El-Sherbini, M.H., Lotfy, A.A., et al., 2009. Great toe metatarsophalangeal arthrodesis for hallux valgus deformity in ambulatory adolescents with spastic cerebral palsy. Journal of Children's Orthopaedics 3 (1), 47–52.

Blackmore, A.M., Boettcher-Hunt, E., Jordan, M., et al., 2007. A systematic review of the effects of casting on equinus in children with cerebral palsy: an evidence report of the AACPDM. Developmental Medicine and Child Neurology 49 (10), 781–790.

Blair, E., 2010. Epidemiology of the cerebral palsies. Orthopedic Clinics of North America 41 (4), 441–455.

Blair, E., Stanley, F., 1985. Interobserver agreement in the classification of cerebral palsy. Developmental Medicine and Child Neurology 27 (5), 615–622.

Blood, A.J., Kuster, J.K., Woodman, S.C., et al., 2012. Evidence for altered basal ganglia–brainstem connections in cervical dystonia. PLoS ONE 7 (2), e31654.

Bodkin, A.W., Robinson, C., Perales, F.P., 2003. Reliability and validity of the gross motor function classification system for cerebral palsy. Pediatric Physical Therapy 15 (4), 247–252.

Bohannon, R.W., Smith, M.B., 1987. Interrater reliability of a modified Ashworth scale of muscle spasticity. Physical Therapy 67 (2), 206–207.

Borton, D.C., Walker, K., Pirpiris, M., et al., 2001. Isolated calf lengthening in cerebral palsy: outcome analysis of risk factors. Journal of Bone and Joint Surgery, British Volume 83B (3), 364–370.

Bosanquet, M., Copeland, L., Ware, R., et al., 2013. A systematic review of tests to predict cerebral palsy in young children. Developmental Medicine and Child Neurology 55 (5), 418–426.

Boyd, R.N., 2012. Functional progressive resistance training improves muscle strength but not walking ability in children with cerebral palsy. Journal of Physiotherapy 58 (3), 197.

Brooke, M.H., Engel, W.K., 1969. The histographic analysis of human muscle biopsies with regard to fiber types. 4. Children's biopsies. Neurology 19 (6), 591–605.

Brunnekreef, J.J., van Uden, C.J., van Moorsel, S., et al., 2005. Reliability of videotaped observational gait analysis in patients with orthopedic impairments. BMC Musculoskeletal Disorders 6, 17.

Buckon, C.E., Thomas, S.S., Jakobson-Huston, S., et al., 2004. Comparison of three ankle–foot orthosis configurations for children with spastic diplegia. Developmental Medicine and Child Neurology 46 (9), 590–598.

Burger, M., Louw, Q.A., 2009. The predictive validity of general movements – a systematic review. European Journal of Paediatric Neurology 13 (5), 408–420.

Burke, R.E., Fahn, S., Gold, A.P., 1980. Delayed-onset dystonia in patients with static encephalopathy. Journal of Neurology, Neurosurgery, and Psychiatry 43 (9), 789–797.

Butler, C., Darrah, J., Adams, R., et al., 2001. Effects of neurodevelopmental treatment (NDT) for cerebral palsy: an AACPDM evidence report. Developmental Medicine and Child Neurology 43 (11), 778–790.

Butler, P.B., Farmer, S.E., Stewart, C., et al., 2007. The effect of fixed ankle foot orthoses in children with cerebral palsy. Disability and rehabilitation. Assistive Technology 2 (1), 51–58.

Cascade Orthotics, 2013. Cascade Orthotics Ltd. Online. Available: <http://www.cascadeorthotics.com/>.

Caty, G.D., Arnould, C., Thonnard, J.L., et al., 2008. ABILOCO-Kids: a Rasch-built 10-item questionnaire for assessing locomotion ability in children with cerebral palsy. Journal of Rehabilitation Medicine 40 (10), 823–830.

Cauraugh, J.H., Naik, S.K., Hsu, W.H., et al., 2010. Children with cerebral palsy: a systematic review and meta-analysis on gait and electrical stimulation. Clinical Rehabilitation 24 (11), 963–978.

Chen, C.S., Phillips, K.D., Grist, S., et al., 2006. Congenital hypertrophy of the retinal pigment epithelium (CHRPE) in familial colorectal cancer. Familial Cancer 5 (4), 397–404.

Chiu, M.C., Wu, H.C., Chang, L.Y., 2013. Gait speed and gender effects on center of pressure progression during normal walking. Gait and Posture 37 (1), 43–48.

Chong, J., Mackey, A.H., Broadbent, E., et al., 2011. Relationship between walk tests and parental reports of walking abilities in children with cerebral palsy. Archives of Physical Medicine and Rehabilitation 92 (2), 265–270.

Clopton, N., Dutton, J., Featherston, T., et al., 2005. Interrater and intrarater reliability of the Modified Ashworth Scale in children with hypertonia. Pediatric Physical Therapy 17 (4), 268–274.

Cottalorda, J., Violas, P., Seringe, R., 2012. Neuro-orthopaedic evaluation of children and adolescents: A simplified algorithm. Orthopaedics and Traumatology, Surgery and Research 98 (6 Suppl.), S146–S153. [Epub 2012 Aug 30].

Couillard-Despres, S., Winkler, J., Uyanik, G., et al., 2001. Molecular mechanisms of neuronal migration disorders, quo vadis? Current Molecular Medicine 1 (6), 677–688.

Cousins, S.D., Morrison, S.C., Drechsler, W.I., 2012. The reliability of plantar pressure assessment during barefoot level walking in children aged 7–11 years. Journal of Foot and Ankle Research 5 (1), 8.

Crenshaw, S., Herzog, R., Castagno, P., et al., 2000. The efficacy of tone-reducing features in orthotics on the gait of children with spastic diplegic cerebral palsy. Journal of Pediatric Orthopedics 20 (2), 210–216.

Cronin, J., Nash, M., Whatman, C., 2006. Assessing dynamic knee joint range of motion using siliconcoach. Physical Therapy in Sport 7 (4), 191–194.

Damiano, D.L., 2006. Activity, activity, activity: rethinking our physical therapy approach to cerebral palsy. Physical Therapy 86 (11), 1534–1540.

Damiano, D.L., Abel, M.F., 1998. Functional outcomes of strength training in spastic cerebral palsy. Archives of Physical Medicine and Rehabilitation 79 (2), 119–125.

Damiano, D.L., Quinlivan, J., Owen, B.F., et al., 2001. Spasticity versus strength in cerebral palsy: relationships among involuntary resistance, voluntary torque, and motor function. European Journal of Neurology 8 (Suppl. 5), 40–49.

Darrah, J., Watkins, B., Chen, L., et al., 2004. Conductive education intervention for children with cerebral palsy: an AACPDM evidence report. Developmental Medicine and Child Neurology 46 (3), 187–203.

Davids, J.R., 2010. The foot and ankle in cerebral palsy. Orthopedic Clinics of North America 41 (4), 579–593.

Davids, J.R., Mason, T.A., Danko, A., et al., 2001. Surgical management of hallux valgus deformity in children with cerebral palsy. Journal of Pediatric Orthopedics 21 (1), 89–94.

Davids, J.R., Rowan, F., Davis, R.B., 2007. Indications for orthoses to improve gait in children with cerebral palsy. Journal of the American Academy of Orthopaedic Surgeons 15 (3), 178–188.

Davis, E., Mackinnon, A., Waters, E., 2012. Parent proxy-reported quality of life for children with cerebral palsy: is it related to parental psychosocial distress? Child: Care, Health and Development 38 (4), 553–560.

Davis, E., Mackinnon, A., Davern, M., et al., 2013. Description and psychometric properties of the CP QOL-Teen: a quality of life questionnaire for adolescents with cerebral palsy. Research in Developmental Disabilities 34 (1), 344–352.

Dennyson, W.G., Fulford, G.E., 1976. Subtalar arthrodesis by cancellous grafts and metallic internal fixation. Journal of Bone and Joint Surgery, British Volume 58-B (4), 507–510.

Desloovere, K., De Cat, J., Molenaers, G., et al., 2012. The effect of different physiotherapy interventions in post-BTX-A treatment of children with cerebral palsy. European Journal of Paediatric Neurology 16 (1), 20–28.

Dickinson, H.O., Rapp, M., Arnaud, C., et al., 2012. Predictors of drop-out in a multi-centre longitudinal study of participation and quality of life of children with cerebral palsy. BMC Research Notes 5, 300.

Dodd, K.J., Taylor, N.F., Damiano, D.L., 2002. A systematic review of the effectiveness of strength-training programs for people with cerebral palsy. Archives of Physical Medicine and Rehabilitation 83 (8), 1157–1164.

Doucet, B.M., Lam, A., Griffin, L., 2012. Neuromuscular electrical stimulation for skeletal muscle function. Yale Journal of Biology and Medicine 85 (2), 201–215.

Eek, M.N., Beckung, E., 2008. Walking ability is related to muscle strength in children with cerebral palsy. Gait and Posture 28 (3), 366–371.

Eek, M.N., Kroksmark, A.K., Beckung, E., 2006. Isometric muscle torque in children 5 to 15 years of age:normative data. Archives of Physical Medicine and Rehabilitation 87 (8), 1091–1099.

Eek, M.N., Tranberg, R., Zugner, R., et al., 2008. Muscle strength training to improve gait function in children with cerebral palsy. Developmental Medicine and Child Neurology 50 (10), 759–764.

Elveru, R.A., Rothstein, J.M., Lamb, R.L., et al., 1988. Methods for taking subtalar joint measurements. A clinical report. Physical Therapy 68 (5), 678–682.

Eyre, J.A., Smith, M., Dabydeen, L., et al., 2007. Is hemiplegic cerebral palsy equivalent to amblyopia of the corticospinal system? Annals of Neurology 62 (5), 493–503.

Faigenbaum, A.D., Kraemer, W.J., Blimkie, C.J., et al., 2009. Youth resistance training: updated position statement paper from the national strength and conditioning association. Journal of Strength and Conditioning Research 23 (5 Suppl.), S60–S79.

Ferrari, F., Cioni, G., Einspieler, C.J., et al., 2002. Cramped synchronized general movements in preterm infants as an early marker for cerebral palsy. Archives of Pediatrics and Adolescent Medicine 156 (5), 460–467.

Ferriero, D.M., 2004. Neonatal brain injury. New England Journal of Medicine 351 (19), 1985–1995.

Figueiredo, E.M., Ferreira, G.B., Maia Moreira, R.C., et al., 2008. Efficacy of ankle–foot orthoses on gait of children with cerebral palsy: systematic review of literature. Pediatric Physical Therapy 20 (3), 207–223.

Firth, G.B., Passmore, E., Sangeux, M., et al., 2013. Multilevel surgery for equinus gait in children with spastic diplegic cerebral palsy: medium-term follow-up with gait analysis. Journal of Bone and Joint Surgery, American Volume 95 (10), 931–938.

Fosang, A.L., Galea, M.P., McCoy, A.T., et al., 2003. Measures of muscle and joint performance in the lower limb of children with cerebral palsy. Developmental Medicine and Child Neurology 45 (10), 664–670.

Franki, I., Desloovere, K., De Cat, J., et al., 2012. The evidence-base for conceptual approaches and additional therapies targeting lower limb function in children with cerebral palsy: a systematic review using the ICF as a framework. Journal of Rehabilitation Medicine 44 (5), 396–405.

Gage, J.R., 2004. Treatment of gait problems in cerebral palsy. Mac Kieth Press, Minnesota.

Gajdosik, R.L., Allred, J.D., Gabbert, H.L., et al., 2007. A stretching program increases the dynamic passive length and passive resistive properties of the calf muscle–tendon unit of unconditioned younger women. European Journal of Applied Physiology 99 (4), 449–454.

Gaskin, C.J., Morris, T., 2008. Physical activity, health-related quality of life, and psychosocial functioning of adults with cerebral palsy. Journal of Physical Activity and Health 5 (1), 146–157.

Gibson, N., Graham, H.K., Love, S., 2007. Botulinum toxin A in the management of focal muscle overactivity in children with cerebral palsy. Disability and Rehabilitation 29 (23), 1813–1822.

Gorton, G.E. 3rd, Stout, J.L., Bagley, A.M., et al., 2011. Gillette Functional Assessment Questionnaire 22-item skill set: factor and Rasch analyses. Developmental Medicine and Child Neurology 53 (3), 250–255.

Gracies, J.M., Burke, K., Clegg, N.J., et al., 2010. Reliability of the Tardieu Scale for assessing spasticity in children with cerebral palsy. Archives of Physical Medicine and Rehabilitation 91 (3), 421–428.

Grant, P.E., Barkovich, A.J., 1998. Neuroimaging in CP: issues in pathogenesis and diagnosis. Mental Retardation and Developmental Disabilities Research Reviews 3 (2), 118–128.

Gunn, A.J., Bennet, L., 2008. Timing of injury in the fetus and neonate. Current Opinion in Obstetrics and Gynecology 20 (2), 175–181.

Gurney, J.K., Kersting, U.G., Rosenbaum, D., 2008. Between-day reliability of repeated plantar pressure distribution measurements in a normal population. Gait and Posture 27 (4), 706–709.

Hagglund, G., Wagner, P., 2008. Development of spasticity with age in a total population of children with cerebral palsy. BMC Musculoskeletal Disorders 9, 150.

Hagglund, G., Wagner, P., 2011. Spasticity of the gastrosoleus muscle is related to the development of reduced passive dorsiflexion of the ankle in children with cerebral palsy:a registry analysis of 2,796 examinations in 355 children. Acta Orthopaedica 82 (6), 744–748.

Han, T.R., Paik, N.J., Im, M.S., 1999. Quantification of the path of center of pressure (COP) using an F-scan in-shoe transducer. Gait and Posture 10 (3), 248–254.

Hanna, S.E., Bartlett, D.J., Rivard, L.M., et al., 2008. Reference curves for the Gross Motor Function Measure: percentiles for clinical description and tracking over time among children with cerebral palsy. Physical Therapy 88 (5), 596–607.

Harvey, A., 2010. Stability of parent-reported manual ability and gross motor function classification of cerebral palsy. Developmental Medicine and Child Neurology 52 (2), 114–115.

Harvey, A., Robin, J., Morris, M.E., et al., 2008. A systematic review of measures of activity limitation for children with cerebral palsy. Developmental Medicine and Child Neurology 50 (3), 190–198.

Harvey, A.R., Morris, M.E., Graham, H.K., et al., 2010. Reliability of the functional mobility scale for children with cerebral palsy. Physical and Occupational Therapy in Pediatrics 30 (2), 139–149.

Haugh, A.B., Pandyan, A.D., Johnson, G.R., 2006. A systematic review of the Tardieu Scale for the measurement of spasticity. Disability and Rehabilitation 28 (15), 899–907.

Hennig, E.M., Staats, A., Rosenbaum, D., 1994. Plantar pressure distribution patterns of young school children in comparison to adults. Foot and Ankle International 15 (1), 35–40.

Himmelmann, K., Ahlin, K., Jacobsson, B., et al., 2011. Risk factors for cerebral palsy in children born at term. Acta Obstetricia et Gynecologica Scandinavica 90 (10), 1070–1081.

Hjern, A., Thorngren-Jerneck, K., 2008. Perinatal complications and socio-economic differences in cerebral palsy in Sweden – a national cohort study. BMC Pediatrics 8, 49.

Hnatyszyn, G., Cyrylowski, L., Czeszynska, M.B., et al., 2010. The role of magnetic resonance imaging in early prediction of cerebral palsy. Turkish Journal of Pediatrics 52 (3), 278–284.

Hoffer, M.M., Reiswig, J.A., Garrett, A.M., et al., 1974. The split anterior tibial tendon transfer in the treatment of spastic varus hindfoot of childhood. Orthopedic Clinics of North America 5 (1), 31–38.

Holmefur, M., Kits, A., Bergstrom, J., et al., 2013. Neuroradiology can predict the development of hand function in children with unilateral cerebral palsy. Neurorehabilitation and Neural Repair 27 (1), 72–78.

Hombergen, S.P., Huisstede, B.M., Streur, M.F., et al., 2012. Impact of cerebral palsy on health-related physical fitness in adults: systematic review. Archives of Physical Medicine and Rehabilitation 93 (5), 871–881.

Horsman, M., Suto, M., Dudgeon, B., et al., 2010. Ageing with cerebral palsy: psychosocial issues. Age and Ageing 39 (3), 294–299.

Huh, K., Rethlefsen, S.A., Wren, T.A., et al., 2010. Development of calcaneal gait without prior triceps surae lengthening: an examination of predictive factors. Journal of Pediatric Orthopedics 30 (3), 240–243.

Hvidtjorn, D., Grove, J., Schendel, D.E., et al., 2006. Cerebral palsy among children born after in vitro fertilization: the role of preterm delivery – a population-based, cohort study. Pediatrics 118 (2), 475–482.

Jahnsen, R., Villien, L., Stanghelle, J.K., et al., 2003. Fatigue in adults with cerebral palsy in Norway compared with the general population. Developmental Medicine and Child Neurology 45 (5), 296–303.

Jahnsen, R., Aamodt, G., Rosenbaum, P., 2006. Gross Motor Function Classification System used in adults with cerebral palsy: agreement of self-reported versus professional rating. Developmental Medicine and Child Neurology 48 (9), 734–738.

Jenter, M., Lipton, G.E., Miller, F., 1998. Operative treatment for hallux valgus in children with cerebral palsy. Foot and Ankle International 19 (12), 830–835.

Jethwa, A., Mink, J., Macarthur, C., et al., 2010. Development of the Hypertonia Assessment Tool (HAT): a discriminative tool for hypertonia in children. Developmental Medicine and Child Neurology 52 (5), e83–e87.

Jewell, A.T., Stokes, A.I., Bartlett, D.J., 2011. Correspondence of classifications between parents of children with cerebral palsy aged 2 to 6 years and therapists using the Gross Motor Function Classification System. Developmental Medicine and Child Neurology 53 (4), 334–337.

Johnston, M.V., 2009. Plasticity in the developing brain: implications for rehabilitation. Developmental Disabilities Research Reviews 15 (2), 94–101.

Johnston, T.E., Wainwright, S.F., 2011. Cycling with functional electrical stimulation in an adult with spastic diplegic cerebral palsy. Physical Therapy 91 (6), 970–982.

Jones, G.C., 2009. Aging with cerebral palsy and other disabilities: personal reflections and recommendations. Developmental Medicine and Child Neurology 51 (Suppl. 4), 12–15.

Kadaba, M.P., Ramakrishnan, H.K., Wootten, M.E., 1990. Measurement of lower extremity kinematics during level walking. Journal of Orthopaedic Research 8 (3), 383–392.

Kazon, S., Grecco, L.A., Pasini, H., et al., 2012. Static balance and function in children with cerebral palsy submitted to neuromuscular block and neuromuscular electrical stimulation: study protocol for prospective, randomized, controlled trial. BMC Pediatrics 12, 53.

Kilgour, G., McNair, P., Stott, N.S., 2002. Lower limb sagittal range of motion reliability of measures and normative values. New Zealand Journal of Physiology 30, 8–24.

Kilgour, G., McNair, P., Stott, N.S., 2003. Intrarater reliability of lower limb sagittal range-of-motion measures in children with spastic diplegia. Developmental Medicine and Child Neurology 45 (6), 391–399.

Koog, Y.H., Min, B.I., 2010. Effects of botulinum toxin A on calf muscles in children with cerebral palsy: a systematic review. Clinical Rehabilitation 24 (8), 685–700.

Korzeniewski, S.J., Birbeck, G., DeLano, M.C., et al., 2008. A systematic review of neuroimaging for cerebral palsy. Journal of Child Neurology 23 (2), 216–227.

Krageloh-Mann, I., Cans, C., 2009. Cerebral palsy update. Brain Development 31 (7), 537–544.

Krageloh-Mann, I., Horber, V., 2007. The role of magnetic resonance imaging in furthering understanding of the pathogenesis of cerebral palsy. Developmental Medicine and Child Neurology 49 (12), 948.

Lance, J.W., 1980. The control of muscle tone, reflexes, and movement: Robert Wartenberg Lecture. Neurology 30 (12), 1303–1313.

Leidinger, B., Heyse, T.J., Fuchs-Winkelmann, S., et al., 2011. Grice-Green procedure for severe hindfoot valgus in ambulatory patients with cerebral palsy. Journal of Foot and Ankle Surgery 50 (2), 190–196.

Little, W., 1861. On the influence of abnormal parturition, difficult labor, premature birth, and asphyxia neonatorum, on the mental and physical condition of the child, especially in relation to deformities. Transactions of the London Obstetric Society 3, 293–344.

Liu, J.S., 2011. Molecular genetics of neuronal migration disorders. Current Neurology and Neuroscience Reports 11 (2), 171–178.

Livingston, M.H., Rosenbaum, P.L., Russell, D.J., et al., 2007. Quality of life among adolescents with cerebral palsy: what does the literature tell us? Developmental Medicine and Child Neurology 49 (3), 225–231.

Love, S.C., Novak, I., Kentish, M., et al., 2010. Botulinum toxin assessment, intervention and after-care for lower limb spasticity in children with cerebral palsy: international consensus statement. European Journal of Neurology 17 (Suppl. 2), 9–37.

Lundkvist Josenby, A., Jarnlo, G.B., Gummesson, C., et al., 2009. Longitudinal construct validity of the GMFM-88 total score and goal total score and the GMFM-66 score in a 5-year follow-up study. Physical Therapy 89 (4), 342–350.

Maanum, G., Jahnsen, R., Froslie, J.K., et al., 2010. Walking ability and predictors of performance on the 6-minute walk test in adults with spastic cerebral palsy. Developmental Medicine and Child Neurology 52 (6), e126–e132.

Maanum, G., Jahnsen, R., Stanghelle, K.F., et al., 2012. Face and construct validity of the Gait Deviation Index in adults with spastic cerebral palsy. Journal of Rehabilitation Medicine 44 (3), 272–275.

Maas, J.C., Dallmeijer, A.J., Huijing, P.A., et al., 2012. Splint: the efficacy of orthotic management in rest to prevent equinus in children with cerebral palsy, a randomised controlled trial. BMC Pediatrics 12, 38.

MacKeith, R., Polani, P., 1959. The Little Club: memorandum on terminology and classification of cerebral palsy. Cerebral Palsy Bulletin 5, 27–35.

Mackey, A.H., Lobb, G.L., Walt, S.E., et al., 2003. Reliability and validity of the Observational Gait Scale in children with spastic diplegia. Developmental Medicine and Child Neurology 45 (1), 4–11.

Mackey, A.H., Walt, S.E., Lobb, G.L., et al., 2004. Intraobserver reliability of the modified Tardieu scale in the upper limb of children with hemiplegia. Developmental Medicine and Child Neurology 46 (4), 267–272.

Mackey, A.H., Walt, S.E., Lobb, G.L., et al., 2005. Reliability of upper and lower limb three-dimensional kinematics in children with hemiplegia. Gait and Posture 22 (1), 1–9.

Maher, C.A., Williams, M.T., Olds, T.S., 2008. The six-minute walk test for children with cerebral palsy. International Journal of Rehabilitation Research 31 (2), 185–188.

Maltais, D.B., Robitaille, N.M., Dumas, F., et al., 2012. Measuring steady-state oxygen uptake during the 6-min walk test in adults with cerebral palsy: feasibility and construct validity. International Journal of Rehabilitation Research 35 (2), 181–183.

Mathur, A., Inder, T., 2009. Magnetic resonance imaging – insights into brain injury and outcomes in premature infants. Journal of Communication Disorders 42 (4), 248–255.

Maurer, J.D., Ward, V., Mayson, T.A., et al., 2013. A kinematic description of dynamic midfoot break in children using a multi-segment foot model. Gait and Posture 2, 287–292. [Epub 2012 Dec 28].

McCormick, A., Brien, M., Plourde, J., et al., 2007. Stability of the Gross Motor Function Classification System in adults with cerebral palsy. Developmental Medicine and Child Neurology 49 (4), 265–269.

McIntyre, S., Taitz, D., Keogh, J., et al., 2013. A systematic review of risk factors for cerebral palsy in children born at term in developed countries. Developmental Medicine and Child Neurology 55 (6), 499–508. [Epub 2012 Nov 26].

Medical Research Council, 1943. Aids to the investigation of the peripheral nervous injuries. Her Majesty's Stationary Office, London.

Ment, L.R., Hirtz, D., Huppi, P.S., 2009. Imaging biomarkers of outcome in the developing preterm brain. Lancet Neurology 8 (11), 1042–1055.

Michlitsch, M.G., Rethlefsen, S.A., Kay, R.M., 2006. The contributions of anterior and posterior tibialis dysfunction to varus foot deformity in patients with cerebral palsy. Journal of Bone and Joint Surgery, American Volume 88 (8), 1764–1768.

Mockford, M., Caulton, J.M., 2008. Systematic review of progressive strength training in children and adolescents with cerebral palsy who are ambulatory. Pediatric Physical Therapy 20 (4), 318–333.

Morris, C., Bartlett, D., 2004. Gross Motor Function Classification System: impact and utility. Developmental Medicine and Child Neurology 46 (1), 60–65.

Mosca, V.S., 1995. Calcaneal lengthening for valgus deformity of the hindfoot. Results in children who had severe, symptomatic flatfoot and skewfoot. Journal of Bone and Joint Surgery, American Volume 77 (4), 500–512.

Murphy, K.P., 2009. Cerebral palsy lifetime care – four musculoskeletal conditions. Developmental Medicine and Child Neurology 51 (Suppl. 4), 30–37.

Mutlu, A., Livanelioglu, A., Gunel, M.K., 2008. Reliability of Ashworth and Modified Ashworth scales in children with spastic cerebral palsy. BMC Musculoskeletal Disorders 9, 44.

Nelson, K.B., Ellenberg, J.H., 1982. Children who "outgrew" cerebral palsy. Pediatrics 69 (5), 529–536.

Nosek, M.A., Howland, C.A., 1997. Breast and cervical cancer screening among women with physical disabilities. Archives of Physical Medicine and Rehabilitation 78 (12 Suppl. 5), S39–S44.

Novak, I., Hines, M., Goldsmith, S., et al., 2012. Clinical prognostic messages from a systematic review on cerebral palsy. Pediatrics 130 (5), e1285–e1312.

Nsenga Leunkeu, A., Shephard, R.J., Ahmaidi, S., 2012. Six-minute walk test in children with cerebral palsy gross motor function classification system levels I and II: reproducibility, validity, and training effects. Archives of Physical Medicine and Rehabilitation 93 (12), 2333–2339.

Numanoglu, A., Gunel, M.K., 2012. Intraobserver reliability of modified Ashworth scale and modified Tardieu scale in the assessment of spasticity in children with cerebral palsy. Acta Orthopaedica et Traumatologica Turcica 46 (3), 196–200.

O'Callaghan, M.E., Maclennan, A.H., Gibson, C.S., et al., 2012. Fetal and maternal candidate single nucleotide polymorphism associations with cerebral palsy: a case-control study. Pediatrics 129 (2), e414–e423.

O'Connell, P.A., D'Souza, L., Dudeney, S., et al., 1998. Foot deformities in children with cerebral palsy. Journal of Pediatric Orthopedics 18 (6), 743–747.

Oberhofer, K., Stott, N.S., Mithraratne, K., et al., 2010. Subject-specific modelling of lower limb muscles in children with cerebral palsy. Clinical Biomechanics (Bristol, Avon) 25 (1), 88–94.

Odding, E., Roebroeck, M.E., Stam, H.J., 2006. The epidemiology of cerebral palsy: incidence, impairments and risk factors. Disability and Rehabilitation 28 (4), 183–191.

Olver, J., Esquenazi, A., Fung, V.S., et al., 2010. Botulinum toxin assessment, intervention and aftercare for lower limb disorders of movement and muscle tone in adults: international consensus statement. European Journal of Neurology 17 (Suppl. 2), 57–73.

Opheim, A., Jahnsen, R., Olsson, E., et al., 2011. Physical and mental components of health-related quality of life and musculoskeletal pain sites over seven years in adults with spastic cerebral palsy. Journal of Rehabilitation Medicine 43 (5), 382–387.

Ounpuu, S., Bell, K.J., Davis, R.B., et al., 1996. An evaluation of the posterior leaf spring orthosis using joint kinematics and kinetics. Journal of Pediatric Orthopedics 16 (3), 378–384.

Palisano, R.J., Cameron, D., Rosenbaum, P.L., et al., 2006. Stability of the gross motor function classification system. Developmental Medicine and Child Neurology 48 (6), 424–428.

Palisano, R.J., Rosenbaum, P., Bartlett, D., et al., 2008. Content validity of the expanded and revised Gross Motor Function Classification System. Developmental Medicine and Child Neurology 50 (10), 744–750.

Palisano, R., Rosenbaum, P., Walter, S., et al., 1997. Development and reliability of a system to classify gross motor function in children with cerebral palsy. Developmental Medicine and Child Neurology 39 (4), 214–223.

Paneth, N., Hong, T., Korzeniewski, S., 2006. The descriptive epidemiology of cerebral palsy. Clinics in Perinatology 33 (2), 251–267.

Park, E.S., Kim, H.W., Park, C.I., et al., 2006. Dynamic foot pressure measurements for assessing foot deformity in persons with spastic cerebral palsy. Archives of Physical Medicine and Rehabilitation 87 (5), 703–709.

Park, K.B., Park, H.W., Lee, K.S., et al., 2008. Changes in dynamic foot pressure after surgical treatment of valgus deformity of the hindfoot in cerebral palsy. Journal of Bone and Joint Surgery, American Volume 90 (8), 1712–1721.

Parkinson, K.N., Gibson, L., Dickinson, H.O., et al., 2010. Pain in children with cerebral palsy: a cross-sectional multicentre European study. Acta Paediatrica 99 (3), 446–451.

Pedowitz, W.J., Kovatis, P., 1995. Flatfoot in the adult. Journal of the American Academy of Orthopaedic Surgeons 3 (5), 293–302.

Persson-Bunke, M., Hagglund, G., Lauge-Pedersen, H., et al., 2012. Scoliosis in a total population of children with cerebral palsy. Spine 37 (12), E708–E713.

Peterson, M.D., Gordon, P.M., Hurvitz, E.A., 2013. Chronic disease risk among adults with cerebral palsy: the role of premature sarcopoenia, obesity and sedentary behaviour. Obesity Reviews 14 (2), 171–182.

Pimm, P., 1992. Cerebral palsy: a non-progressive disorder? Educational and Child Psychology 9 (1), 27–33.

Pin, T., Dyke, P., Chan, M., et al., 2006. The effectiveness of passive stretching in children with cerebral palsy. Developmental Medicine and Child Neurology 48 (10), 855–862.

Pohl, M., Ruckriem, S., Mehrholz, et al., 2002. Effectiveness of serial casting in patients with severe cerebral spasticity: a comparison study. Archives of Physical Medicine and Rehabilitation 83 (6), 784–790.

Prechtl, H.F., 2001. General movement assessment as a method of developmental neurology: new paradigms and their consequences. The 1999 Ronnie MacKeith lecture. Developmental Medicine and Child Neurology 43 (12), 836–842.

Razak, A.H., Zayegh, A., Begg, R.K., et al., 2012. Foot plantar pressure measurement system: a review. Sensors (Basel) 12 (7), 9884–9912.

Reid, S.M., Carlin, J.B., Reddihough, D.S., 2011. Classification of topographical pattern of spasticity in cerebral palsy: a registry perspective. Research in Developmental Disabilities 32 (6), 2909–2915.

Rezaie, P., Dean, A., 2002. Periventricular leukomalacia, inflammation and white matter lesions within the developing nervous system. Neuropathology 22 (3), 106–132.

Rice, J., Russo, R., Halbert, J., et al., 2009. Motor function in 5-year-old children with cerebral palsy in the South Australian population. Developmental Medicine and Child Neurology 51 (7), 551–556.

Roebroeck, M.E., Jahnsen, R., Carona, C., et al., 2009. Adult outcomes and lifespan issues for people with childhood-onset physical disability. Developmental Medicine and Child Neurology 51 (8), 670–678.

Rose, S., Guzzetta, A., Pannek, K., et al., 2011. MRI structural connectivity, disruption of primary sensorimotor pathways, and hand function in cerebral palsy. Brain Connectivity 1 (4), 309–316.

Rosenbaum, P., Paneth, N., Leviton, A., et al., 2007. A report: the definition and classification of cerebral palsy April 2006. Developmental Medicine and Child Neurology. Supplement 109, 8–14.

Rosenbaum, P.L., Palisano, R.J., Bartlett, D.J., et al., 2008. Development of the Gross Motor Function Classification System for cerebral palsy. Developmental Medicine and Child Neurology 50 (4), 249–253.

Ross, S.A., Engsberg, J.R., 2007. Relationships between spasticity, strength, gait, and the GMFM-66 in persons with spastic diplegia cerebral palsy. Archives of Physical Medicine and Rehabilitation 88 (9), 1114–1120.

Russell, D.J., Rosenbaum, P.L., Cadman, D.T., et al., 1989. The gross motor function measure: a means to evaluate the effects of physical therapy. Developmental Medicine and Child Neurology 31 (3), 341–352.

Russell, D.J., Avery, L.M., Rosenbaum, P.L., et al., 2000. Improved scaling of the gross motor function measure for children with cerebral palsy: evidence of reliability and validity. Physical Therapy 80 (9), 873–885.

Russman, B.S., Ashwal, S., 2004. Evaluation of the child with cerebral palsy. Seminars in Pediatric Neurology 11 (1), 47–57.

Russo, R.N., Miller, M.D., Haan, E., et al., 2008. Pain characteristics and their association with quality of life and self-concept in children with hemiplegic cerebral palsy identified from a population register. Clinical Journal of Pain 24 (4), 335–342.

Sadnicka, A., Hoffland, B.S., Bhatia, K.P., et al., 2012. The cerebellum in dystonia – help or hindrance? Clinical Neurophysiology 123 (1), 65–70.

Sagawa, Y. Jr., Watelain, E., De Coulon, G., et al., 2013. Are clinical measurements linked to the Gait Deviation Index in cerebral palsy patients? Gait and Posture 38 (2), 276–280. [Epub 2012 Dec 21].

Satila, H., Huhtala, H., 2010. Botulinum toxin type A injections for treatment of spastic equinus in cerebral palsy: a secondary analysis of factors predictive of favorable response. American Journal of Physical Medicine and Rehabilitation 89 (11), 865–872.

Scheck, S.M., Boyd, R.N., Rose, S.E., 2012. New insights into the pathology of white matter tracts in cerebral palsy from diffusion magnetic resonance imaging: a systematic review. Developmental Medicine and Child Neurology 54 (8), 684–696.

Scholtes, V.A., Becher, J.G., Janssen-Potten, Y.J., et al., 2012. Effectiveness of functional progressive resistance exercise training on walking ability in children with cerebral palsy: a randomized controlled trial. Research in Developmental Disabilities 33 (1), 181–188.

Schwartz, M.H., Rozumalski, A., 2008. The Gait Deviation Index: a new comprehensive index of gait pathology. Gait and Posture 28 (3), 351–357.

Schwartz, M.H., Viehweger, E., Stout, J., et al., 2004. Comprehensive treatment of ambulatory children with cerebral palsy: an outcome assessment. Journal of Pediatric Orthopedics 24 (1), 45–53.

Scianni, A., Butler, J.M., Ada, L., et al., 2009. Muscle strengthening is not effective in children and adolescents with cerebral palsy: a systematic review. Australian Journal of Physiotherapy 55 (2), 81–87.

Sellier, E., Horber, V., Krageloh-Mann, I., et al., 2012. Interrater reliability study of cerebral palsy diagnosis, neurological subtype, and gross motor function. Developmental Medicine and Child Neurology 54 (9), 815–821.

Sheridan, K.J., 2009. Osteoporosis in adults with cerebral palsy. Developmental Medicine and Child Neurology 51 (Suppl. 4), 38–51.

Shore, B.J., White, N., Kerr Graham, H., 2010. Surgical correction of equinus deformity in children with cerebral palsy: a systematic review. Journal of Children's Orthopaedics 4 (4), 277–290.

Shore, B., Spence, D., Graham, H., 2012. The role for hip surveillance in children with cerebral palsy. Current Reviews in Musculoskeletal Medicine 5 (2), 126–134.

Shortland, A., 2009. Muscle deficits in cerebral palsy and early loss of mobility: can we learn something from our elders? Developmental Medicine and Child Neurology 51 (Suppl. 4), 59–63.

Sienko Thomas, S., Buckon, C.E., Jakobson-Huston, S., et al., 2002. Stair locomotion in children with spastic hemiplegia: the impact of three different ankle foot orthosis (AFOs) configurations. Gait and Posture 16 (2), 180–187.

Silfverskiold, N., 1924. Reduction of the uncrossed two-joints muscles of the leg to one-joint muscles in spastic conditions. Acta Chirurgica Scandinavica 56, 315–328.

Smith, L.R., Chambers, H.G., Lieber, R.L., et al., 2013. Reduced satellite cell population may lead to contractures in children with cerebral palsy. Developmental Medicine and Child Neurology 55 (3), 264–270. [Epub 2012 Dec 5].

Spalice, A., Parisi, P., Nicita, F., et al., 2009. Neuronal migration disorders: clinical, neuroradiologic and genetics aspects. Acta Paediatrica 98 (3), 421–433.

Stanger, M., Oresic, S., 2003. Rehabilitation approaches for children with cerebral palsy:overview. Journal of Child Neurology 18 (Suppl. 1), S79–S88.

Stark, T., Walker, B., Phillips, J.K., et al., 2011. Hand-held dynamometry correlation with the gold standard isokinetic dynamometry: a systematic review. Physical Medicine and Rehabilitation 3 (5), 472–479.

Stebbins, J., Harrington, M., Thompson, N., et al., 2006. Repeatability of a model for measuring multi-segment foot kinematics in children. Gait and Posture 23 (4), 401–410.

Steinwender, G., Saraph, V., Scheiber, S., et al., 2000. Intrasubject repeatability of gait analysis data in normal and spastic children. Clinical Biomechanics (Bristol, Avon) 15 (2), 134–139.

Stolp, H., Neuhaus, A., Sundramoorthi, R., et al., 2012. The long and the short of it: gene and environment interactions during early cortical development and consequences for long-term neurological disease. Frontiers in Psychiatry 3, 50.

Swiggum, M., Hamilton, M.L., Gleeson, P., et al., 2010. Pain assessment and management in children with neurologic impairment: a survey of pediatric physical therapists. Pediatric Physical Therapy 22 (3), 330–335.

Tamura, Y., Shibukawa, Y., Shintani, M., et al., 2008. Oral structure representation in human somatosensory cortex. Neuroimage 43 (1), 128–135.

Tardieu, C., Lespargot, A., Tabary, C., et al., 1988. For how long must the soleus muscle be stretched each day to prevent contracture? Developmental Medicine and Child Neurology 30 (1), 3–10.

Taylor, N.F., Dodd, K.J., Larkin, H., 2004. Adults with cerebral palsy benefit from participating in a strength training programme at a community gymnasium. Disability and Rehabilitation 26 (19), 1128–1134.

Terjesen, T., 2012. The natural history of hip development in cerebral palsy. Developmental Medicine and Child Neurology 54 (10), 951–957.

Thorngren-Jerneck, K., Herbst, A., 2006. Perinatal factors associated with cerebral palsy in children born in Sweden. Obstetrics and Gynecology 108 (6), 1499–1505.

Tiberio, D., 1987. Evaluation of functional ankle dorsiflexion using subtalar neutral position. A clinical report. Physical Therapy 67 (6), 955–957.

Turk, M.A., 2009. Health, mortality, and wellness issues in adults with cerebral palsy. Developmental Medicine and Child Neurology 51 (Suppl. 4), 24–29.

van der Ploeg, R.J., Fidler, V., Oosterhuis, H.J., 1991. Hand-held myometry: reference values. Journal of Neurology, Neurosurgery, and Psychiatry 54 (3), 244–247.

van der Slot, W.M., Nieuwenhuijsen, C., van den Berg-Emons, R.J., et al., 2010. Participation and health-related quality of life in adults with spastic bilateral cerebral palsy and the role of self-efficacy. Journal of Rehabilitation Medicine 42 (6), 528–535.

Varni, J.W., Burwinkle, T.M., Sherman, S.A., et al., 2005. Health-related quality of life of children and adolescents with cerebral palsy: hearing the voices of the children. Developmental Medicine and Child Neurology 47 (9), 592–597.

Vattanasilp, W., Ada, L., Crosbie, J., 2000. Contribution of thixotropy, spasticity, and contracture to ankle stiffness after stroke. Journal of Neurology, Neurosurgery, and Psychiatry 69 (1), 34–39.

Verschuren, O., Ada, L., Maltais, D.B., et al., 2011. Muscle strengthening in children and adolescents with spastic cerebral palsy: considerations for future resistance training protocols. Physical Therapy 91 (7), 1130–1139.

Vogtle, L.K., 2009. Pain in adults with cerebral palsy: impact and solutions. Developmental Medicine and Child Neurology 51 (Suppl. 4), 113–121.

Volpe, J.J., 2009. Electroencephalography may provide insight into timing of premature brain injury. Pediatrics 124 (3), e542–e544.

Waters, E., Davis, E., Ronen, G.M., et al., 2009. Quality of life instruments for children and adolescents with neurodisabilities: how to choose the appropriate instrument. Developmental Medicine and Child Neurology 51 (8), 660–669.

Wei, S., Su-Juan, W., Yuan-Gui, L., et al., 2006. Reliability and validity of the GMFM-66 in 0- to 3-year-old children with cerebral palsy. American Journal of Physical Medicine and Rehabilitation 85 (2), 141–147.

Westberry, D.E., Davids, J.R., Shaver, J.C., et al., 2007. Impact of ankle-foot orthoses on static foot alignment in children with cerebral palsy. Journal of Bone and Joint Surgery, American Volume 89 (4), 806–813.

White, H., Jenkins, J., Neace, W.P., et al., 2002. Clinically prescribed orthoses demonstrate an increase in velocity of gait in children with cerebral palsy: a retrospective study. Developmental Medicine and Child Neurology 44 (4), 227–232.

Williams, N., Love, S.C., Gibson, N., et al., 2008. Reliability of the Australian Spasticity Assessment Scale. Developmental Medicine and Child Neurology 50 (Suppl 113), 4–4.

Wren, T.A., Cheatwood, A.P., Rethlefsen, S.A., et al., 2010. Achilles tendon length and medial gastrocnemius architecture in children with cerebral palsy and equinus gait. Journal of Pediatric Orthopedics 30 (5), 479–484.

Wright, P.A., Durham, S., Ewins, D.J., et al., 2012. Neuromuscular electrical stimulation for children with cerebral palsy: a review. Archives of Disease in Childhood 97 (4), 364–371.

Wu, Y.W., Croen, L.A., Vanderwerf, D.J., et al., 2011. Candidate genes and risk for CP: a population-based study. Pediatric Research 70 (6), 642–646.

Yam, W.K., Leung, M.S., 2006. Interrater reliability of Modified Ashworth Scale and Modified Tardieu Scale in children with spastic cerebral palsy. Journal of Child Neurology 21 (12), 1031–1035.

Zwiren, L.D., Bar-Or, O., 1975. Responses to exercise of paraplegics who differ in conditioning level. Medicine and Science in Sports 7 (2), 94–98.

Index

Page numbers followed by 'f' indicate figures, 't' indicate tables, and 'b' indicate boxes.